a LANGE medica

CURRENT
ESSENTIALS
of MEDICINE

Fourth Edition

Edited by

Lawrence M. Tierney, Jr., MD
Professor of Medicine
University of California, San Francisco
Associate Chief of Medical Services
Veterans Affairs Medical Center
San Francisco, California

Sanjay Saint, MD, MPH
Associate Chief of Medicine, Ann Arbor VA Medical Center
Director, VA/UM Patient Safety Enhancement Program
Professor of Internal Medicine, University of Michigan Medical School
Ann Arbor, Michigan

Mary A. Whooley, MD
Professor of Medicine, Epidemiology and Biostatistics
University of California, San Francisco
Department of Veterans Affairs Medical Center
San Francisco, California

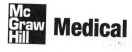 **Medical**

New York   Chicago   San Francisco   Lisbon   London   Madrid   Mexico City
Milan   New Delhi   San Juan   Seoul   Singapore   Sydney   Toronto

Current Essentials of Medicine, Fourth Edition

1 2 3 4 5 6 7 8 9 0   DOC/DOC   14 13 12 11 10

ISSN 97-70188
ISBN 978-0-07-163790-9
MHID 0-07-163790-7

Notice

This book was set in Times by Glyph International.
The editors were Lindsey Zahuranec and Karen Edmondson.
The production supervisor was Catherine H. Saggese.
Project management was provided by Deepti Narwat at Glyph International.
RR Donnelley was printer and binder.

This book is printed on acid-free paper.

International Edition ISBN 978-0-07-174275-7; MHID 0-07-174275-1. Copyright © 2011. Exclusive rights by The McGraw-Hill Companies, Inc., for manufacture and export. This book cannot be re-exported from the country to which it is consigned by McGraw-Hill. The International Edition is not available in North America.

To Katherine Tierney: a sister whose absolute commitment to her parents at the end of their lives provides a model for anyone fortunate enough to know her.

Lawrence M. Tierney, Jr.

To my father, Prem Saint, and father-in-law, James McCarthy, whose commitment to education will inspire generations.

Sanjay Saint

In memory of my mother, Mary Aquinas Whooley (1940–2003).

Mary A. Whooley

Contents

Contributors

Timir Baman, MD
Cardiolology Fellow, University of Michigan Medical School, Ann Arbor, Michigan
Cardiovascular Diseases

Alex Benson, MD
Fellow, Department of Pulmonary and Critical Care Medicine, University of Colorado Hospital, Aurora, Colorado
Pulmonary Diseases

Aaron Berg, MD
Clinical Lecturer and Hospitalist, Department of Internal Medicine, University of Michigan Medical School, Ann Arbor, Michigan
Fluid, Acid–Base, and Electrolyte Disorders

Jeffrey Critchfield, MD
Associate Professor of Clinical Medicine, Department of Medicine, San Francisco General Hospital, University of California, San Francisco School of Medicine, San Francisco, California
Rheumatologic & Autoimmune Disorders

Vanja Douglas, MD
Assistant Clinical Professor, Department of Neurology, University of California, San Francisco, California
Neurologic Disorders

Rebecca A. Jackson, MD
Associate Professor & Chief, Obstetrics, Gynecology and Reproductive Sciences, San Francisco General Hospital, University of California, San Francisco, California
Gynecologic, Obstetric, and Breast Disorders

Kirsten Neudoerffer Kangelaris, MD
Research Fellow, Division of Hospital Medicine, University of
California, San Francisco, California
Selected Genetic Disorders

Helen Kao, MD
Assistant Professor, Division of Geriatrics, Department of Medicine,
University of California, San Francisco, San Francisco, California
Geriatrics

Kewchang Lee, MD
Associate Clinical Professor of Psychiatry, University of California,
San Francisco; Director of Psychiatry Consultation, San Francisco
Veterans Affairs Medical Center, San Francisco, California
Psychiatric Disorders

Joan C. Lo, MD
Research Scientist, Division of Research, Kaiser Permanente
Northern California; Associate Clinical Professor of Medicine,
University of California, San Francisco, Oakland, California
Endocrine Disorders

Michael P. Lukela, MD
Director, Medicine-Pediatrics Residency Program, University of
Michigan Medical School, Ann Arbor, Michigan
Common Pediatric Disorders

Read G. Pierce, MD
Chief Resident, Internal Medicine, University of California, San
Francisco, San Francisco, California
References

Jack Resneck, Jr., MD
Associate Professor of Dermatology and Health Policy, Department
of Dermatology and Phillip R. Lee Institute for Health Policy
Studies, University of California, San Francisco School of
Medicine, San Francisco, California
Dermatologic Disorders

Michael Rizen, MD, PhD, and Stephanie T. Phan, MD
Eye Clinic of Bellevue, Ltd, P.S., Bellevue, Washington
Common Disorders of the Eye

Amandeep Shergill, MD
Assistant Clinical Professor of Medicine, Division of
Gastroenterology, Department of Medicine, San Francisco Veterans
Affairs Medical Center & University of California, San Francisco,
San Francisco, California
Gastrointestinal Diseases
Hepatobiliary Disorders

Sanjay Shewarkramani, MD
Clinical Assistant Professor, Department of Emergency Medicine,
Georgetown University Hospital, Washington, DC
Poisoning

Emily Shuman, MD
Clinical Lecturer, Department of Internal Medicine, Division of
Infectious Diseases, University of Michigan, Ann Arbor, Michigan
Infectious Diseases

Jennifer F. Waljee, MD, MS
Department of Surgery, University of Michigan, Ann Arbor, Michigan
Common Surgical Disorders

Sunny Wang, MD
Assistant Clinical Professor of Medicine, Hematology/Oncology,
University of California, San Francisco & San Francisco VA
Medical Center, San Francisco, California
Hematologic Diseases
Oncologic Diseases

Suzanne Watnick, MD
Medical Director, VA Dialysis Unit, Associate Professor of Medicine,
Portland VA Medical Center and Oregon Health & Science
University, Portland, Oregon
Genitourinary and Renal Disorders

Katherine C. Yung, MD
Assistant Professor, Department of Otolaryngology-Head and Neck
Surgery, Division of Laryngology, University of California, San
Francisco, California
Common Disorders of the Ear, Nose, and Throat

Preface

The fourth edition of *Current Essentials of Medicine* (originally titled *Essentials of Diagnosis & Treatment*) continues a feature introduced in the second edition: a Clinical Pearl for each diagnosis. Pearls are timeless. Learners at every level, and in many countries, remember them as crucial adjuncts to more detailed information about disorders of every type. Ideally, a Pearl is succinct, witty, and often colloquial; it is stated with a certitude suggesting 100% accuracy. Of course, nothing in medicine is so, yet a Pearl such as "If you diagnose multiple sclerosis over the age of fifty, diagnose something else" is easily committed to memory. Thus, Pearls should be accepted as offered. Many have been changed since the previous editions, and we urge readers to come up with Pearls of their own, which may prove to be more useful than our own.

The fourth edition, like its predecessors, uses a single page to consider each disease, providing the reader with a concise yet usable summary about most of the common diseases seen in clinical practice. For readers seeking more detailed information, a current reference has been provided for each disease. We have expanded the number of diseases from the previous edition and updated the clinical manifestations, diagnostic tests, and treatment considerations with the help of our contributing subject-matter experts.

We hope that you enjoy this edition as much as, if not more than, the previous ones.

Lawrence M. Tierney, Jr., MD
San Francisco, California

Sanjay Saint, MD, MPH
Ann Arbor, Michigan

Mary A. Whooley, MD
San Francisco, California

1

Cardiovascular Diseases

Acute Coronary Syndrome

- **Essentials of Diagnosis**
  - Classified as ST-segment elevation (Q wave) myocardial infarction (MI), non–ST-segment elevation (non-Q wave) MI, or unstable angina
  - Prolonged (> 30 minutes) chest pain, associated with shortness of breath, nausea, left arm or neck pain, and diaphoresis; can be painless in diabetics
  - S_4 common; S_3, mitral insufficiency on occasion
  - Cardiogenic shock, ventricular arrhythmias may complicate
  - Unrelenting chest pain may mean ongoing jeopardized myocardium

- **Differential Diagnosis**
  - Stable angina; aortic dissection; pulmonary emboli
  - Tietze's syndrome (costochondritis)
  - Cervical or thoracic radiculopathy, including pre-eruptive zoster
  - Esophageal spasm or reflux; cholecystitis
  - Pericarditis; myocarditis; Takotsubo's (stress-induced) cardiomyopathy
  - Pneumococcal pneumonia; pneumothorax

- **Treatment**
  - Monitoring, oxygen, aspirin, oral beta-blockers, and heparin if not contraindicated; consider clopidogrel
  - Reperfusion by thrombolysis early or percutaneous coronary intervention (PCI) in selected patients with either ST-segment elevation or new left bundle-branch block on ECG
  - Glycoprotein IIb/IIIa inhibitors considered for ST-segment elevation MI in patients undergoing PCI
  - Nitroglycerin and morphine for recurrent ischemic pain; also useful for relieving pulmonary congestion, decreasing sympathetic tone, and reducing blood pressure
  - Angiotensin-converting enzyme (ACE) inhibitors, angiotensin II receptor blockers, and aldosterone blockers such as eplerenone improve ventricular remodeling after infarcts

- **Pearl**

Proceed rapidly to reperfusion in ST-segment elevation MI as time equals muscle.

Reference

Kumar A, Cannon CP. Acute coronary syndromes: diagnosis and management, part II. Mayo Clin Proc 2009;84:1021. [PMID: 19880693]

Acute Pericarditis

- **Essentials of Diagnosis**
  - Inflammation of the pericardium due to viral infection, drugs, recent myocardial infarction, autoimmune syndromes, renal failure, cardiac surgery, trauma, or neoplasm
  - Common symptoms include pleuritic chest pain radiating to the shoulder (trapezius ridge) and dyspnea; pain improves with sitting up and expiration
  - Examination may reveal fever, tachycardia, and an intermittent friction rub; cardiac tamponade may occur in any patient
  - Electrocardiography usually shows PR depression, diffuse concave ST-segment elevation followed by T-wave inversions; no reciprocal changes are seen
  - Echocardiography may reveal pericardial effusion

- **Differential Diagnosis**
  - Acute myocardial infarction
  - Aortic dissection
  - Pulmonary embolism
  - Pneumothorax
  - Pneumonia
  - Cholecystitis and pancreatitis

- **Treatment**
  - Aspirin or nonsteroidal anti-inflammatory agents such as ibuprofen or indomethacin to relieve symptoms; colchicine has been shown to reduce recurrence; rarely, steroids for recurrent cases
  - Hospitalization for patients with symptoms suggestive of significant effusions, cardiac tamponade, elevated biomarkers, or recent trauma or surgery

- **Pearl**

Patients with pericarditis often present with chest pain that is worse when lying flat.

Reference

Imazio M, Cecchi E, Demichelis B, et al. Myopericarditis versus viral or idiopathic acute pericarditis. Heart 2008;94:498. [PMID: 17575329]

Acute Rheumatic Fever

■ Essentials of Diagnosis

- A systemic immune process complicating group A beta-hemolytic streptococcal pharyngitis
- Usually affects children between the ages of 5 and 15; rare after 25
- Occurs 1–5 weeks after throat infection
- Diagnosis based on Jones' criteria (two major or one major and two minor) and confirmation of recent streptococcal infection
- Major criteria: Erythema marginatum, migratory polyarthritis, subcutaneous nodules, carditis, and Sydenham's chorea; the latter is the most specific, least sensitive
- Minor criteria: Fever, arthralgias, elevated erythrocyte sedimentation rate, elevated C-reactive protein, PR prolongation on ECG, and history of pharyngitis

■ Differential Diagnosis

- Juvenile or adult rheumatoid arthritis
- Endocarditis
- Osteomyelitis
- Systemic lupus erythematosus
- Lyme disease
- Disseminated gonococcal infection

■ Treatment

- Bed rest until vital signs and ECG become normal
- Salicylates and nonsteroidal anti-inflammatory drugs reduce fever and joint complaints but do not affect the natural course of the disease; rarely, corticosteroids may be used
- If streptococcal infection is still present, penicillin is indicated
- Prevention of recurrent streptococcal pharyngitis until 18 years old (a monthly injection of benzathine penicillin is most commonly used)

■ Pearl

Inappropriate tachycardia in a febrile child with a recent sore throat suggests this diagnosis.

Reference

van Bemmel JM, Delgado V, Holman ER, et al. No increased risk of valvular heart disease in adult poststreptococcal reactive arthritis. Arthritis Rheum 2009;60:987. [PMID: 19333942]

1

Angina Pectoris

- **Essentials of Diagnosis**
  - Generally caused by atherosclerotic coronary artery disease and severe coronary obstruction; cigarette smoking, diabetes mellitus, hypertension, hypercholesterolemia, and family history are established risk factors
  - Stable angina characterized by pressure-like episodic precordial chest discomfort, precipitated by exertion or stress, relieved by rest or nitrates; unstable angina can occur with less exertion or at rest
  - Stable angina is predictable in initiation and termination; unstable angina is not
  - S_4, S_3, mitral murmur, paradoxically split S_2 may occur transiently with pain
  - Electrocardiography usually normal between episodes (or may show evidence of old infarction); electrocardiography with pain may show evidence of ischemia, classically ST depression
  - Diagnosis from history and stress tests; confirmed by coronary arteriography

- **Differential Diagnosis**
  - Other coronary syndromes (myocardial infarction, vasospasm)
  - Tietze's syndrome (costochondritis)
  - Intercostal neuropathy, especially caused by herpes zoster
  - Cervical or thoracic radiculopathy, including pre-eruptive zoster
  - Esophageal spasm or reflux disease; cholecystitis
  - Pneumothorax; pulmonary embolism; pneumonia

- **Treatment**
  - Address risk factors; sublingual nitroglycerin for episodes
  - Ongoing treatment includes aspirin, long-acting nitrates, beta-blockers, and calcium channel blockers
  - Angioplasty with stenting considered in patients with anatomically suitable stenoses who remain symptomatic on medical therapy
  - Bypass grafting for patients with refractory angina on medical therapy, three-vessel disease (or two-vessel disease with proximal left anterior descending artery disease) and decreased left ventricular function, or left main coronary artery disease

- **Pearl**

Many patients with angina will not say they are having pain; they will deny it but say they have discomfort, heartburn, or pressure.

Reference

Poole-Wilson PA, Vokó Z, Kirwan BA, de Brouwer S, Dunselman PH, Lubsen J; ACTION investigators. Clinical course of isolated stable angina due to coronary heart disease. Eur Heart J 2007;28:1928. [PMID: 17562665]

Aortic Coarctation

- **Essentials of Diagnosis**
  - Elevated blood pressure in the aortic arch and its branches with reduced blood pressure distal to the left subclavian artery
  - Lower extremity claudication or leg weakness with exertion in young adults is characteristic
  - Systolic blood pressure is higher in the arms than in the legs, but diastolic pressure is similar compared with radial
  - Femoral pulses delayed and decreased, with pulsatile collaterals in the intercostal areas; a harsh, late systolic murmur may be heard in the back; an aortic ejection murmur suggests concomitant bicuspid aortic valve
  - Electrocardiography with left ventricular hypertrophy; chest x-ray may show rib notching inferiorly due to collaterals
  - Transesophageal echo with Doppler or MRI is diagnostic; angiography confirms gradient across the coarctation

- **Differential Diagnosis**
  - Essential hypertension
  - Renal artery stenosis
  - Renal parenchymal disease
  - Pheochromocytoma
  - Mineralocorticoid excess
  - Oral contraceptive use
  - Cushing's syndrome

- **Treatment**
  - Surgery is the mainstay of therapy; balloon angioplasty in selected patients
  - Twenty-five percent of patients remain hypertensive after surgery

- **Pearl**

Intermittent claudication in a young person with no vascular disease should suggest this problem; listen to the back for the characteristic murmur.

Reference

Tomar M, Radhakrishanan S. Coarctation of aorta: intervention from neonates to adult life. Indian Heart J 2008;60(suppl D):D22. [PMID: 19845083]

1

Aortic Dissection

- **Essentials of Diagnosis**
  - Most patients between age 50 and 70; risks include hypertension, Marfan's syndrome, bicuspid aortic valve, coarctation of the aorta, and pregnancy
  - Type A involves the ascending aorta or arch; type B does not
  - Sudden onset of chest pain with interscapular radiation in at-risk patient
  - Unequal blood pressures in upper extremities, new diastolic murmur of aortic insufficiency occasionally seen in type A
  - Chest x-ray nearly always abnormal; ECG unimpressive unless coronary artery compromised
  - CT, transesophageal echocardiography, MRI, or aortography usually diagnostic

- **Differential Diagnosis**
  - Acute myocardial infarction
  - Angina pectoris
  - Acute pericarditis
  - Pneumothorax
  - Pulmonary embolism
  - Boerhaave's syndrome

- **Treatment**
  - Nitroprusside and beta-blockers to lower systolic blood pressure to approximately 100 mm Hg, pulse to 60/min
  - Emergent surgery for type A dissection; medical therapy for type B is reasonable, with surgery or percutaneous intra-aortic stenting reserved for high-risk patients

- **Pearl**

The pain of dissection starts abruptly; that of ischemic heart disease increases to maximum over several minutes.

Reference

Tran TP, Khoynezhad A. Current management of type B aortic dissection. Vasc Health Risk Manag 2009;5:53. [PMID: 19436678]

Aortic Regurgitation

- ■ Essentials of Diagnosis
  - Causes include congenital bicuspid valve, endocarditis, rheumatic heart disease, Marfan's syndrome, aortic dissection, ankylosing spondylitis, reactive arthritis, and syphilis
  - Acute aortic regurgitation: Abrupt onset of pulmonary edema
  - Chronic aortic regurgitation: Asymptomatic until middle age, when symptoms of left heart failure develop insidiously
  - Soft, high-pitched, decrescendo holodiastolic murmur in chronic aortic regurgitation; occasionally, an accompanying apical low-pitched diastolic rumble (Austin Flint murmur) in nonrheumatic patients; in acute aortic regurgitation, the diastolic murmur can be short (or not even heard) and harsh
  - Acute aortic regurgitation: Reduced S_1 and an S_3; rales
  - Chronic aortic regurgitation: Reduced S_1, wide pulse pressure, water-hammer pulse, subungual capillary pulsations (Quincke's sign), rapid rise and fall of pulse (Corrigan's pulse), and a diastolic murmur over a partially compressed femoral artery (Duroziez's sign)
  - ECG shows left ventricular hypertrophy
  - Echo Doppler confirms diagnosis, estimates severity

- ■ Differential Diagnosis
  - Pulmonary hypertension with Graham Steell murmur
  - Mitral, or rarely, tricuspid stenosis
  - Left ventricular failure due to other cause
  - Dock's murmur of left anterior descending artery stenosis

- ■ Treatment
  - Vasodilators (eg, nifedipine and ACE inhibitors) do not delay the progression to valve replacement in patients with mild to moderate aortic regurgitation
  - In chronic aortic regurgitation, surgery reserved for patients with symptoms or ejection function < 50% on echocardiography
  - Acute regurgitation caused by aortic dissection or endocarditis requires surgical replacement of the valve

- ■ Pearl

The Hodgkin-Key murmur of aortic regurgitation is harsh and raspy, caused by leaflet eventration typical of luetic aortopathy.

Reference

Kamath AR, Varadarajan P, Turk R, Sampat U, Patel R, Khandhar S, Pai RG. Survival in patients with severe aortic regurgitation and severe left ventricular dysfunction is improved by aortic valve replacement. Circulation 2009; 120(suppl):S134. [PMID: 19752358]

1

Aortic Stenosis

- ■ Essentials of Diagnosis
  - • Causes include congenital bicuspid valve and progressive calcification with aging of a normal three-leaflet valve; rheumatic fever rarely, if ever, causes isolated aortic stenosis
  - • Dyspnea, angina, and syncope singly or in any combination; sudden death in less than 1% of asymptomatic patients
  - • Weak and delayed carotid pulses (pulsus parvus et tardus); a soft, absent, or paradoxically split S_2; a harsh diamond-shaped systolic ejection murmur to the right of the sternum, often radiating to the neck, but on occasion heard apically (Gallavardin's phenomenon)
  - • Left ventricular hypertrophy by ECG and chest x-ray may show calcification in the aortic valve
  - • Echo confirms diagnosis and estimates valve area and gradient; cardiac catheterization confirms severity if there is discrepancy between physical exam and echo; concomitant coronary atherosclerotic disease present in 50%

- ■ Differential Diagnosis
  - • Mitral regurgitation
  - • Hypertrophic obstructive or dilated cardiomyopathy
  - • Atrial or ventricular septal defect
  - • Syncope due to other causes
  - • Ischemic heart disease without valvular abnormality

- ■ Treatment
  - • Surgery is indicated for all patients with severe aortic stenosis (mean aortic valve gradient > 40 mm Hg or valve area ≤ 1.0 cm^2) and the presence of symptoms or ejection fraction < 50%
  - • Percutaneous balloon valvuloplasty for temporary (6 months) relief of symptoms in poor surgical candidates

- ■ Pearl

In many cases, the softer the murmur, the worse the stenosis.

Reference

Dal-Bianco JP, Khandheria BK, Mookadam F, Gentile F, Sengupta PP. Management of asymptomatic severe aortic stenosis. J Am Coll Cardiol 2008;52:1279. [PMID: 18929238]

Atrial Fibrillation

- ■ Essentials of Diagnosis
  - The most common chronic arrhythmia
  - Causes include mitral valve disease, hypertensive and ischemic heart disease, dilated cardiomyopathy, alcohol use, hyperthyroidism, pericarditis, cardiac surgery; many idiopathic ("lone" atrial fibrillation)
  - Complications include precipitation of cardiac failure, arterial embolization
  - Palpitations, dyspnea, chest pain; commonly asymptomatic
  - Irregularly irregular heartbeat, variable intensity S_1, occasional S_3; S_4 absent in all
  - Electrocardiography shows ventricular rate of 80–170/min in untreated patients; if associated with an accessory pathway (ie, Wolff-Parkinson-White), the ventricular rate can be > 200/min with wide QRS and antegrade conduction through the pathway

- ■ Differential Diagnosis
  - Multifocal atrial tachycardia; sinus arrhythmia
  - Atrial flutter or tachycardia with variable block
  - Normal sinus rhythm with multiple premature contractions

- ■ Treatment
  - Control ventricular response with AV-nodal blockers such as digoxin, beta-blocker, calcium channel blocker—choice depending on contractile state of left ventricle and blood pressure
  - Cardioversion in unstable patients with acute atrial fibrillation; elective cardioversion in stable patients once a left atrial thrombus has been ruled out or effectively treated
  - Antiarrhythmic agents (eg, propafenone, procainamide, amiodarone, sotalol) for highly symptomatic patients despite rate control
  - Chronic warfarin or aspirin in all patients
  - With elective cardioversion, documented therapeutic anticoagulation for 4 weeks prior to the procedure unless transesophageal echocardiography excludes a left atrial thrombus; all patients require anticoagulation during and after cardioversion
  - Radiofrequency ablation of pulmonary vein sources of atrial fibrillation increasingly used in symptomatic patients who fail antiarrhythmic therapy

- ■ Pearl

In 2010, electrophysiology has allowed pathway or nodal ablation in increasing numbers of patients; remember this option.

Reference

Hart RG, Pearce LA. Current status of stroke risk stratification in patients with atrial fibrillation. Stroke 2009;40:2607. [PMID: 19461020]

Atrial Flutter

- **Essentials of Diagnosis**
  - Common in chronic obstructive pulmonary disease (COPD); also seen in dilated cardiomyopathy, especially in alcoholics
  - Atrial rate between 250 and 350 beats/min with every second, third, or fourth impulse conducted by the ventricle; 2:1 most common
  - Patients may be asymptomatic, complain of palpitations, or have evidence of congestive heart failure
  - Flutter (*a*) waves visible in the neck in occasional patients
  - Electrocardiography shows "sawtooth" P waves in V_1 and the inferior leads; ventricular response usually regular; less commonly, irregular due to variable atrioventricular block

- **Differential Diagnosis**

  With regular ventricular rate:
  - Automatic atrial tachycardia
  - Atrioventricular nodal reentry tachycardia
  - Atrioventricular reentry tachycardia with accessory pathway
  - Sinus tachycardia

  With irregular ventricular rate:
  - Atrial fibrillation
  - Multifocal atrial tachycardia
  - Sinus rhythm with frequent premature atrial contractions

- **Treatment**
  - Often spontaneously converts to atrial fibrillation
  - Electrical cardioversion is reliable and safe
  - Conversion may also be achieved by drugs (eg, ibutilide)
  - Risk of embolization is lower than for atrial fibrillation, but anticoagulation still recommended
  - Radiofrequency ablation is highly successful (> 90%) in patients with chronic atrial flutter

- **Pearl**

  A regular heart rate of 140–150 in a patient with COPD is flutter until proven otherwise.

Reference

Rodgers M, McKenna C, Palmer S, et al. Curative catheter ablation in atrial fibrillation and typical atrial flutter: systematic review and economic evaluation. Health Technol Assess 2008;12:iii-iv, xi-xiii, 1-198. [PMID: 19036232]

Atrial Myxoma

1

■ Essentials of Diagnosis

- Most common cardiac tumor, usually originating in the interatrial septum, with 80% growing into the left atrium; 5–10% bilateral
- Symptoms fall into one of three categories: (1) systemic—fever, malaise, weight loss; (2) obstructive—positional dyspnea and syncope; and (3) embolic—acute vascular or neurologic deficit
- Diastolic "tumor plop" or mitral stenosis-like murmur; signs of congestive heart failure and systemic embolization in many
- Episodic pulmonary edema, classically when patient assumes an upright position
- Leukocytosis, anemia, accelerated erythrocyte sedimentation rate
- MRI or echocardiogram demonstrates tumor

■ Differential Diagnosis

- Subacute infective endocarditis
- Lymphoma
- Autoimmune disease
- Mitral stenosis
- Cor triatriatum
- Parachute mitral valve
- Other causes of congestive heart failure
- Renal carcinoma involving the inferior vena cava

■ Treatment

- Surgery usually curative (recurrence rate is approximately 5%)

■ Pearl

One of the three causes of inflow obstruction to the left ventricle, with mitral stenosis and cor triatriatum being the other two.

Reference

Kuroczyński W, Peivandi AA, Ewald P, Pruefer D, Heinemann M, Vahl CF. Cardiac myxomas: short- and long-term follow-up. Cardiol J 2009;16:447. [PMID: 19753524]

1

Atrial Septal Defect

- ■ Essentials of Diagnosis
  - Patients with small defects are usually asymptomatic and have a normal life span
  - Large shunts symptomatic by age 40, including exertional dyspnea, fatigue, and palpitations
  - Paradoxical embolism may occur (ie, upper or lower extremity venous thrombus embolizing to brain or extremity rather than lung) with transient shunt reversal
  - Right ventricular lift, widened and fixed splitting of S_2, and systolic flow murmur in the pulmonary area
  - ECG may show right ventricular hypertrophy and right axis deviation (in ostium secundum defects), left anterior hemiblock (in ostium primum defects); complete or incomplete right bundle-branch block in 95%
  - Atrial fibrillation commonly complicates
  - Echo Doppler with agitated saline contrast injection is diagnostic; radionuclide angiogram or cardiac catheterization estimates ratio of pulmonary flow to systemic flow (Q_P:Q_S)

- ■ Differential Diagnosis
  - Left ventricular failure
  - Left-sided valvular disease
  - Primary pulmonary hypertension
  - Chronic pulmonary embolism
  - Sleep apnea
  - Chronic obstructive pulmonary disease
  - Eisenmenger's syndrome
  - Pulmonary stenosis

- ■ Treatment
  - Small defects do not require surgical correction
  - Surgery or percutaneous closure devices indicated for patients with symptoms or Q_P:$Q_S > 1.5$
  - Surgery contraindicated in patients with pulmonary hypertension and right-to-left shunting

- ■ Pearl

Prophylaxis for endocarditis is unnecessary; the low interatrial gradient is the reason.

Reference

Rosas M, Attie F. Atrial septal defect in adults. Timely Top Med Cardiovasc Dis 2007;11:E34. [PMID: 18301787]

Atrioventricular Block

■ Essentials of Diagnosis

- First-degree block: Delayed conduction at the level of the atrioventricular node; PR interval > 0.20 seconds
- Second-degree block: Mobitz I—progressive prolongation of the PR interval and decreasing R-R interval prior to a blocked sinus impulse as well as "group beating"; Mobitz II—fixed PR intervals before a beat is dropped
- Third-degree block: Complete block at or below the node; P waves and QRS complexes occur independently of one another, both at fixed rates with atrial rate > ventricular rate
- Clinical manifestations of third-degree block include chest pain, syncope, and shortness of breath; cannon *a* waves in neck veins; first heart sound varies in intensity

■ Differential Diagnosis

Causes of first-degree and Mobitz I atrioventricular block:
- Increased vagal tone
- Drugs that prolong atrioventricular conduction
- All causes of second- and third-degree block

Causes of Mobitz II and third-degree atrioventricular block:
- Chronic degenerative conduction system disease (Lev's and Lenègre's syndromes)
- Acute myocardial infarction: Inferior myocardial infarction causes complete block at the node, anterior myocardial infarction below it
- Acute myocarditis (eg, Lyme disease, viral myocarditis, rheumatic fever)
- Digitalis toxicity
- Aortic valve abscess
- Congenital

■ Treatment

- In symptomatic patients with Mobitz I, permanent pacing; asymptomatic patients with Mobitz I do not need therapy
- For some with Mobitz II and all with infranodal third-degree atrioventricular block, permanent pacing unless a reversible cause (eg, drug toxicity, inferior myocardial infarction, Lyme disease) is present

■ Pearl

A "circus of atrial sounds" may be created by atrial contractions at different rates than ventricular, in any cause of AV dissociation.

Reference

Dovgalyuk J, Holstege C, Mattu A, Brady WJ. The electrocardiogram in the patient with syncope. Am J Emerg Med 2007;25:688. [PMID: 17606095]

1

Cardiac Tamponade

- **Essentials of Diagnosis**
  - Life-threatening disorder occurring when pericardial fluid accumulates under pressure; effusions rapidly increasing in size may cause an elevated intrapericardial pressure (> 15 mm Hg), leading to impaired cardiac filling and decreased cardiac output
  - Common causes include metastatic malignancy, uremia, viral or idiopathic pericarditis, and cardiac trauma; however, any cause of pericarditis can cause tamponade
  - Clinical manifestations include dyspnea, cough, tachycardia, hypotension, pulsus paradoxus, jugular venous distention, and distant heart sounds
  - Electrocardiography usually shows low QRS voltage and occasionally electrical alternans; chest x-ray shows an enlarged cardiac silhouette with a "water-bottle" configuration if a large (> 250 mL) effusion is present—which it need not be if effusion develops rapidly
  - Echocardiography delineates effusion and its hemodynamic significance, eg, atrial collapse; cardiac catheterization confirms the diagnosis if equalization of diastolic pressures in all four chambers occurs with loss of the normal y descent

- **Differential Diagnosis**
  - Tension pneumothorax
  - Right ventricular infarction
  - Severe left ventricular failure
  - Constrictive pericarditis
  - Restrictive cardiomyopathy
  - Pneumonia with septic shock

- **Treatment**
  - Immediate pericardiocentesis if hemodynamic compromise is noted
  - Volume expansion until pericardiocentesis is performed
  - Definitive treatment for reaccumulation may require surgical anterior and posterior pericardiectomy

- **Pearl**

Pulsus paradoxus is in fact not paradoxical: it merely exaggerates a normal phenomenon.

Reference

Jacob S, Sebastian JC, Cherian PK, Abraham A, John SK. Pericardial effusion impending tamponade: a look beyond Beck's triad. Am J Emerg Med 2009;27:216. [PMID: 19371531]

Congestive Heart Failure

- ■ Essentials of Diagnosis
  - • Two pathophysiologic categories: Systolic dysfunction and diastolic dysfunction
  - • Systolic: The ability to pump blood is compromised; ejection fraction is decreased; causes include coronary artery disease, dilated cardiomyopathy, myocarditis, "burned-out" hypertensive heart disease, and regurgitant valvular heart disease
  - • Diastolic: Heart unable to relax and allow adequate diastolic filling; normal ejection fraction; causes include ischemia, hypertension with left ventricular hypertrophy, aortic stenosis, hypertrophic cardiomyopathy, restrictive cardiomyopathy, and small-vessel disease (especially diabetes)
  - • Evidence of both common in the typical heart failure patient, but up to 50% of patients will have isolated diastolic dysfunction
  - • Symptoms and signs can result from left-sided failure, right-sided failure, or both
  - • Left ventricular failure: Exertional dyspnea, orthopnea, paroxysmal nocturnal dyspnea, pulsus alternans, rales, gallop rhythm; pulmonary venous congestion on chest x-ray
  - • Right ventricular failure: Fatigue, malaise, elevated venous pressure, hepatomegaly, abdominojugular reflux, and dependent edema
  - • Diagnosis confirmed by echo, pulmonary capillary wedge measurement, or elevated levels of brain natriuretic peptide (BNP)

- ■ Differential Diagnosis
  - • Constrictive pericarditis; nephrosis; cirrhosis
  - • Hypothyroidism or hyperthyroidism; beriberi
  - • Noncardiogenic causes of pulmonary edema

- ■ Treatment
  - • Systolic dysfunction: Vasodilators (ACE inhibitors, angiotensin II receptor blockers, or combination of hydralazine and isosorbide dinitrate), beta-blockers, spironolactone, and low-sodium diet; for symptoms, use diuretics and digoxin; anticoagulation perhaps in high-risk patients with apical akinesis even with sinus rhythm; look for ischemia, valvular disease, alcohol use, or hypothyroidism as causes
  - • Diastolic dysfunction: A negative inotrope (beta-blocker or calcium channel blocker), low-sodium diet, and diuretics for symptoms

- ■ Pearl

Remember that a normal ejection fraction is the rule in flash pulmonary edema; severe diastolic dysfunction is the problem.

Reference

Donlan SM, Quattromani E, Pang PS, Gheorghiade M. Therapy for acute heart failure syndromes. Curr Cardiol Rep 2009;11:192. [PMID: 19379639]

1

Constrictive Pericarditis

- **Essentials of Diagnosis**
  - A thickened fibrotic pericardium impairing cardiac filling and decreasing cardiac output
  - May follow tuberculosis, cardiac surgery, radiation therapy, or viral, uremic, or neoplastic pericarditis
  - Gradual onset of dyspnea, fatigue, weakness, pedal edema, and abdominal swelling; right-sided heart failure symptoms often predominate, with ascites sometimes disproportionate to pedal edema
  - Physical examination reveals tachycardia, elevated jugular venous distention with rapid y descent, Kussmaul's sign, hepatosplenomegaly, ascites, "pericardial knock" following S_2, and peripheral edema
  - Pericardial calcification on chest film in less than half; electrocardiography may show low QRS voltage; liver function tests abnormal from passive congestion
  - Echocardiography can demonstrate a thick pericardium and normal left ventricular function; CT or MRI is more sensitive in revealing pericardial pathology; cardiac catheterization demonstrates ventricular discordance with respiration in contrast to restrictive cardiomyopathy

- **Differential Diagnosis**
  - Cardiac tamponade
  - Right ventricular infarction
  - Restrictive cardiomyopathy
  - Cirrhosis with ascites (most common misdiagnosis)

- **Treatment**
  - Acute treatment usually includes gentle diuresis
  - Definitive therapy is surgical stripping of the pericardium; effective in up to half of patients
  - Evaluation for tuberculosis

- **Pearl**

The most overlooked cause of new-onset ascites.

Reference

Marnejon T, Kassis H, Gemmel D. The constricted heart. Postgrad Med 2008;120:8. [PMID: 18467803]

Cor Pulmonale

- ■ **Essentials of Diagnosis**
  - • Heart failure resulting from pulmonary disease
  - • Most commonly due to COPD; other causes include pulmonary fibrosis, pneumoconioses, recurrent pulmonary emboli, primary pulmonary hypertension, sleep apnea, and kyphoscoliosis
  - • Clinical manifestations are due to both the underlying pulmonary disease and the right ventricular failure
  - • Chest x-ray reveals an enlarged right ventricle and pulmonary artery; electrocardiography may show right axis deviation, right ventricular hypertrophy, and tall, peaked P waves (P pulmonale) in the face of low QRS voltage
  - • Pulmonary function tests usually confirm the presence of underlying lung disease, and echocardiography will show right ventricular dilation but normal left ventricular function and elevated right ventricular systolic pressures

- ■ **Differential Diagnosis**

  Other causes of right ventricular failure:
  - • Left ventricular failure (due to any cause)
  - • Pulmonary stenosis
  - • Left-to-right shunt causing Eisenmenger's syndrome

- ■ **Treatment**
  - • Treatment is primarily directed at the pulmonary process causing the right heart failure (eg, oxygen if hypoxia is present)
  - • In frank right ventricular failure, include salt restriction, diuretics, and oxygen
  - • For primary pulmonary hypertension, cautious use of vasodilators (calcium channel blockers) or continuous-infusion prostacyclin may benefit some patients

- ■ **Pearl**

  Oxygen is the furosemide of the right ventricle.

Reference

Weitzenblum E, Chaouat A. Cor pulmonale. Chron Respir Dis 2009;6:177. [PMID: 19643833]

1

Deep Venous Thrombosis

- **Essentials of Diagnosis**
  - Dull pain or tight feeling in the calf or thigh
  - Up to half of patients are asymptomatic in the early stages
  - Increased risk: Congestive heart failure, recent major surgery, neoplasia, oral contraceptive use by smokers, prolonged inactivity, varicose veins, hypercoagulable states (eg, protein C, protein S, other anticoagulant deficiencies, nephrotic syndrome)
  - Physical signs unreliable
  - Doppler ultrasound and impedance plethysmography are initial tests of choice (less sensitive in asymptomatic patients); venography is definitive but difficult to perform
  - Pulmonary thromboembolism, especially with proximal, above-the-knee deep vein thrombosis, is a life-threatening complication

- **Differential Diagnosis**
  - Calf strain or contusion; ruptured Baker's cyst
  - Cellulitis; lymphatic obstruction
  - Congestive heart failure, especially right-sided

- **Treatment**
  - Anticoagulation with heparin followed by oral warfarin for 3–6 months
  - Subcutaneous low-molecular-weight heparin may be substituted for intravenous heparin
  - NSAIDs for associated pain and swelling
  - For idiopathic and recurrent cases, hypercoagulable conditions should be considered, although factor V Leiden should be sought on a first episode without risk factors in patients of European ethnicity
  - Postphlebitic syndrome (chronic venous insufficiency) is common following an episode of deep venous thrombosis and should be treated with graduated compression stockings, local skin care, and in many, chronic warfarin administration

- **Pearl**

The left leg is 1 cm greater in circumference than the right, as the left common iliac vein courses under the aorta; remember this in evaluating suspected deep venous thrombosis.

Reference

Blann AD, Khoo CW. The prevention and treatment of venous thromboembolism with LMWHs and new anticoagulants. Vasc Health Risk Manag 2009;5:693. [PMID: 19707288]

Dilated Cardiomyopathy

- **Essentials of Diagnosis**
  - A cause of systolic dysfunction, this represents a group of disorders that lead to congestive heart failure
  - Symptoms and signs of congestive heart failure: Exertional dyspnea, cough, fatigue, paroxysmal nocturnal dyspnea, cardiac enlargement, rales, gallop rhythm, elevated venous pressure, hepatomegaly, and dependent edema
  - Electrocardiography may show nonspecific repolarization abnormalities and atrial or ventricular ectopy, but is not diagnostic
  - Echocardiography reveals depressed contractile function and cardiomegaly
  - Cardiac catheterization useful to exclude ischemia as a cause

- **Differential Diagnosis**

  Causes of dilated cardiomyopathy:
  - Alcoholism
  - Infectious (including postviral) myocarditis, human immunodeficiency virus, and Chagas' disease
  - Sarcoidosis
  - Postpartum
  - Doxorubicin toxicity
  - Endocrinopathies (hyperthyroidism, acromegaly, pheochromocy-toma)
  - Hemochromatosis
  - Idiopathic

- **Treatment**
  - Treat the underlying disorder when identifiable
  - Abstention from alcohol and NSAIDs
  - Routine management of systolic dysfunction, including with vasodilators (ACE inhibitors, angiotensin II receptor blockers, and/or a combination of hydralazine and isosorbide dinitrate), beta-blockers, spironolactone, and low-sodium diet; digoxin and diuretics for symptoms
  - Many empirically employ chronic warfarin if apical akinesis is noted
  - In a patient with ischemic or nonischemic heart disease and a low left ventricular ejection fraction (< 35%), an implantable cardiac defibrillator (ICD) may be warranted even in the absence of documented ventricular tachycardia
  - Cardiac transplant for end-stage patients

- **Pearl**

  Causes of death: one-third pump failure, one-third arrhythmia, and one-third stroke; arrhythmia and stroke are potentially preventable.

Reference

Luk A, Ahn E, Soor GS, Butany J. Dilated cardiomyopathy: a review. J Clin Pathol 2009;62:219. [PMID: 19017683]

Hypertension

- **Essentials of Diagnosis**
  - In most patients (95% of cases), no cause can be found
  - Chronic elevation in blood pressure (> 140/90 mm Hg) occurs in 23% of non-Hispanic white adults and 32% of non-Hispanic black adults in the United States; onset is usually between ages 20 and 55
  - The pathogenesis is multifactorial: Environmental, dietary, genetic, and neurohormonal factors all contribute
  - Most patients are asymptomatic; some, however, complain of headache, epistaxis, or blurred vision if hypertension is severe
  - Most diagnostic study abnormalities are referable to "target organ" damage: heart, kidney, brain, retina, and peripheral arteries

- **Differential Diagnosis**

  Secondary causes of hypertension:
  - Coarctation of the aorta
  - Renal insufficiency
  - Renal artery stenosis
  - Pheochromocytoma
  - Cushing's syndrome
  - Primary hyperaldosteronism
  - Chronic use of oral contraceptive pills or alcohol

- **Treatment**
  - Decrease blood pressure with a single agent (if possible) while minimizing side effects; however, those with blood pressure > 160/100 may require combination therapy
  - Many recommend diuretics, beta-blockers, ACE inhibitors, or calcium channel blockers as initial therapy, but considerable latitude is allowed for individual patients; these agents can be used alone or in combination; α1-blockers are considered second-line agents
  - If hypertension is unresponsive to medical treatment, evaluate for secondary causes

- **Pearl**

  Increasingly a condition diagnosed by the patient; sphygmomanometers are widely available in pharmacies and supermarkets.

Reference

Fuchs FD. Diuretics: still essential drugs for the management of hypertension. Expert Rev Cardiovasc Ther 2009;7:591. [PMID: 19505274]

Hypertrophic Obstructive Cardiomyopathy (HOCM)   1

- ■ Essentials of Diagnosis
    - Asymmetric myocardial hypertrophy causing dynamic obstruction to left ventricular outflow below the aortic valve
    - Sporadic or dominantly inherited
    - Obstruction is worsened by increasing left ventricular contractility or decreasing filling
    - Symptoms are dyspnea, chest pain, and syncope; a subgroup of younger patients is at high risk for sudden cardiac death (1% per year), especially with exercise
    - Sustained, bifid (rarely trifid) apical impulse, S_4
    - Electrocardiography shows exaggerated septal Q waves suggestive of myocardial infarction; supraventricular and ventricular arrhythmias may also be seen
    - Echocardiography with hypertrophy, evidence of dynamic obstruction from abnormal systolic motion of the anterior mitral valve leaflet
    - Role for genetic testing including familial screening, but current tests only identify 50–60% of mutations

- ■ Differential Diagnosis
    - Hypertensive or ischemic heart disease
    - Restrictive cardiomyopathy (eg, amyloidosis)
    - Aortic stenosis; athlete's heart

- ■ Treatment
    - Beta-blockers or calcium channel blockers are the initial drugs of choice in symptomatic patients
    - Avoid afterload reducers such as ACE inhibitors
    - Surgical myectomy, percutaneous transcoronary septal reduction with alcohol, or dual-chamber pacing is considered in some
    - Implantable cardiac defibrillator in patients at high risk for sudden death; risk factors include left ventricle thickness > 30 mm, family history of sudden death, nonsustained ventricular tachycardia on Holter, hypotensive blood pressure response on treadmill, previous cardiac arrest, and syncope
    - Natural history is unpredictable; sports requiring high cardiac output should be discouraged
    - All first-degree relatives should be evaluated with echocardiography every 5 years if > 18 years of age; every year if < 18 years of age

- ■ Pearl

Hypertrophic obstructive cardiomyopathy is the most common cause of sudden cardiac death in athletes.

Reference

Elliott P, Spirito P. Prevention of hypertrophic cardiomyopathy-related deaths: theory and practice. Heart 2008;94:1269. [PMID: 18653582]

1

Mitral Regurgitation

- **Essentials of Diagnosis**
  - Causes include rheumatic heart disease, infectious endocarditis, mitral valve prolapse, ischemic papillary muscle dysfunction, torn chordae tendineae
  - Acute: Immediate onset of symptoms of pulmonary edema
  - Chronic: Asymptomatic for years, then exertional dyspnea and fatigue
  - S_1 usually reduced; a blowing, high-pitched apical pansystolic murmur increased by finger squeeze is characteristic; S_3 common in chronic cases; murmur is not pansystolic and less audible in acute
  - Left atrial abnormality and often left ventricular hypertrophy on ECG; atrial fibrillation typical with chronicity
  - Echo Doppler confirms diagnosis, estimates severity

- **Differential Diagnosis**
  - Aortic stenosis or sclerosis
  - Tricuspid regurgitation
  - Hypertrophic obstructive cardiomyopathy
  - Atrial septal defect
  - Ventricular septal defect

- **Treatment**
  - Acute mitral regurgitation due to endocarditis or torn chordae may require immediate surgical repair
  - Surgical repair or replacement for severe mitral regurgitation in patients with symptoms, left ventricular dysfunction (eg, ejection fraction < 60%), or left ventricular systolic dimension > 40 mm
  - There are no data supporting the use of vasodilators in patients with asymptomatic chronic mitral regurgitation; digoxin, beta-blockers, and calcium channel blockers control ventricular response with atrial fibrillation, and warfarin anticoagulation should be given

- **Pearl**

The rapid up-and-down carotid pulse may be decisive in separating this murmur from that of aortic stenosis.

Reference

Mehra MR, Reyes P, Benitez RM, Zimrin D, Gammie JS. Surgery for severe mitral regurgitation and left ventricular failure: what do we really know? J Card Fail 2008;14:145. [PMID: 18325462]

Mitral Stenosis

- ■ Essentials of Diagnosis
  - Always caused by rheumatic heart disease, but 30% of patients have no history of rheumatic fever
  - Dyspnea, orthopnea, paroxysmal nocturnal dyspnea, even hemoptysis—often precipitated by volume overload (pregnancy, salt load) or tachycardia
  - Right ventricular lift in many; opening snap occasionally palpable
  - Crisp S_1, increased P_2, opening snap; these sounds often easier to appreciate than the characteristic low-pitched apical diastolic murmur
  - Electrocardiography shows left atrial abnormality, and commonly, atrial fibrillation; echo confirms diagnosis, quantifies severity

- ■ Differential Diagnosis
  - Left ventricular failure due to any cause
  - Mitral valve prolapse (if systolic murmur present)
  - Pulmonary hypertension due to other cause
  - Left atrial myxoma
  - Cor triatriatum (in patients under 30)
  - Tricuspid stenosis

- ■ Treatment
  - Heart failure symptoms may be treated with diuretics and sodium restriction
  - With atrial fibrillation, ventricular rate controlled with beta-blockers, calcium channel blockers such as verapamil or digoxin; long-term anticoagulation instituted with warfarin
  - Balloon valvuloplasty or surgical valve replacement in patients with mitral orifice of < 1.5 cm^2 and symptoms or evidence of pulmonary hypertension; valvuloplasty preferred in noncalcified and pliable valves

- ■ Pearl

Think of the crisp first heart sound as the "closing snap" of the mitral valve.

Reference

American College of Cardiology/American Heart Association Task Force on Practice Guidelines; Society of Cardiovascular Anesthesiologists; Society for Cardiovascular Angiography and Interventions; Society of Thoracic Surgeons, Bonow RO, Carabello BA, Kanu C, de Leon AC, et al. ACC/AHA 2006 guidelines for the management of patients with valvular heart disease: a report of the American College of Cardiology/American Heart Association Task Force on Practice Guidelines. Circulation 2006;114:e84. [PMID: 16880336]

1

Multifocal Atrial Tachycardia

- **Essentials of Diagnosis**
  - Classically seen in patients with severe COPD; electrolyte abnormalities (especially hypomagnesemia or hypokalemia) occasionally responsible
  - Symptoms include those of the underlying disorder, but some may complain of palpitations
  - Irregularly irregular heart rate
  - Electrocardiography shows at least three different P-wave morphologies with varying PR intervals
  - Ventricular rate usually between 100 and 140 beats/min; if < 100, rhythm is wandering atrial pacemaker

- **Differential Diagnosis**
  - Normal sinus rhythm with multiple premature atrial contractions
  - Atrial fibrillation
  - Atrial flutter with variable block
  - Reentry tachycardia with variable block

- **Treatment**
  - Treatment of the underlying disorder is most important
  - Verapamil particularly useful for rate control; digitalis ineffective
  - Intravenous magnesium and potassium administered slowly may convert some patients to sinus rhythm even if serum levels are within normal range; be sure renal function is normal
  - Medications causing atrial irritability, such as theophylline, should be avoided
  - Atrioventricular nodal ablation with permanent pacing is used in rare cases that are highly symptomatic and refractory to pharmacologic therapy

- **Pearl**

Multifocal atrial tachycardia is the paradigm COPD arrhythmia, electrocardiographically defined and increasingly treated electrophysiologically.

Reference

Spodick DH. Multifocal atrial arrhythmia. Am J Geriatr Cardiol 2005;14:162. [PMID: 15886545]

Myocarditis

- ■ Essentials of Diagnosis
  - Focal or diffuse inflammation of the myocardium due to various infections, toxins, drugs, or immunologic reactions; viral infection, particularly with coxsackieviruses, is the most common cause
  - Other infectious causes include Rocky Mountain spotted fever, Q fever, Chagas' disease, Lyme disease, HIV, trichinosis, and toxoplasmosis
  - Symptoms include fever, fatigue, palpitations, chest pain, or symptoms of congestive heart failure, often following an upper respiratory tract infection
  - Electrocardiography may reveal ST-T wave changes, conduction blocks
  - Echocardiography shows diffusely depressed left ventricular function and enlargement
  - Routine myocardial biopsy usually not recommended since inflammatory changes are often focal and nonspecific

- ■ Differential Diagnosis
  - Acute myocardial ischemia or infarction due to coronary artery disease
  - Pneumonia
  - Congestive heart failure due to other causes

- ■ Treatment
  - Bed rest
  - Specific antimicrobial treatment if an infectious agent can be identified
  - Immunosuppressive therapy is controversial
  - Appropriate treatment of systolic dysfunction: vasodilators (ACE inhibitors, angiotensin II receptor blockers, or combination of hydralazine and isosorbide dinitrate), beta-blockers, spironolactone, digoxin, low-sodium diet, and diuretics
  - Inotropes and cardiac transplant for severe cases

- ■ Pearl

In viral myocarditis, remember the following: one-third return to normal, one-third have stable left ventricular dysfunction, and one-third have a severe cardiomyopathy.

Reference

Schultz JC, Hilliard AA, Cooper LT Jr, Rihal CS. Diagnosis and treatment of viral myocarditis. Mayo Clin Proc 2009;84:1001. [PMID: 19880690]

1

Paroxysmal Supraventricular Tachycardia (PSVT)

- **Essentials of Diagnosis**
  - A group of arrhythmias including atrioventricular nodal reentrant, atrioventricular reentrant tachycardias, automatic atrial tachycardia, and junctional tachycardia
  - Attacks usually begin and end abruptly, last seconds to hours
  - Patients often asymptomatic with transient episodes but may complain of palpitations, mild dyspnea, or chest pain
  - Electrocardiography between attacks normal unless the patient has Wolff-Parkinson-White syndrome or a very short PR interval
  - Unless aberrant conduction occurs, the QRS complexes are regular and narrow; P wave location helps determine the origin; electrophysiologic study establishes the exact diagnosis

- **Differential Diagnosis**
  No P:
  - Atrioventricular nodal reentry tachycardia
  Short RP:
  - Typical atrioventricular reentrant tachycardia
  - Orthodromic atrioventricular reentrant tachycardia
  - Atrial tachycardia with 1st degree AV delay
  - Junctional tachycardia
  Long RP:
  - Atrial tachycardia
  - Sinus tachycardia
  - Atypical atrioventricular nodal reentry tachycardia
  - Permanent junctional reciprocating tachycardia

- **Treatment**
  - Many attacks resolve spontaneously; if not, first try vagal maneuvers such as carotid sinus massage or adenosine to transiently block the AV node and break the reentrant circuit
  - Prevention of frequent attacks can be achieved by calcium channel blockers, beta-blockers, or antiarrhythmics if necessary
  - Electrophysiologic study and ablation of the abnormal reentrant circuit or focus, when available, is the treatment of choice

- **Pearl**

  If "Q-wave MI" is the computer readout with a short PR interval, consider this: erroneous interpretation may make your patient ineligible for life insurance, when the innocent WPW is the diagnosis.

Reference

Holdgate A, Foo A. Adenosine versus intravenous calcium channel antagonists for the treatment of supraventricular tachycardia in adults. Cochrane Database Syst Rev 2006;(4):CD005154. [PMID: 17054240]

Patent Ductus Arteriosus

- Essentials of Diagnosis
  - Caused by failure of closure of embryonic ductus arteriosus with continuous blood flow from aorta to pulmonary artery (ie, left-to-right shunt)
  - Symptoms are those of left ventricular failure or pulmonary hypertension; many cases are complaint-free
  - Widened pulse pressure, a loud S_2, and a continuous, "machinery" murmur loudest over the pulmonary area but heard posteriorly
  - Echo Doppler helpful, but contrast or MR aortography is the study of choice

- Differential Diagnosis

  In patients presenting with left heart failure:
  - Mitral regurgitation
  - Aortic stenosis
  - Ventricular septal defect

  If pulmonary hypertension dominates the picture:
  - Primary pulmonary hypertension
  - Chronic pulmonary embolism
  - Eisenmenger's syndrome

- Treatment
  - Pharmacologic closure in premature infants, using indomethacin or aspirin
  - Surgical or percutaneous closure in patients with large shunts, symptoms, or previous endocarditis; controversial in other settings

- Pearl

Patients usually remain asymptomatic as adults if problems have not developed by age 10 years.

Reference

Schneider DJ, Moore JW. Patent ductus arteriosus. Circulation 2006;114:1873. [PMID: 17060397]

1

Prinzmetal's Angina

- **Essentials of Diagnosis**
  - Caused by intermittent focal spasm of an otherwise normal coronary artery
  - Associated with migraine, Raynaud's phenomenon
  - The chest pain resembles typical angina, but often is more severe and occurs at rest
  - Affects women under 50, occurs in the early morning, and typically involves the right coronary artery
  - Electrocardiography shows ST-segment elevation, but enzyme studies are normal
  - Diagnosis can be confirmed by ergonovine challenge during cardiac catheterization

- **Differential Diagnosis**
  - Typical angina pectoris; myocardial infarction; unstable angina
  - Tietze's syndrome (costochondritis)
  - Cervical or thoracic radiculopathy, including pre-eruptive zoster
  - Esophageal spasm or reflux disease
  - Cholecystitis
  - Pericarditis
  - Pneumothorax
  - Pulmonary embolism
  - Pneumococcal pneumonia

- **Treatment**
  - Statins, smoking cessation, nitrates, and calcium channel blockers acutely effective and are the mainstay of chronic therapy
  - Prognosis excellent given absence of atherosclerosis

- **Pearl**

In its classic iteration, vasospasm of the right coronary artery, mostly women, nonexertional, no atherosclerosis, ST elevation at the same time of the day; in 2010, consider cocaine or methamphetamine use.

Reference

Stern S, Bayes de Luna A. Coronary artery spasm: a 2009 update. Circulation 2009;119:2531. [PMID: 19433770]

Pulmonary Stenosis

- ■ Essentials of Diagnosis
  - Exertional dyspnea and chest pain due to right ventricular ischemia; sudden death occurs in severe cases
  - Jugular venous distention, parasternal lift, systolic click and ejection murmur, delayed and soft pulmonary component of S_2
  - Right ventricular hypertrophy on ECG; poststenotic dilation of the main and left pulmonary arteries on chest x-ray
  - Echo Doppler is diagnostic
  - May be associated with Noonan's syndrome

- ■ Differential Diagnosis
  - Left ventricular failure due to any cause
  - Left-sided valvular disease
  - Primary pulmonary hypertension
  - Chronic pulmonary embolism
  - Sleep apnea
  - Chronic obstructive pulmonary disease
  - Eisenmenger's syndrome

- ■ Treatment
  - Symptomatic patients with peak gradient > 30 mm Hg: Percutaneous balloon or surgical valvuloplasty
  - Asymptomatic patients with peak gradient > 40 mm Hg: Percutaneous balloon or surgical valvuloplasty
  - Prognosis for those with mild disease is good

- ■ Pearl

If contemplating this as the cause of a murmur, be sure to inquire about flushing; carcinoid syndrome is one of the few causes of right-sided valvular disease.

Reference

Kogon B, Plattner C, Kirshbom P, et al. Risk factors for early pulmonary valve replacement after valve disruption in congenital pulmonary stenosis and tetralogy of Fallot. J Thorac Cardiovasc Surg 2009;138:103. [PMID: 19577064]

1

Restrictive Cardiomyopathy

- **Essentials of Diagnosis**
    - Characterized by impaired diastolic filling with preserved left ventricular function
    - Causes include amyloidosis, sarcoidosis, hemochromatosis, scleroderma, carcinoid syndrome, endomyocardial fibrosis, and postradiation or postsurgical fibrosis
    - Clinical manifestations are those of the underlying disorder; congestive heart failure with right-sided symptoms and signs usually predominates
    - Electrocardiography may show low voltage and nonspecific ST-T wave abnormalities in amyloidosis; supraventricular and ventricular arrhythmias may also be seen
    - Echo Doppler shows increased wall thickness with preserved contractile function and mitral and tricuspid inflow velocity patterns consistent with impaired diastolic filling
    - Cardiac catheterization shows ventricular concordance with respiration as compared with constrictive pericarditis

- **Differential Diagnosis**
    - Constrictive pericarditis
    - Hypertensive heart disease
    - Hypertrophic obstructive cardiomyopathy
    - Aortic stenosis
    - Ischemic heart disease

- **Treatment**
    - Sodium restriction and diuretic therapy for patients with evidence of fluid overload; diuresis must be cautious, as volume depletion may worsen this disorder
    - Digitalis should be used with caution due to increase in intracellular calcium
    - Treatment of underlying disease causing the restriction if possible

- **Pearl**

In a patient with this condition, if the right upper quadrant appears dense on plain chest x-ray, consider hemochromatosis; hepatic iron deposition is responsible.

Reference

Whalley GA, Gamble GD, Doughty RN. The prognostic significance of restrictive diastolic filling associated with heart failure: a meta-analysis. Int J Cardiol 2007;116:70. [PMID: 16901562]

Sudden Cardiac Death

- ■ Essentials of Diagnosis
  - Death in a well patient within 1 hour of symptom onset
  - Can be due to cardiac or noncardiac disease
  - Most common cause (> 80% of cases) is ventricular fibrillation or tachycardia in the setting of coronary artery disease
  - Ventricular fibrillation is almost always the terminal rhythm

- ■ Differential Diagnosis
  Noncardiac causes of sudden death:
  - Pulmonary embolism
  - Asthma
  - Aortic dissection
  - Ruptured aortic aneurysm
  - Intracranial hemorrhage
  - Tension pneumothorax
  - Anaphylaxis

- ■ Treatment
  - Aggressive approach obligatory if coronary artery disease is suspected; see below
  - Electrolyte abnormalities, digitalis toxicity, or implantable cardiac defibrillator malfunction can be the precipitant and is treated accordingly
  - Without obvious cause, echocardiography and cardiac catheterization are indicated; if normal, electrophysiologic studies thereafter
  - An automatic implantable cardiac defibrillator should be used in all patients surviving an episode of sudden cardiac death secondary to ventricular fibrillation or tachycardia without a transient or reversible cause

- ■ Pearl

In resuscitated ventricular fibrillation in adults, if myocardial infarction is ruled out, the prognosis is paradoxically worse than if ruled in; it suggests that active ischemia or significant structural heart disease is present.

Reference

Mudawi TO, Albouaini K, Kaye GC. Sudden cardiac death: history, aetiology and management. Br J Hosp Med (Lond) 2009;70:89. [PMID: 19229149]

1

Tricuspid Regurgitation

- **Essentials of Diagnosis**
  - Causes include infective endocarditis, right ventricular heart failure of any cause, carcinoid syndrome, systemic lupus erythematosus, Ebstein's anomaly, and leaflet disruption due to cardiac device leads
  - Most cases secondary to dilation of the right ventricle from left-sided heart disease
  - Edema, abdominal discomfort, anorexia; otherwise, symptoms of associated disease
  - Prominent (*v*) waves in jugular venous pulse; pulsatile liver, abdominojugular reflux
  - Characteristic high-pitched blowing holosystolic murmur along the left sternal border increasing with inspiration
  - Echo Doppler is diagnostic

- **Differential Diagnosis**
  - Mitral regurgitation
  - Aortic stenosis
  - Pulmonary stenosis
  - Atrial septal defect
  - Ventricular septal defect

- **Treatment**
  - Diuretics and dietary sodium restriction in patients with evidence of fluid overload
  - If tricuspid regurgitation is functional and surgery is performed for multivalvular disease, then tricuspid valve annuloplasty can be considered

- **Pearl**

Ninety percent of right heart failure is caused by left heart failure.

Reference

Chang BC, Song SW, Lee S, Yoo KJ, Kang MS, Chung N. Eight-year outcomes of tricuspid annuloplasty using autologous pericardial strip for functional tricuspid regurgitation. Ann Thorac Surg 2008;86:1485. [PMID: 19049736]

Tricuspid Stenosis

- ■ Essentials of Diagnosis
  - Usually rheumatic in origin; rarely, seen in carcinoid heart disease
  - Almost always associated with mitral stenosis when rheumatic
  - Evidence of right-sided failure: Hepatomegaly, ascites, peripheral edema, jugular venous distention with prominent (*a*) wave
  - A diastolic rumbling murmur along the left sternal border, increasing with inspiration
  - Echo Doppler is diagnostic

- ■ Differential Diagnosis
  - Atypical aortic regurgitation
  - Mitral stenosis
  - Pulmonary hypertension due to any cause with right heart failure
  - Constrictive pericarditis
  - Liver cirrhosis
  - Right atrial myxoma

- ■ Treatment
  - Valve replacement in severe cases
  - Balloon valvuloplasty may prove to be useful in many patients

- ■ Pearl

Almost never encountered in the United States with the wane of rheumatic heart disease; the rare patient with carcinoid syndrome may have it.

Reference

Guenther T, Noebauer C, Mazzitelli D, Busch R, Tassani-Prell P, Lange R. Tricuspid valve surgery: a thirty-year assessment of early and late outcome. Eur J Cardiothorac Surg 2008;34:402. [PMID: 18579403]

Unstable Angina

- **Essentials of Diagnosis**
  - Spectrum of illness between chronic stable angina and acute myocardial infarction
  - Characterized by accelerating angina, pain at rest, or pain less responsive to medications
  - Usually due to atherosclerotic plaque rupture, spasm, hemorrhage, or thrombosis
  - Chest pain resembles typical angina but is more severe and lasts longer (up to 30 minutes)
  - ECG may show dynamic ST-segment depression or T-wave changes during pain, but normalizes when symptoms abate; a normal ECG, however, does not exclude the diagnosis

- **Differential Diagnosis**
  - Typical angina pectoris; myocardial infarction
  - Coronary vasospasm; aortic dissection
  - Tietze's syndrome (costochondritis)
  - Cervical or thoracic radiculopathy, including pre-eruptive zoster
  - Esophageal spasm or reflux disease
  - Cholecystitis; pneumonia; pericarditis
  - Pneumothorax
  - Pulmonary embolism

- **Treatment**
  - Hospitalization with bed rest, telemetry, and treatment similar to acute coronary syndrome
  - Low-dose aspirin (81–325 mg) immediately on admission for all; intravenous heparin of benefit
  - Beta-blockers to keep heart rate and blood pressure in the low-normal range
  - In high-risk patients, glycoprotein IIb/IIIa inhibitors effective, especially if percutaneous intervention likely
  - Nitroglycerin, either in paste or intravenously
  - Cardiac catheterization and consideration of revascularization in appropriate candidates

- **Pearl**

  This condition requires aggressive anticoagulation; give aortic dissection a thought before writing the orders for same.

Reference

Hitzeman N. Early invasive therapy or conservative management for unstable angina or NSTEMI? Am Fam Physician 2007;75:47. [PMID: 17225702]

Ventricular Septal Defect

- ■ Essentials of Diagnosis
  - Many congenital ventricular septal defects close spontaneously during childhood
  - Symptoms depend on the size of the defect and the magnitude of the left-to-right shunt
  - Small defects in adults are usually asymptomatic except for complicating endocarditis, but may be associated with a loud murmur (maladie de Roger)
  - Large defects usually associated with softer murmurs, but commonly lead to Eisenmenger's syndrome
  - Echo Doppler diagnostic; radionuclide angiogram or cardiac catheterization quantifies the ratio of pulmonary flow to systemic flow (Q_P:Q_S)

- ■ Differential Diagnosis
  - Mitral regurgitation
  - Aortic stenosis
  - Cardiomyopathy due to various causes

- ■ Treatment
  - Small shunts in asymptomatic patients may not require surgery
  - Mild dyspnea treatable with diuretics and preload reduction
  - Q_P:Q_S shunts over 1.5 are repaired to prevent irreversible pulmonary vascular disease, but decision to close needs to be tailored to individual patient
  - Surgery if patient has developed shunt reversal (Eisenmenger's syndrome) without fixed pulmonary hypertension

- ■ Pearl

Small defects have a higher risk of endocarditis than large ones; endothelial injury is favored by a small, localized jet.

Reference

Butera G, Chessa M, Carminati M. Percutaneous closure of ventricular septal defects. State of the art. J Cardiovasc Med (Hagerstown) 2007;8:39. [PMID: 17255815]

1

Ventricular Tachycardia

- ### Essentials of Diagnosis
  - Three or more consecutive premature ventricular beats; nonsustained (lasting < 30 seconds) or sustained
  - Mechanisms are reentry or automatic focus; may occur spontaneously or with myocardial infarction
  - Other causes include acute or chronic ischemia, cardiomyopathy, and drugs (eg, antiarrhythmics)
  - Most patients symptomatic; syncope, palpitations, shortness of breath, and chest pain are common
  - S_1 of variable intensity; S_3 present
  - Electrocardiography shows a regular, wide-complex tachycardia (usually between 140 and 220 beats/min); between attacks, the ECG often reveals evidence of prior myocardial infarction

- ### Differential Diagnosis
  - Any cause of supraventricular tachycardia with aberrant conduction (but a history of myocardial infarction or low ejection fraction indicates ventricular tachycardia until proved otherwise)
  - Atrial flutter with aberrant conduction

- ### Treatment
  - Depends on whether the patient is stable or unstable
  - If stable: intravenous lidocaine, procainamide, or amiodarone can be used initially
  - If unstable (hypotension, congestive heart failure, or angina): immediate synchronized cardioversion
  - Implantable cardiac defibrillator placement should be strongly considered
  - In a patient with ischemic or nonischemic heart disease and a low left ventricular ejection fraction (< 35%), an implantable cardiac defibrillator is warranted, even in the absence of documented ventricular tachycardia
  - Ablation for those with repetitive shocks from defibrillator

- ### Pearl
  All wide-complex tachycardia should be treated as ventricular tachycardia until proven otherwise.

Reference

Aronow WS. Treatment of ventricular arrhythmias in the elderly. Cardiol Rev 2009;17:136. [PMID: 19384088]

2

Pulmonary Diseases

Acute Bacterial Pneumonia

- **Essentials of Diagnosis**
    - Fever, chills, dyspnea, cough with purulent sputum production; early pleuritic pain suggests pneumococcal etiology
    - Tachycardia, tachypnea; bronchial breath sounds with percussive dullness and egophony over involved lungs
    - Leukocytosis; WBC < 5000 or > 25,000 worrisome
    - Patchy or lobar infiltrate by chest x-ray
    - Diagnosis is clinical, but pathogen can be determined from proper sputum Gram stain and/or culture of sputum, blood (positive in ~10%, or pleural fluid; pathogen only determined in 30–60%
    - Principal causes include *Streptococcus pneumoniae*, *Haemophilus influenzae*, *Legionella* (elderly, smokers), gram-negative rods (alcoholics and aspirators), *Staphylococcus (postviral)*

- **Differential Diagnosis**
    - Atypical or viral pneumonia
    - Pulmonary embolism with infarct
    - Congestive heart failure; acute respiratory distress syndrome (ARDS)
    - Interstitial lung disease
    - Bronchoalveolar cell carcinoma

- **Treatment**
    - Empiric antibiotics for common organisms after obtaining cultures; initial dose given in the emergency department
    - Hospitalize selected patients: ≥ 2 of the following CURB-65 criteria: **c**onfusion, blood **u**rea nitrogen > 20 mg/dL, **r**espiratory rate > 30, systolic **b**lood pressure ≤ 90 mm Hg, age ≥ 65, or patients with significant comorbidities or a vital sign, laboratory, or radiographic abnormality
    - Pneumococcal vaccine to prevent or lessen severity of pneumococcal infections

- **Pearl**

When diplococci thrive within neutrophils on Gram stain, think staphylococci, not pneumococci.

Reference

Niven DJ, Laupland KB. Severe community-acquired pneumonia in adults: current antimicrobial chemotherapy. Expert Rev Anti Infect Ther 2009;7:69. [PMID: 19622058]

Acute Pulmonary Venous Thromboembolism

2

- ■ Essentials of Diagnosis
  - Seen in immobilized patients, congestive heart failure, malignancies, hypercoagulable states, and after pelvic trauma or surgery
  - Abrupt onset of dyspnea and anxiety, with or without pleuritic chest pain, cough with hemoptysis; syncope rare
  - Tachycardia, tachypnea most common; loud P_2 with right-sided S_3 characteristic but unusual
  - Acute respiratory alkalosis and hypoxemia
  - Elevations in brain natriuretic peptide (eg, BNP > 100 pg/mL) and/or troponins portend a worse prognosis and should prompt an echocardiographic evaluation of right ventricular function
  - Quantitative D-dimer has excellent negative predictive value in patients with low clinical pretest probability
  - CT angiogram is the new gold standard and essentially rules out clinically significant pulmonary embolism
  - A ventilation-perfusion scan can be done in patients who cannot tolerate contrast dye; results rely on pretest probability
  - Lower-extremity ultrasound demonstrates deep venous thrombosis (DVT) in half of patients
  - Rarely, pulmonary angiography required

- ■ Differential Diagnosis
  - Pneumonia; myocardial infarction
  - Any cause of acute respiratory distress
  - Systemic inflammatory response syndrome (SIRS)

- ■ Treatment
  - Anticoagulation: Acutely with heparin, start warfarin concurrently and continue for a minimum of 6 months (for reversible cause) to lifelong (unprovoked or irreversible cause)
  - Thrombolytic therapy in selected patients with hemodynamic compromise
  - Intravenous filter placement for selected patients; consider temporary filter if risk of anticoagulation is time-limited

- ■ Pearl

Ten percent of pulmonary emboli originate from upper-extremity veins; there is more endothelial thromboplastin activity than in the leg veins.

Reference
Todd JL, Tapson VF. Thrombolytic therapy for acute pulmonary embolism: a critical appraisal. Chest 2009;135:1321. [PMID: 19420199]

Acute Respiratory Distress Syndrome (ARDS)

■ Essentials of Diagnosis

- Rapid onset of dyspnea and respiratory distress, commonly in setting of trauma, shock, aspiration, or sepsis
- Tachypnea, fever; crackles heard by auscultation
- Arterial hypoxemia refractory to supplemental oxygen, frequently requiring positive pressure ventilation; hypercapnia and respiratory acidosis due to increase in dead space fraction and decrease in tidal volume (lungs become stiff and difficult to expand)
- Diffuse alveolar and interstitial infiltrates by radiography, often sparing costophrenic angles
- No clinical evidence of left atrial hypertension; pulmonary capillary wedge pressure < 18 mm Hg
- Acute lung injury defined by a $Pao_2:Fio_2$ ratio < 300; ARDS is defined by $Pao_2:Fio_2$ ratio < 200

■ Differential Diagnosis

- Cardiogenic pulmonary edema
- Primary pneumonia due to any cause
- Diffuse alveolar hemorrhage
- Acute interstitial pneumonia (ie, Hamman-Rich syndrome)
- Cryptogenic organizing pneumonia

■ Treatment

- Mechanical ventilation with supplemental oxygen; positive end-expiratory pressure often required
- Low-tidal-volume ventilation, using 6 mL/kg predicted body weight, may reduce mortality
- A conservative fluid strategy targeting an even total body fluid balance (requires daily diuretics) decreases both time on the ventilator and time in the ICU
- Supportive therapy including adequate nutrition, vigilance for other organ dysfunction, and prevention of nosocomial complications (eg, catheter-related infection, UTI, ventilator-associated pneumonia, venous thromboembolism, stress gastritis)
- Mortality rate is 30–60%

■ Pearl

As the Swan-Ganz catheter falls from favor, the cardiac echo becomes increasingly important in ruling out a cardiogenic cause of this problem.

Reference

Tang BM, Craig JC, Eslick GD, Seppelt I, McLean AS. Use of corticosteroids in acute lung injury and acute respiratory distress syndrome: a systematic review and meta-analysis. Crit Care Med 2009;37:1594. [PMID: 19325471]

Acute Tracheobronchitis

2

- ■ Essentials of Diagnosis
  - Poorly defined but common condition characterized by inflammation of the trachea and bronchi
  - Due to infectious agents (bacteria or viruses) or irritants (eg, dust and smoke)
  - Consider nasal swab for influenza if constitutional symptoms present
  - Cough is most common symptom; purulent sputum production and malaise common; hemoptysis occasionally
  - Variable rhonchi and wheezing; fever often absent but may be prominent in cases caused by *Haemophilus influenzae*
  - Chest x-ray normal
  - Increased incidence in smokers

- ■ Differential Diagnosis
  - Asthma
  - Pneumonia
  - Foreign body aspiration
  - Inhalation pneumonitis
  - Viral croup

- ■ Treatment
  - Symptomatic therapy with inhaled bronchodilators, cough suppressants
  - Antibiotics not recommended in most; they shorten the disease course by less than 1 day
  - Treat patients with influenza according to guideline recommendations
  - Patients encouraged to quit smoking

- ■ Pearl

Haemophilus influenzae and Pseudomonas *have a tropism for large airways; study the Gram stain carefully in this syndrome, especially absent underlying lung disease.*

Reference

Wenzel RP, Fowler AA 3rd. Clinical practice. Acute bronchitis. N Engl J Med 2006;355:2125. [PMID: 17108344]

Allergic Bronchopulmonary Mycosis (Formerly Allergic Bronchopulmonary Aspergillosis)

- ■ Essentials of Diagnosis
  - Caused by allergy to antigens of *Aspergillus* species or other fungi colonizing the tracheobronchial tree
  - Recurrent dyspnea, unmasked by corticosteroid withdrawal, with history of asthma; cough productive of brownish plugs of sputum
  - Physical examination as in asthma
  - Peripheral eosinophilia, elevated serum IgE level, precipitating antibody to *Aspergillus* antigen present; positive skin hypersensitivity to *Aspergillus* antigen
  - Infiltrate (often fleeting) and central bronchiectasis by chest radiography

- ■ Differential Diagnosis
  - Asthma
  - Bronchiectasis
  - Invasive aspergillosis
  - Churg-Strauss syndrome
  - Chronic obstructive pulmonary disease

- ■ Treatment
  - Oral corticosteroids often required for several months
  - Inhaled bronchodilators as for attacks of asthma
  - Treatment with itraconazole (for 16 weeks) improves disease control
  - Complications include hemoptysis, severe bronchiectasis, and pulmonary fibrosis

- ■ Pearl

One of at least three ways this fungus causes illness—all different pathophysiologically.

Reference

de Oliveira E, Giavina-Bianchi P, Fonseca LA, França AT, Kalil J. Allergic bronchopulmonary aspergillosis' diagnosis remains a challenge. Respir Med 2007;101:2352. [PMID: 17689062]

Asbestosis

2

- ■ Essentials of Diagnosis
  - History of exposure to dust containing asbestos particles (eg, from work in mining, insulation, construction, shipbuilding)
  - Progressive dyspnea that appears 20–40 years after exposure, rarely pleuritic chest pain
  - Dry inspiratory crackles and clubbing are common; cyanosis and signs of cor pulmonale occasionally seen
  - Interstitial fibrosis is characteristic (lower lung greater than upper); pleural thickening and diaphragmatic calcification common but nonspecific; however, the three together with exposure history establish the diagnosis
  - Exudative pleural effusion develops before parenchymal disease
  - High-resolution CT scan often confirmatory
  - Pulmonary function testing shows a restrictive defect; diminished diffusion lung capacity for carbon monoxide (DLCO) often the earliest abnormality

- ■ Differential Diagnosis
  - Other inhalation pneumoconioses (eg, silicosis)
  - Fungal disease
  - Sarcoidosis
  - Idiopathic pulmonary fibrosis
  - Hypersensitivity pneumonitis

- ■ Treatment
  - Supportive care; chronic oxygen supplementation for sustained hypoxemia
  - Screen for other respiratory diseases associated with asbestos exposure (diffuse pleural thickening, plaques, effusions, rounded atelectasis, mesothelioma, bronchogenic carcinoma)
  - Legal counseling regarding compensation for occupational exposure using above diagnostic criteria

- ■ Pearl

Remember that the highest exposure on ships comes from sweeping the floor; this history may aid a patient in being compensated for pulmonary disability.

Reference

Centers for Disease Control and Prevention (CDC). Asbestosis-related years of potential life lost before age 65 years—United States, 1968-2005. MMWR Morb Mortal Wkly Rep 2008;57:1321. [PMID: 19078920]

Asthma

■ Essentials of Diagnosis

- Episodic wheezing, cough, and dyspnea; poorly controlled chronic dyspnea or chest tightness; can present as nighttime cough
- Triggers include: allergens (pets), irritants (smoke), infections (viral), drugs (aspirin), cold air, exercise, stress
- Prolonged expiratory time, wheezing; if severe, pulsus paradoxus
- Peripheral eosinophilia; mucus casts, eosinophils in sputum
- Obstructive pattern by spirometry supports diagnosis, though may be normal between attacks
- With methacholine challenge, absence of bronchial hyperreactivity makes diagnosis unlikely

■ Differential Diagnosis

- Congestive heart failure; vocal cord dysfunction
- Chronic obstructive pulmonary disease
- Foreign body aspiration
- Allergic bronchopulmonary mycosis
- Churg-Strauss syndrome

■ Treatment

- Avoidance of known precipitants, inhaled corticosteroids in persistent asthma, inhaled bronchodilators for symptoms
- Goal of treatment is to "step up" drug treatment until patient has achieved complete control of symptoms then "step down" as tolerated
- In patients not well controlled on inhaled corticosteroids, add a long-acting inhaled β-agonist (eg, salmeterol); do not use long-acting β-agonists in patients not using inhaled glucocorticoids
- Treatment of exacerbations: Oxygen, inhaled bronchodilators (β_2-agonists > anticholinergics), systemic corticosteroids (5 days)
- Leukotriene modifiers (eg, montelukast) may provide a second option for long-term therapy in mild to moderate disease
- Nedocromil/cromolyn is effective for exercise-induced asthma
- For difficult-to-control asthma, consider exacerbating factors such as gastroesophageal reflux disease and chronic sinusitis

■ Pearl

All that wheezes is not asthma; remember conditions like heart failure and vocal cord dysfunction in patients with "steroid-resistant" asthma.

Reference

Ni Chroinin M, Greenstone I, Lasserson TJ, Ducharme FM. Addition of inhaled long-acting beta2-agonists to inhaled steroids as first line therapy for persistent asthma in steroid-naive adults and children. Cochrane Database Syst Rev 2009;4:CD005307. [PMID: 19821344]

Atypical Pneumonia

2

- **Essentials of Diagnosis**
  - Pathogens include *Legionella*, *Mycoplasma*, *Chlamydia*, viruses
  - Cough with scant sputum, fever, malaise, headache; gastrointestinal symptoms variable
  - Physical examination of lungs may be unimpressive
  - Mild leukocytosis; cold agglutinins sometimes positive but not diagnostic for *Mycoplasma*
  - Patchy, nonlobar infiltrate by chest x-ray often surprisingly extensive
  - Typical and atypical pneumonia are not reliably distinguishable clinically or radiographically

- **Differential Diagnosis**
  - Typical bacterial pneumonia
  - *Pneumocystis jiroveci* pneumonia
  - Congestive heart failure
  - Diffuse alveolar hemorrhage
  - Interstitial lung disease (hypersensitivity pneumonitis, nonspecific interstitial fibrosis, cryptogenic organizing pneumonitis)

- **Treatment**
  - Empiric antibiotic treatment with doxycycline, erythromycin or other macrolide (eg, azithromycin), fluoroquinolone (eg, levofloxacin)
  - Hospitalize as for bacterial pneumonia

- **Pearl**

Bullous myringitis is encountered in 5% of patients with Mycoplasma pneumonia; it's as diagnostically specific as serology and takes seconds rather than days to verify.

Reference

Robenshtok E, Shefet D, Gafter-Gvili A, Paul M, Vidal L, Leibovici L. Empiric antibiotic coverage of atypical pathogens for community acquired pneumonia in hospitalized adults. Cochrane Database Syst Rev 2008;1:CD004418. [PMID: 18254049]

Bronchiectasis

- **Essentials of Diagnosis**

  - A congenital or acquired disorder, affecting the large bronchi causing permanent abnormal dilation and destruction of bronchial walls; may be a consequence of untreated pneumonia
  - Chronic cough with copious purulent sputum, hemoptysis; weight loss, recurrent pneumonias
  - Coarse, midinspiratory moist crackles; clubbing
  - Hypoxemia; obstructive pattern by spirometry
  - Chest x-rays variable, may show tram-tracking (best seen on lateral films) and multiple cystic lesions at bases in advanced cases
  - High-resolution CT scan necessary for diagnosis in many cases
  - Often associated with underlying systemic disorder (eg, cystic fibrosis, hypogammaglobulinemia, IgA deficiency, common variable immunodeficiency, primary ciliary dyskinesia), allergic bronchopulmonary mycosis, HIV, or chronic pulmonary infection (eg, tuberculosis, other mycobacterioses, lung abscess)
  - Complications include massive hemoptysis, cor pulmonale, amyloidosis, and secondary visceral abscesses (eg, brain abscess)

- **Differential Diagnosis**

  - Chronic obstructive pulmonary disease
  - Tuberculosis
  - Hypogammaglobulinemia
  - Ciliary dysmotility
  - Cystic fibrosis
  - Pneumonia due to any cause

- **Treatment**

  - Antibiotics selected by sputum culture and sensitivities
  - Chest physiotherapy
  - Inhaled bronchodilators
  - Inhaled glucocorticoids in selected patients especially during exacerbation
  - Mucolytics and airway hydration
  - Surgical resection in selected patients with unresponsive localized disease or massive hemoptysis

- **Pearl**

Largely a disappearing condition given antibiotic use, but it remains the only cause in medicine of three-layered sputum.

Reference
Kapur N, Bell S, Kolbe J, Chang AB. Inhaled steroids for bronchiectasis. Cochrane Database Syst Rev 2009;1:CD000996. [PMID: 19160186]

Chronic Cough

2

- **Essentials of Diagnosis**
  - One of the most common reasons for seeking medical attention
  - Defined as a cough persisting for at least 4 weeks
  - Nasal and oral examination for signs of postnasal drip (eg, cobblestone appearance or erythema of mucosa), chest auscultation for wheezing
  - Chest x-ray to exclude specific parenchymal lung diseases
  - Consider spirometry before and after bronchodilator, methacholine challenge, sinus CT scan, and 24-hour esophageal pH monitoring
  - Bronchoscopy in selected cases

- **Differential Diagnosis**
  - Bronchitis
  - Respiratory bronchiolitis (smoking-related)
  - Angiotensin-converting enzyme (ACE) inhibitor
  - Postnasal drip
  - Sinusitis
  - Asthma
  - Gastroesophageal reflux
  - Postinfectious cough
  - Chronic obstructive pulmonary disease
  - Congestive heart failure
  - Interstitial lung disease
  - Bronchogenic carcinoma
  - Psychogenic cough

- **Treatment**
  - Smoking cessation
  - Treat underlying condition if present
  - Trial of inhaled β-agonist (eg, albuterol)
  - For postnasal drip: Antihistamines (H_1-antagonists or may add nasal ipratropium bromide)
  - For suspected gastroesophageal reflux disease, proton pump inhibitors (eg, omeprazole)

- **Pearl**

Commonly caused by ACE inhibitors, but don't forget esophageal reflux and aspiration.

Reference

Pavord ID, Chung KF. Management of chronic cough. Lancet 2008;371:1375. [PMID: 18424326]

Chronic Eosinophilic Pneumonia

- ■ Essentials of Diagnosis
  - • Fever, dry cough, wheezing, dyspnea, and weight loss—all variable from transient to severe and progressive
  - • Wheezing, dry crackles occasionally appreciated by auscultation
  - • Peripheral blood eosinophilia (> 1000 μL) present in most, but not all
  - • Peripheral pulmonary infiltrates on radiographs in many cases (the "radiologic negative" of pulmonary edema); > 25% eosinophils by bronchoalveolar lavage; lung biopsy shows abundant eosinophils

- ■ Differential Diagnosis
  - • Infectious pneumonia
  - • Asthma
  - • Idiopathic pulmonary fibrosis
  - • Cryptogenic organizing pneumonitis
  - • Allergic bronchopulmonary mycosis
  - • Churg-Strauss syndrome
  - • Other eosinophilic pulmonary syndromes (eg, drug- or parasite-related, acute eosinophilic pneumonia)

- ■ Treatment
  - • Moderate-dose corticosteroid therapy often results in dramatic improvement, but recurrence is common (~50%)
  - • Most patients require corticosteroids for a year, others indefinitely

- ■ Pearl

Consider the epidemiology before giving steroids to a patient with asthma and eosinophilia; you may cause commonly fatal hyper-infestation syndrome of Strongyloides.

Reference

Marchand E, Cordier JF. Idiopathic chronic eosinophilic pneumonia. Orphanet J Rare Dis 2006;1:11. [PMID: 16722612]

Chronic Obstructive Pulmonary Disease (COPD)

2

■ Essentials of Diagnosis

- Primarily consisting of emphysema and chronic bronchitis
- Dyspnea or chronic productive cough or both are characteristic; COPD is nearly always a disease of heavy smokers (80–90%)
- Tachypnea, barrel chest, distant breath sounds, wheezes or rhonchi, cyanosis; clubbing unusual
- Hypoxemia and hypercapnia more pronounced with chronic bronchitis than with emphysema, whereas pulmonary hypertension is more common in patients with emphysema
- Hyperexpansion with decreased markings by chest radiography
- Airflow obstruction by spirometry (FEV_1/FVC ratio < 0.70); reduced diffusing capacity (DLCO) in emphysema

■ Differential Diagnosis

- Asthma
- Bronchiectasis
- β_1-Antitrypsin deficiency
- Bronchiolitis

■ Treatment

- Stopping smoking is most important intervention
- Inhaled anticholinergic agents improve symptoms and decrease exacerbations (inhaled tiotropium may be superior to ipratropium)
- Long-acting β-agonists decrease exacerbations
- Chronic inhaled glucocorticoids may increase pneumonia risk; use only if patient has clear symptomatic improvement
- Pneumococcal vaccination; yearly influenza vaccination
- Supplemental oxygen for hypoxemic patients (Pao_2 < 55 mm Hg or O_2 saturation < 88%) reduces mortality
- For exacerbations, treat with bronchodilators, antibiotics, systemic glucocorticoids with taper over 2 weeks
- Inpatients with ventilatory failure have a mortality benefit from the institution of early noninvasive positive pressure ventilation
- Lung reduction surgery in selected patients with emphysema

■ Pearl

The blue bloater pushes the pink puffer's wheelchair; the bronchitis patient has better exercise tolerance.

Reference

El Moussaoui R, Roede BM, Speelman P, Bresser P, Prins JM, Bossuyt PM. Short-course antibiotic treatment in acute exacerbations of chronic bronchitis and COPD: a meta-analysis of double-blind studies. Thorax 2008;63:415. [PMID: 18234905]

Cryptogenic Organizing Pneumonia (Idiopathic Bronchiolitis Obliterans with Organizing Pneumonia [BOOP])

2

- ■ Essentials of Diagnosis
    - Cryptogenic organizing pneumonia (COP) and idiopathic BOOP are synonymous
    - COP may follow infections (eg, *Mycoplasma*, viral infection), may be due to toxic fume inhalation or associated with connective tissue disease or organ transplantation
    - Affects patients of all ages (mean is 50 years), no sex predilection, smoking not a precipitant
    - Presentation often similar to community-acquired pneumonia; up to half have abrupt onset of flulike symptoms such as fever, malaise, nonproductive cough, fatigue, and dyspnea
    - Weight loss (often > 10 lb) commonly observed
    - Dry crackles by auscultation; wheezing and clubbing are both unusual
    - Restrictive abnormalities with pulmonary function studies; hypoxemia typical
    - Chest radiograph shows patchy alveolar infiltrates bilaterally
    - Open or thoracoscopic lung biopsy necessary for precise diagnosis

- ■ Differential Diagnosis
    - Pneumonia due to bacteria, fungi, or tuberculosis
    - Diffuse alveolar hemorrhage
    - Acute interstitial pneumonia
    - ARDS
    - AIDS-related lung infections (eg, *Pneumocystis*)
    - Congestive heart failure
    - Hypersensitivity pneumonitis
    - Chronic eosinophilic pneumonia
    - Pulmonary toxicity due to drugs or autoimmune disorder

- ■ Treatment
    - Corticosteroids effective in two-thirds of cases; cytotoxic agents (eg, cyclophosphamide) in steroid failures
    - Relapse common after short (< 6 months) steroid courses

- ■ Pearl

COP is a leading diagnosis when "community-acquired pneumonia" persists despite antibiotics.

Reference

Vasu TS, Cavallazzi R, Hirani A, Sharma D, Weibel SB, Kane GC. Clinical and radiologic distinctions between secondary bronchiolitis obliterans organizing pneumonia and cryptogenic organizing pneumonia. Respir Care 2009;54:1028. [PMID: 19650943]

Cystic Fibrosis

2

- **Essentials of Diagnosis**
  - A generalized autosomal-recessive disorder of the exocrine glands more common than was once believed
  - Cough, dyspnea, recurrent pulmonary infections often due to *Pseudomonas*; symptoms of malabsorption, infertility
  - Distant breath sounds, rhonchi, clubbing, nasal polyps
  - Hypoxemia; obstructive or mixed pattern by spirometry; decreased diffusion capacity
  - Chest radiograph reveals bronchiectasis, upper lobe volume loss, and cystic disease
  - Sweat chloride > 60 mEq/L is characteristic, but false-negative results can occur
  - Testing for genetic mutations can confirm diagnosis when sweat test is negative

- **Differential Diagnosis**
  - Asthma
  - Bronchiectasis (primary ciliary dysmotility)
  - Congenital emphysema (α_1-antiprotease deficiency)
  - Atypical mycobacterial disease with bronchiectasis
  - Pancreatic insufficiency; other causes of malabsorption

- **Treatment**
  - Comprehensive multidisciplinary therapy required, including genetic and occupational counseling
  - Inhaled bronchodilators and chest physiotherapy
  - Antibiotics for recurrent airway infections targeted at resistant *Pseudomonas aeruginosa* and *Staphylococcus aureus* species
  - Pneumococcal vaccination; yearly influenza vaccinations
  - Inhaled recombinant human deoxyribonuclease (a mucolytic agent) and hypertonic saline decrease sputum viscosity and may facilitate airway clearance
  - Chest physiotherapy with a variety of devices improves airway clearance
  - Lung transplantation is the definitive treatment in selected patients

- **Pearl**

Consider this in adults with recurrent pulmonary infections; antibiotics have led to longer life spans and have shown that formes frustes are surprisingly common.

Reference

Langton Hewer SC, Smyth AR. Antibiotic strategies for eradicating Pseudomonas aeruginosa in people with cystic fibrosis. Cochrane Database Syst Rev 2009;4:CD004197. [PMID: 19821321]

Foreign Body Aspiration

- ■ Essentials of Diagnosis
  - • Sudden onset of cough, wheeze, and dyspnea; in children may be witnessed at onset of symptoms
  - • Localized wheezing, hyperresonance, stridor, and diminished breath sounds
  - • Localized air trapping or atelectasis on end-expiratory chest radiograph
  - • Diagnostic fiberoptic bronchoscopy usually identifies and localizes the foreign body

- ■ Differential Diagnosis
  - • Mucus plugging due to asthma or chronic bronchitis
  - • Bronchiectasis
  - • Endobronchial tumor
  - • Pyogenic upper airway process (eg, Ludwig's angina, soft tissue abscess, epiglottitis)
  - • Laryngospasm associated with anaphylaxis
  - • Bronchial compression from mass lesion
  - • Substernal goiter
  - • Tracheal cystadenoma

- ■ Treatment
  - • Bronchoscopic or surgical removal of foreign body, often by rigid bronchoscopy
  - • Emergency attention to airway—may require endotracheal intubation

- ■ Pearl

Remember this in a restaurant when a patron collapses and cannot speak; the Heimlich maneuver has saved many lives in this setting.

Reference

Boyd M, Chatterjee A, Chiles C, Chin R Jr. Tracheobronchial foreign body aspiration in adults. South Med J 2009;102:171. [PMID: 19139679]

2

Hypersensitivity Pneumonitis (Extrinsic Allergic Alveolitis)

■ Essentials of Diagnosis

- Work and environmental history suggesting link between activities and symptoms
- Caused by exposure to microbial agents (eg, thermophilic *Actinomyces* in farmer's lung, bagassosis, sequoiosis), animal proteins (eg, bird fancier's lung), with resultant IgG complement deposition, and chemical sensitizers (eg, isocyanates, trimellitic anhydride)
- Acute form: 4–12 hours after exposure, cough, dyspnea, fever, chills, myalgias; tachypnea, tachycardia, inspiratory crackles; leukocytosis with lymphopenia and neutrophilia; eosinophilia unusual
- Subacute or chronic form: Exertional dyspnea, cough, fatigue, anorexia, weight loss; basilar crackles
- Presence of IgG precipitating antibodies against above antigens indicates exposure but does not make diagnosis
- Skin testing not useful
- Pulmonary function tests reveal either airflow limitation or a restrictive pattern and decreased DLCO
- High-resolution thoracic CT scan reveals upper lobe predominant fine diffuse ground-glass abnormality with centrilobular nodules; expiratory images reveal mosaicism
- Bronchoalveolar lavage reveals marked lymphocytosis
- Transbronchial or thoracoscopic lung biopsy can confirm diagnosis in unclear cases

■ Differential Diagnosis

- Idiopathic pulmonary fibrosis
- Sarcoidosis
- Asthma
- Atypical pneumonia
- Bronchiolitis of alternative etiology
- Collagen vascular disease (eg, systemic lupus erythematosus)

■ Treatment

- Identification and removal of exposure
- Consider systemic corticosteroids in subacute or chronic forms

■ Pearl

A disorder with many colorful names, such as bagassosis—bagasse is the French word for sugar cane—and many antigens produce the identical clinical picture.

Reference

Lacasse Y, Cormier Y. Hypersensitivity pneumonitis. Orphanet J Rare Dis 2006;1:25. [PMID: 16817954]

Idiopathic Pulmonary Arterial Hypertension

- ■ Essentials of Diagnosis
  - A rare disorder seen primarily in young and middle-aged women
  - Defined as pulmonary hypertension (mean pulmonary artery pressure > 25 mm Hg) absent lung or left heart disease
  - Progressive dyspnea, malaise, chest pain, exertional syncope
  - Tachycardia, right ventricular lift, increased P_2, pulmonary and/or tricuspid regurgitation murmurs, right-sided S_3; evidence of right-sided heart failure (jugular venous distention, peripheral edema, hepatomegaly, ascites) common
  - Right axis deviation, right bundle-branch block, right ventricular strain or hypertrophy by electrocardiography
  - Echocardiographic evidence of elevated right ventricular (RV) systolic pressure with or without evidence of RV dilation or dysfunction

- ■ Differential Diagnosis
  - Pulmonary venous hypertension (mitral stenosis, left heart failure from any etiology)
  - Sleep apnea and obesity hypoventilation syndromes
  - Chronic thromboembolic disease
  - Parenchymal lung disease; autoimmune lung disease
  - Chronic obstructive pulmonary disease
  - Anorexic (Fen-phen) or sympathomimetic (methamphetamine) drug-induced pulmonary hypertension
  - HIV-associated pulmonary hypertension
  - Portopulmonary hypertension (cirrhosis and portal hypertension)

- ■ Treatment
  - A minority of patients (~5%) respond well to calcium channel blockers over the long term; response seen only in patients who respond to vasodilator challenge during right heart catheterization
  - Continuous intravenous prostacyclin analogues are the best studied agents and are generally initiated in more severe cases
  - Endothelin receptor blockers and phosphodiesterase 5 inhibitors improve symptoms in mild or moderately severe cases
  - Empiric anticoagulation may confer survival benefit
  - Combinations of agents are generally more beneficial than any agent alone: clinical benefit versus side effects must be considered
  - Lung or heart-lung transplantation should be considered

- ■ Pearl

"Primary pulmonary hypertension" with a left atrial abnormality on ECG is mitral stenosis until shown otherwise.

Reference

Saggar R, Saggar R, Aboulhosn J, Belperio JA, Zisman DA, Lynch JP 3rd. Diagnosis and hemodynamic assessment of pulmonary arterial hypertension. Semin Respir Crit Care Med 2009;30:399. [PMID: 19634079]

Idiopathic Pulmonary Fibrosis

2

■ Essentials of Diagnosis

- Insidious onset of exertional dyspnea and dry cough in patients, usually in their sixth or seventh decades
- Definition requires the histopathologic pattern of usual interstitial pneumonia
- Inspiratory crackles by auscultation; clubbing
- Hypoxemia, especially exertional
- Predominantly lower lobe, bilateral reticular abnormality by chest x-ray, which may progress to honeycombing pattern
- Restrictive pattern with decreased total lung capacity and diffusing capacity (DLCO)
- High-resolution thoracic CT scan may confidently establish diagnosis in many
- Biopsy via visually assisted thoracoscopic surgery (VATS) is the best method for definitive diagnosis, demonstrating usual interstitial pneumonia

■ Differential Diagnosis

- Nonspecific interstitial pneumonia
- Cryptogenic organizing pneumonia (COP)
- Interstitial lung disease due to collagen vascular disease
- Drug-induced fibrosis (eg, bleomycin, nitrofurantoin)
- Sarcoidosis
- Pneumoconiosis
- Asbestosis
- Hypersensitivity pneumonitis

■ Treatment

- Supportive therapy, including supplemental oxygen
- Combined high-dose corticosteroids and cytotoxic therapy largely ineffective
- Oral acetylcysteine (600 mg three times daily) may slow physiologic progression, though no clear functional outcome benefit
- Early referral to lung transplantation center is critical for good candidates

■ Pearl

With the right history and high resolution CT scan imaging characteristics, the diagnosis can be made without biopsy.

Reference

Meltzer EB, Noble PW. Idiopathic pulmonary fibrosis. Orphanet J Rare Dis 2008;3:8. [PMID: 18366757]

Lung Abscess

2

- ■ Essentials of Diagnosis
  - Cough producing foul-smelling sputum; hemoptysis; fever, weight loss, malaise
  - Patients with periodontal disease, alcoholism, impaired deglutition (eg, neurologic or esophageal disorder or altered consciousness) predisposed
  - Usual cause is mixed aerobic/anaerobic infection
  - Bronchial breath sounds with dullness and egophony over involved lung; succussion splash and amphoric breathing indicate air-fluid level
  - Leukocytosis; hypoxemia
  - Chest x-ray density, often with central lucency or air-fluid level

- ■ Differential Diagnosis
  - Tuberculosis
  - Bronchogenic carcinoma
  - Pulmonary mycoses
  - Bronchiectasis
  - Pulmonary infarct from pulmonary embolism or from vasculitis (eg, Wegener's granulomatosis)

- ■ Treatment
  - Clindamycin or high-dose penicillin (treatment for 6 or more weeks, until abscess resolves)
  - Surgery in selected cases (particularly large abscess; massive or persistent hemoptysis)
  - Supplemental oxygen as needed
  - Bronchoscopic exclusion of airway obstruction due to carcinoma or foreign body in patients with atypical features, especially edentulous patients

- ■ Pearl

A lung abscess without teeth is lung cancer until proven otherwise.

Reference

Moreira Jda S, Camargo Jde J, Felicetti JC, Goldenfun PR, Moreira AL, Porto Nda S. Lung abscess: analysis of 252 consecutive cases diagnosed between 1968 and 2004. J Bras Pneumol 2006;32:136. [PMID: 17273583]

Pandemic H1N1 Influenza A

2

- **Essentials of Diagnosis**
  - A novel H1N1 influenza A virus created by reassortment of two swine, one human, and one avian strain; first noted in summer of 2009
  - Unlike seasonal influenza, pandemic H1N1 strain disproportionately causes severe infection in patients aged 20-40
  - Human-to-human transmissibility, primarily through sneezing and coughing, appears higher compared with seasonal influenza
  - Most common symptoms are those of seasonal influenza (fever, cough, sore throat, malaise, headache), though nausea, vomiting, and diarrhea may also be present
  - Less than 1% of patients require hospitalization; common risk factors for complications are COPD, immunosuppression, heart disease, pregnancy, diabetes, obesity
  - Diagnostic testing recommended on hospitalized patients and those at risk for complications
  - Rapid antigen testing has poor sensitivity; confirmation of pandemic infection can only be made by polymerase chain reaction or culture

- **Differential Diagnosis**
  - Acute bronchitis (noninfluenza)
  - Cryptogenic organizing pneumonia (COP)
  - Acute respiratory distress syndrome
  - Atypical pneumonia (eg, *Mycoplasma*, *Chlamydia*)

- **Treatment**
  - The neuraminidase inhibitors (oseltamivir and zanamivir) are likely most beneficial if used within 48 hours of symptom onset and continued for 5 days
  - In hospitalized and high-risk patients as well as those with lower respiratory tract involvement, neuraminidase inhibitors should be initiated past the 48-hour window
  - Pandemic H1N1 influenza A is resistant to the antiviral medications amantadine and rimantadine

- **Pearl**

There is no risk of acquiring pandemic H1N1 influenza A (eg, swine flu) from eating pork.

Reference

Scalera NM, Mossad SB. The first pandemic of the 21st century: a review of the 2009 pandemic variant influenza A (H1N1) virus. Postgrad Med 2009;121:43. [PMID: 19820273]

Pleural Effusion

- ■ Essentials of Diagnosis
  - Many asymptomatic; pleuritic chest pain, dyspnea in some
  - Decreased breath sounds and percussive dullness; bronchial breathing above effusion
  - Layering on decubitus chest x-rays; ultrasonography or chest CT scan occasionally required for confirmation
  - Exudative effusion commonly due to malignancy, infection, autoimmune disease, pulmonary embolism, asbestosis
  - Transudative effusion caused by congestive heart failure, cirrhosis with ascites, nephrotic syndrome, hypothyroidism
  - Exudative effusions have at least one of the following: pleural fluid protein:serum protein ratio > 0.5; pleural fluid lactate dehydrogenase (LDH):serum LDH ratio > 0.6; or pleural fluid LDH > two-thirds the upper limit of normal serum LDH
  - An exudative effusion is considered complicated if any of the following are present: pH < 7.20, glucose < 60 mg/dL, Gram stain or culture positive, effusion > 1/2 hemithorax on chest x-ray, loculations or pleural enhancement seen on CT scan, pleural fluid LDH > 3 times upper limit of normal serum LDH
  - Markedly reduced glucose in empyema, rheumatoid effusion

- ■ Differential Diagnosis
  - Atelectasis
  - Lobar consolidation
  - Chronic pleural thickening
  - Elevated hemidiaphragm

- ■ Treatment
  - Diagnostic thoracentesis for evaluating cause, with pleural fluid glucose, protein, red and white cells counts with differential, cholesterol, LDH, and relevant cultures
  - Complicated parapneumonic pleural effusions usually require chest tube drainage or surgical decortication to achieve resolution
  - Therapy guided by suspected cause
  - Talc sclerosis for symptomatic malignant pleural effusions

- ■ Pearl

Why is transudative unilateral effusion more common on the right? There's more lung and pleura there.

Reference

Seyhan EC, Altin S, Cetinkaya E, Sokucu S, Gunluoglu MZ, Demir A, Korkmaz P, Issever H. The importance of pleural fluid and serum NT-proBNP levels in differentiating pleural effusion due to heart failure from other causes of effusion. Intern Med 2009;48:287. [PMID: 19252349]

Pulmonary Alveolar Proteinosis

2

■ Essentials of Diagnosis

- Most cases are acquired; idiopathic or associated with several diseases (eg, postinfection, immunocompromised host, hematologic malignancy); congenital also possible (rare)
- Acquired cases are due to production of autoantibodies that prevent granulocyte-macrophage colony-stimulating factor (GM-CSF) from binding to its receptor, resulting in decreased surfactant catabolism in alveolar macrophages
- Congenital cases due to mutations in surfactant B and C
- Typical age 30 and 50; men outnumber women 3:1
- Progressive dyspnea on exertion, low-grade fever, weight loss, fatigue, nonproductive cough; asymptomatic patients common
- Physical examination often normal; rales present in 50%
- Hypoxemia; bilateral alveolar infiltrates suggestive of pulmonary edema on chest radiography; "crazy paving" seen on chest CT scan
- Serum lactate dehydrogenase is typically elevated and can be used to follow disease activity
- Measurement of anti–GM-CSF antibodies in serum or bronchial alveolar lavage has excellent sensitivity for diagnosis
- The gold standard for diagnosis is characteristic intra-alveolar accumulation of lipoproteinaceous material without parenchymal fibrosis seen on surgical lung biopsy, though most diagnoses can be made with a compatible history, CT scan, and bronchoscopy
- Superinfection with *Nocardia* and mycobacteria is common

■ Differential Diagnosis

- Congestive heart failure
- Atypical infection (eg, *P. jiroveci* pneumonia)
- Interstitial lung disease
- Diffuse alveolar hemorrhage

■ Treatment

- Up to 25% remit spontaneously
- Periodic whole-lung lavage via double-lumen endotracheal tube reduces exertional dyspnea in those with limiting symptoms
- Treat underlying cause in secondary forms
- In acquired disease, GM-CSF therapy appears to be beneficial

■ Pearl

One of the few conditions in medicine causing chyloptysis–milky sputum.

Reference

Juvet SC, Hwang D, Waddell TK, Downey GP. Rare lung disease II: pulmonary alveolar proteinosis. Can Respir J. 2008;15:203. [PMID: 18551202]

Pulmonary Langerhans' Cell Histiocytosis

- ■ Essentials of Diagnosis
  - • Uncommon interstitial lung disorder primarily affecting smokers between 20 and 40
  - • The pathologic cell (Langerhans' cell) is a differentiated cell within the monocyte-macrophage line
  - • Mid- to upper-zone lung involvement is common (as opposed to characteristic lower-zone involvement of idiopathic pulmonary fibrosis)
  - • Patients may present asymptomatically on chest radiography or after spontaneous pneumothorax
  - • Symptoms are nonspecific and may include dry cough, dyspnea, fatigue, pleuritic chest pain, weight loss, fever
  - • Physical exam usually normal; however, clubbing and crackles occasionally occur; labs usually normal; no eosinophilia
  - • Complications include recurrent spontaneous pneumothorax, hemoptysis, bone pain (due to bone cysts), diabetes insipidus, malignancy
  - • Reticulonodular infiltrates, stellate nodules, upper zone cysts, absence of pleural effusion, normal lung volume on chest film
  - • High-resolution CT especially helpful; pulmonary function tests usually reveal decreased diffusion capacity; some have restrictive or obstructive findings
  - • Definitive diagnosis requires tissue via bronchoscopy or video-assisted thoracoscopic surgery; bronchoalveolar lavage may be suggestive if 5% or more Langerhans' cells are found
  - • Some patients remit; others progress to chronic lung disease

- ■ Differential Diagnosis
  - • Cystic fibrosis
  - • Pulmonary lymphangioleiomyomatosis
  - • Sarcoidosis
  - • Drug-induced or idiopathic pulmonary fibrosis
  - • Hypersensitivity pneumonitis
  - • Lymphocytic interstitial pneumonia

- ■ Treatment
  - • Smoking cessation is most important intervention
  - • Corticosteroids and cytotoxic agents of limited value
  - • Lung transplantation for advanced disease

- ■ Pearl

In a young smoker with bilateral recurrent pneumothoraces, this is the diagnosis unless proven otherwise.

Reference

Tazi A. Adult pulmonary Langerhans' cell histiocytosis. Eur Respir J. 2006;27:1272. [PMID: 16772390]

Pulmonary Tuberculosis

2

- ■ Essentials of Diagnosis
  - Lassitude, weight loss, fever, cough, night sweats, hemoptysis
  - Cachexia in many; posttussive apical rales occasionally present
  - Apical or subapical infiltrates with cavities classic in reactivation tuberculosis; pleural effusion in primary tuberculosis, likewise mid-lung infiltration, but any radiographic abnormality possible
  - Positive skin test to intradermal purified protein derivative (PPD)
  - Interferon-gamma release assays have good specificity for latent tuberculosis
  - *Mycobacterium tuberculosis* by culture of sputum, gastric washing, or pleural biopsy; pleural fluid culture usually sterile
  - Nucleic acid amplification can rapidly distinguish between *M. tuberculosis* and nontuberculous mycobacterium to guide treatment decisions but culture still needed for susceptibility testing
  - Increasingly encountered antibiotic-resistant strains
  - Granuloma on pleural biopsy in patients with effusions; mesothelial cells usually absent from fluid
  - Miliary tuberculosis (widespread hematogenous spread of organism) has diverse clinical presentations including failure to thrive, fever of unknown origin, multiorgan system failure, ARDS; nearly all have overt pulmonary involvement with numerous small nodules

- ■ Differential Diagnosis
  - Lung carcinoma; fungal infection
  - Bacterial pneumonia or lung abscess; other mycobacterial infections
  - Sarcoidosis; pneumoconiosis

- ■ Treatment
  - Combination antituberculous therapy for 6–9 months; all regimens include isoniazid, but rifampin, ethambutol, pyrazinamide, and streptomycin all have activity
  - Avoid empiric treatment for community-acquired pneumonia with fluoroquinolones if *M. tuberculosis* is suspected as transient use may facilitate development of resistance
  - All cases of suspected *M. tuberculosis* infection should be reported to local health departments
  - Hospitalization considered for those incapable of self-care or likely to expose susceptible individuals

- ■ Pearl

Five percent of tuberculosis is diagnosed postmortem.

Reference

Hall RG, Leff RD, Gumbo T. Treatment of active pulmonary tuberculosis in adults: current standards and recent advances. Pharmacotherapy 2009;29:1468. [PMID: 19947806]

Sarcoidosis

■ Essentials of Diagnosis

- A disease of unknown cause with an increased incidence in North American blacks, Northern European whites, and Japanese
- Malaise, fever, dyspnea of insidious onset; symptoms referable to eyes, skin, nervous system, liver, joints, or heart encountered; often presents asymptomatically
- Iritis, erythema nodosum or granulomatous skin lesions, parotid enlargement, lymphadenopathy, hepatosplenomegaly
- Hypercalcemia (5%) less common than hypercalciuria (20%)
- Pulmonary function testing may show evidence of obstruction, but restriction with decreased DLCO is more common
- Symmetric hilar and right paratracheal adenopathy, interstitial infiltrates, or both seen on chest x-ray
- Tissue reveals noncaseating granuloma; transbronchial biopsy sensitive, even without parenchymal disease on chest film
- Increased angiotensin-converting enzyme levels are neither sensitive nor specific; cutaneous anergy in 70%
- ECG may show heart block of varying degrees

■ Differential Diagnosis

- Tuberculosis
- Lymphoma, including lymphocytic interstitial pneumonitis
- Histoplasmosis or coccidioidomycosis
- Idiopathic pulmonary fibrosis
- Pneumoconiosis
- Berylliosis

■ Treatment

- Systemic corticosteroid therapy for symptomatic pulmonary disease, cardiac involvement, iritis unresponsive to local therapy, hypercalcemia, central nervous system involvement, arthritis, nodular skin lesions
- Asymptomatic patients with normal pulmonary function may not require corticosteroids—they should receive close clinical follow-up

■ Pearl

The only disease in medicine in which steroids reverse anergy.

Reference

Iannuzzi MC, Rybicki BA, Teirstein AS. Sarcoidosis. N Engl J Med 2007;357:2153. [PMID: 18032765]

Silicosis

2

- **Essentials of Diagnosis**
    - A chronic fibrotic lung disease caused by inhalation of dusts containing crystalline silicon dioxide in foundry work, sandblasting, and hard rock mining
    - Progressive dyspnea, often over months to years
    - Dry inspiratory crackles by auscultation
    - Characteristic changes on chest radiograph with bilateral, predominantly upper lobe fibrosis, nodules, and hilar lymphadenopathy with "eggshell" calcification
    - Pulmonary function studies yield mixed obstructive and restrictive pattern
    - Superimposed mycobacterial disease (tuberculosis and nontuberculous) common in patients with silicosis and should be ruled out if there is any clinical or radiographic suspicion
    - Connective tissue diseases commonly (~10%) complicate the clinical course

- **Differential Diagnosis**
    - Other pneumoconioses (eg, asbestosis)
    - Tuberculosis (often complicates silicosis)
    - Sarcoidosis
    - Histoplasmosis
    - Coccidioidomycosis

- **Treatment**
    - Supportive care; chronic oxygen if sustained hypoxemia present
    - Chemoprophylaxis with isoniazid necessary for all silicotic patients with positive tuberculin reactivity

- **Pearl**

One of the few causes of the rare broncholithiasis; if you ask, the patient will tell you there are small stones in his sputum.

Reference

Centers for Disease Control and Prevention (CDC). Silicosis-related years of potential life lost before age 65 years—United States, 1968-2005. MMWR Morb Mortal Wkly Rep 2008;57:771. [PMID: 18636065]

Sleep Apnea

■ Essentials of Diagnosis

- Excessive daytime somnolence or fatigue, morning headache, weight gain, erectile dysfunction; bed partner may report restless sleep, loud snoring, and witnessed apneic episodes
- Obesity, systemic hypertension common; signs of pulmonary hypertension or cor pulmonale may develop over time
- Erythrocytosis common
- Diagnosis confirmed by formal polysomnography
- Most cases of central apnea also have an obstructive component; pure central sleep apnea is rare

■ Differential Diagnosis

- Alcohol or sedative abuse
- Narcolepsy
- Seizure disorder
- Chronic obstructive pulmonary disease
- Hypothyroidism

■ Treatment

- Weight loss and avoidance of hypnotic medications mandatory
- Nocturnal continuous positive airway pressure (CPAP) and supplemental oxygen frequently abolish obstructive apnea
- Oral appliances improve symptoms and reduce apnea-hypopnea episodes, but are not as effective as CPAP; use in patients unable to tolerate CPAP
- Modafinil may be beneficial as adjunctive therapy for excessive daytime sleepiness that persists despite adequate conventional therapy
- Surgical approaches (uvulopalatopharyngoplasty, nasal septoplasty, tracheostomy) reserved for selected cases

■ Pearl

When a plethoric clinic patient nods off during the history, it's sleep apnea until proven otherwise; if the historian does, it's a post-call resident.

Reference

Lévy P, Bonsignore MR, Eckel J. Sleep, sleep-disordered breathing and metabolic consequences. Eur Respir J 2009;34:243. [PMID: 19567607]

Solitary Pulmonary Nodule

2

- ■ Essentials of Diagnosis
  - A round or oval circumscribed lesion < 3 cm in diameter amid normal lung tissue
  - Twenty-five percent of cases of bronchogenic carcinoma present as such; the 5-year survival rate so detected is 50%
  - Factors favoring benign lesion: Age < 35 years, asymptomatic, size < 2 cm, diffuse calcification, and smooth margins
  - Factors suggesting malignancy: Age > 45, symptoms, smoking history, size > 2 cm, lack of calcification, indistinct margins (spiculation)
  - Skin tests, serologies, cytology rarely helpful
  - Comparison with earlier radiographs essential, if available; follow-up with serial plain films or CT scans helpful in appropriate patients
  - Positron emission tomography (PET) scans help distinguish malignancy from benign causes in lesions > 8 mm; sensitivity limited by rare slow-growing malignant lesions (bronchioalveolar cell carcinoma and carcinoid tumors), and specificity limited by inflammatory lesions that "light up"

- ■ Differential Diagnosis
  - Benign causes: Granuloma (eg, tuberculosis or fungal infection), arteriovenous malformation, pseudotumor, lipoma, hamartoma
  - Malignant causes: Primary or metastatic malignancy

- ■ Treatment
  - Fine-needle aspiration (FNA) biopsy, bronchoscopic biopsy, surgical resection, or radiographic follow-up over 2 years; negative FNA or bronchoscopic biopsy does not exclude malignancy due to a high percentage of false negatives unless a specific benign diagnosis is made
  - Thoracic CT scan (with thin cuts through nodule) to look for benign-appearing calcifications and evaluate mediastinum for lymphadenopathy
  - With high-risk clinical or radiographic features, surgical resection (eg, using video-assisted thoracoscopy) recommended
  - In low-risk or intermediate-risk cases, close radiographic follow-up may be justified

- ■ Pearl

The Social Security number helps: if the first digit is zero or one, TB is favored, two, three, or four means histoplasmosis, five and six coccidiomycosis (in calcified lesions); the numbers are assigned by place of birth.

Reference

Truong MT, Sabloff BS, Ko JP. Multidetector CT of solitary pulmonary nodules. Radiol Clin North Am 2010;48:141. [PMID: 19995633]

Spontaneous Pneumothorax

- **Essentials of Diagnosis**
  - Primary spontaneous pneumothorax occurs in the absence of clinical pulmonary disease; secondary pneumothorax complicates a preexisting disease (eg, asthma, COPD)
  - Primary spontaneous pneumothorax generally occurs in tall, thin boys and young men who smoke
  - Abrupt onset of ipsilateral chest/shoulder pain and dyspnea
  - Decreased breath sounds over involved hemithorax, which may be bronchial but distant in 100% pneumothorax; hyperresonance, tachycardia, hypotension, and mediastinal shift toward contralateral side if tension is present
  - Chest x-ray diagnostic with retraction of lung from parietal pleura

- **Differential Diagnosis**
  - Myocardial infarction; pulmonary emboli
  - Pericarditis

- **Treatment**
  - Assessment for cause, eg, *P. jiroveci* pneumonia, lung cancer, COPD, cystic lung disease
  - Immediate decompression by needle if tension suspected
  - Spontaneous pneumothoraces of < 15% (< 3 cm from pleura to chest wall on upright chest x-ray) followed by serial radiographs and 6 hours of observation in the hospital for stability; if > 15%, treat by aspirating pleural air through a small catheter; if unsuccessful, insert chest tube
  - 100% humidified oxygen therapy replaces nitrogen with oxygen in the pleural space and markedly decreases re-absorption time
  - Secondary pneumothoraces (eg, due to COPD, cystic fibrosis) usually require chest tube
  - Recurrence high (up to 50%) in primary spontaneous pneumothorax; smoking cessation decreases rate of recurrence
  - In patients whose jobs or hobbies (eg, pilots and deep sea divers) put them or others at risk of death, consider pleurodesis after the first event
  - Therapy for recurrent pneumothorax includes surgical pleurodesis or stapling of the ruptured blebs

- **Pearl**

Catamenial pneumothorax makes pulmonary endometriosis the diagnosis until proven otherwise.

Reference

Kelly AM. Treatment of primary spontaneous pneumothorax. Curr Opin Pulm Med 2009;15:376. [PMID: 19373088]

Gastrointestinal Diseases

Achalasia

■ Essentials of Diagnosis
  - Progressive dysphagia for both liquids and solids, odynophagia, and regurgitation of undigested food
  - Barium swallow demonstrates a dilated upper esophagus with a narrowed cardioesophageal junction ("bird's beak" esophagus); chest x-ray may reveal a retrocardiac air-fluid level
  - Lack of primary peristalsis by manometry or cineradiography, elevated resting lower esophageal sphincter pressure, and incomplete lower esophageal sphincter relaxation with swallowing

■ Differential Diagnosis
  - Diffuse esophageal spasm
  - Aperistalsis
  - Benign lower esophageal stricture
  - Esophageal or mediastinal tumors (increased risk of esophageal carcinoma with achalasia)
  - Scleroderma of esophagus

■ Treatment
  - Nifedipine, 10–20 mg sublingually or nitrates 30 minutes before meals
  - Botulinum toxin injection endoscopically in patients who are not good surgical candidates
  - Pneumatic esophageal dilation
  - Surgical extramucosal myotomy (esophagocardiomyotomy) in refractory cases
  - Consider periodic endoscopy for esophageal carcinoma surveillance after 15 years

■ Pearl
One of the reasons why the lateral chest x-ray is useful, as it shows the likely esophageal location of the air-fluid level.

Reference

Eckardt AJ, Eckardt VF: Current clinical approach to achalasia. World J Gastroenterol 2009;15:3969. [PMID: 19705490]

Acute Colonic Pseudo-Obstruction (Ogilvie's Syndrome)

- ■ Essentials of Diagnosis
  - • Often seen in elderly hospitalized patients
  - • Associated with a history of trauma, fractures, cardiac disease, infection, or the use of opioids, antidepressants, and anticholinergics
  - • Often detected as a distended, tympanitic abdomen with abdominal x-ray revealing gross colonic dilation (usually right sided, with cecum > 10 cm), scant air-fluid levels, a gradual transition to collapsed bowel, and air and stool present in the rectum
  - • May mimic true obstruction, and obstruction should be evaluated with radiologic studies using diatrizoate (Hypaque) enema
  - • Fevers, marked abdominal tenderness, leukocytosis, and acidosis may be present in advanced cases with impending perforation

- ■ Differential Diagnosis
  - • Mechanical obstruction
  - • Toxic megacolon (ie, *Clostridium difficile*)
  - • Chronic intestinal pseudo-obstruction

- ■ Treatment
  - • Cessation of oral intake, nasogastric and rectal suctioning, intravenous fluids
  - • Correction of electrolyte abnormalities (Ca^{2+}, Mg^{2+}, K^+, PO4)
  - • Discontinue offending medications and treat underlying infections
  - • Tap water enemas and patient repositioning may be of benefit
  - • Neostigmine (2 mg intravenously), in patients failing conservative therapy, can be very effective for decompression. Main side effect is bradycardia.
  - • Colonoscopic decompression for patients failing neostigmine or in whom neostigmine therapy is contraindicated
  - • Surgical consultation for patients with peritoneal signs or impending perforation

- ■ Pearl

Be wary if cecal diameter is >12 cm or if colonic dilatation has been present for > 6 days; perforation may ensue.

Reference

Saunders MD. Acute colonic pseudo-obstruction. Best Pract Res Clin Gastroenterol 2007;21:671. [PMID: 17643908]

Acute Pancreatitis

- ■ Essentials of Diagnosis
  - • Background of alcohol binge or gallstones
  - • Abrupt onset of epigastric pain, often with radiation to the back; nausea, vomiting, low-grade fever, and dehydration
  - • Abdominal tenderness, distention
  - • Leukocytosis, elevated serum amylase and lipase; hypocalcemia and hemoconcentration in severe cases; hypertriglyceridemia (> 1000 mg/dL) may be causative, likewise hypercalcemia
  - • RUQ ultrasound to rule out choledocholithiasis in patients with suspected gallstone pancreatitis. CT for patients highly symptomatic, not improving, or for suspected complications

- ■ Differential Diagnosis
  - • Acute cholecystitis or cholangitis
  - • Penetrating or perforating duodenal ulcer
  - • Mesenteric infarction
  - • Gastritis
  - • Abdominal aortic aneurysm
  - • Small bowel obstruction

- ■ Treatment
  - • Nasogastric suction for nausea or ileus, prompt intravenous fluid and electrolyte replacement, analgesics, and antiemetics
  - • Early enteral feeding orally or by jejunal nasogastric tube if patient able; parenteral nutrition if unable to tolerate
  - • Discontinue drugs capable of causing the disease (eg, thiazides, corticosteroids)
  - • Antibiotics (eg, imipenem) for documented infection; the use of antibiotic prophylaxis to prevent pancreatic infection is debated but not recommended at this time
  - • If patient decompensates, rule out infected pancreatic necrosis with ultrasound or CT-guided fine-needle aspiration of pancreatic tissue. Aggressive debridement is recommended for infected pancreatic necrosis.
  - • Early endoscopic retrograde cholangiopancreatography with sphincterotomy for pancreatitis with associated jaundice and cholangitis resulting from choledocholithiasis

- ■ Pearl

  In "idiopathic" pancreatitis, obtain more history from someone other than the patient; in many, alcohol is in the picture.

Reference

Frossard JL, Steer ML, Pastor CM. Acute pancreatitis. Lancet 2008;371:143. [PMID: 18191686]

Anal Fissure (Fissura-in-Ano, Anal Ulcer)

- ■ Essentials of Diagnosis
  - Linear tear of the anal epithelium usually from local trauma, usually posterior midline
  - Rectal pain with defecation; bleeding and constipation
  - Acute anal tenderness to digital examination
  - Ulceration and stenosis of anal canal, hypertrophic anal papilla, external skin tag on anoscopy

- ■ Differential Diagnosis
  - Rectal syphilis, tuberculosis, herpes, chlamydial infections
  - Crohn's disease
  - Other anorectal disease: Abscess, fistula, hemorrhoids
  - Acute monocytic leukemia
  - Malignant epithelioma leukemia

- ■ Treatment
  - Increase water intake, high-fiber diet, psyllium, bran, stool softeners, sitz baths, hydrocortisone suppositories
  - Topical nitrate therapy or botulinum toxin injection, topical calcium channel blockers
  - Lateral internal sphincterotomy if no improvement with medical therapy

- ■ Pearl

Unexplained anal fissures call for a prompt blood count; it is a characteristic presentation of acute monocytic leukemia.

Reference

Steele SR, Madoff RD. Systematic review: the treatment of anal fissure. Aliment Pharmacol Ther 2006;24:247. [PMID: 16842451]

Barrett's Esophagus

- ■ Essentials of Diagnosis
  - • Barrett's esophagus is asymptomatic, but many patients present with symptoms of gastroesophageal reflux disease (GERD): Dysphagia, heartburn, regurgitation in supine position
  - • Upper endoscopy with biopsy reveals columnar epithelium replacing squamous epithelium
  - • Risk of developing esophageal adenocarcinoma is 0.5% per year

- ■ Differential Diagnosis
  - • GERD
  - • Achalasia
  - • Esophageal or mediastinal tumor
  - • Esophageal web
  - • Benign stricture
  - • Left atrial enlargement or pericardial effusion

- ■ Treatment
  - • Acid suppression (pH > 4) with proton pump inhibitors
  - • Surgical fundoplication in selected patients (for therapy of chronic reflux symptoms)
  - • In patients with neoplastic Barrett's, consider endoscopic mucosal resections (for nodular lesions) and mucosal ablation (for flat neoplasia) using radiofrequency ablation, photodynamic therapy, cryoablation, or argon plasma coagulation. Patients with isolated low- or high-grade dysplasia may be treated with endoscopic therapy alone. However, all those with invasive cancers should be considered for surgery.
  - • Surveillance esophagoscopy with biopsy at 1- to 3-year intervals, depending on presence and degree of dysplasia

- ■ Pearl
  - *When potentially exsanguinating gastrointestinal bleeding occurs in a patient with Barrett's esophagus, it is likely to be the rare cardio-esophageal fistula.*

Reference

Sharma P. Clinical practice. Barrett's esophagus. N Engl J Med 2009;361:2548. [PMID: 20032324]

Benign Stricture of Esophagus

■ Essentials of Diagnosis

- Dysphagia for solids more than liquids; odynophagia
- Smooth narrowing of lumen radiographically; esophagoscopy and biopsy or cytology mandatory to exclude malignancy
- Onset months to years after esophageal insult, including gastroesophageal reflux, indwelling nasogastric tube, corrosive ingestion, infectious esophagitis, postradiation, or endoscopic injury

■ Differential Diagnosis

- Achalasia or other esophageal motility disorders
- Esophageal or mediastinal tumor
- Esophageal web
- Schatzki's ring
- Left atrial enlargement
- Pericardial effusion

■ Treatment

- Repeat bougienage or endoscopic balloon dilation is definitive therapy for most patients; high-dose proton pump inhibitors may increase the interval between dilations
- Surgical therapy required rarely

■ Pearl

Esophageal lumen diameter < 13 mm usually leads to solid food dysphagia; dilation to > 18 mm usually allows for resumption of normal diet.

Reference

Standards of Practice Committee, Egan JV, Baron TH, et al. Esophageal dilation. Gastrointest Endosc 2006;63:755. [PMID: 16650533]

Celiac Sprue

3

- ■ Essentials of Diagnosis
  - Caused by an immune reaction to gluten in diet in genetically susceptible individuals
  - The prevalence of celiac disease in the United States is approximately 1:100 (1%)
  - Main manifestations are of malabsorption: Bulky, pale, frothy, greasy stools (steatorrhea); abdominal distention, flatulence, weight loss, and evidence of fat-soluble vitamin deficiencies; labs may be notable for a hypochromic or megaloblastic anemia; abnormal D-xylose absorption; increased fecal fat on quantitative studies
  - However, clinical manifestations are variable. Patients may present with abdominal pain, constipation, iron deficiency anemia, weight loss, or elevated liver enzymes of unknown etiology. Nongastrointestinal manifestations include neuropsychiatric disease, arthritis, metabolic bone disease, and infertility
  - IgA endomysial antibody and tissue transglutaminase antibody are positive in disease; and if negative, can help exclude the diagnosis.
  - Villous atrophy and increased intraepithelial lymphocytes on small bowel biopsy

- ■ Differential Diagnosis
  - Crohn's disease
  - Lactose intolerance
  - Small bowel bacterial overgrowth
  - Intestinal lymphoma (may also complicate celiac sprue)
  - Whipple's disease
  - Pancreatic insufficiency

- ■ Treatment
  - Strict elimination of gluten from diet (ie, wheat, rye, barley) can be monitored using IgA tissue transglutaminase, IgA anti-endomysial or IgA antigliadin antibody; vitamin supplementation (especially vitamin B_{12} and calcium)

- ■ Pearl
  Antibody testing has caused a greater appreciation for the breadth of this disease; even isolated iron deficiency may be the clinical presentation.

Reference

Green PH, Cellier C. Celiac disease. N Engl J Med 2007;357:1731. [PMID: 17960014]

Chronic Pancreatitis

■ Essentials of Diagnosis

- The three main clinical features are abdominal pain, maldigestion, and diabetes.
- Pancreatic calcification by radiographic study
- Causes: Alcoholism (most common), hereditary pancreatitis, autoimmune pancreatitis, tropical pancreatitis, untreated hyperparathyroidism, cystic fibrosis, secondary to ductal obstruction or after abdominal trauma
- Diagnostic studies include endoscopic ultrasound, magnetic resonance cholangiopancreatography, and an abnormal secretin pancreatic stimulation test. Endoscopic retrograde cholangiopancreatography is usually reserved for cases requiring therapeutic intervention. Lipase and amylase are usually normal.

■ Differential Diagnosis

- Carcinoma of the pancreas
- Malabsorption due to other causes
- Intractable duodenal ulcer
- Gallstones
- Irritable bowel syndrome

■ Treatment

- Low-fat diet, pancreatic enzyme supplements, avoidance of alcohol
- Pain management includes opioids and amitriptyline
- Endoscopic sphincterotomy and pancreatic duct stenting, as well as endoscopic ultrasound-guided celiac block for pain management, have yielded disappointing results
- Treatment of hyperlipidemia if present
- Intravenous fluid and electrolyte replacement for acute exacerbations
- Surgical therapy to restore free flow of bile or to treat intractable pain

■ Pearl

Malabsorption is indicative of advanced disease because it does not occur until pancreatic lipase secretion is reduced to < 10% of normal.

Reference

Witt H, Apte MV, Keim V, Wilson JS. Chronic pancreatitis: challenges and advances in pathogenesis, genetics, diagnosis, and therapy. Gastroenterology 2007;132:1557. [PMID: 17466744]

Clostridium difficile (Pseudomembranous) Colitis

■ Essentials of Diagnosis

- Profuse watery, green, foul-smelling, or bloody diarrhea
- Cramping abdominal pain
- Fecal leukocytes present in more than half of patients
- Fevers, marked abdominal tenderness, marked leukocytosis, hypo-volemia, dehydration, and hypoalbuminemia are common
- History of antibiotic use (especially penicillin family antibiotics and clindamycin), hospitalization, or institutionalization; increasingly recognized as a potential community-acquired infection
- Many cases may be asymptomatic or associated with minimal symptoms
- Diagnosis confirmed by positive stool antigen test or via sigmoi-doscopy or colonoscopy

■ Differential Diagnosis

- Antibiotic-associated diarrhea (without *C. difficile* or pseudomem-branous colitis)
- Other bacterial diarrheas
- Inflammatory bowel disease
- Parasitic (amebiasis) and viral (cytomegalovirus) causes of diar-rhea and colitis

■ Treatment

- Discontinue offending antibiotic therapy
- Replacement of fluid and electrolyte losses
- Oral metronidazole; oral vancomycin reserved for metronidazole-resistant cases or critically ill patients; treatment is for 10–14 days
- Surgical therapy is needed rarely (1–3%) for severe cases with megacolon or impending perforation
- Avoid opioids and antidiarrheal agents

■ Pearl

The cause of the highest benign white count in all of medicine save pertussis.

Reference

Kelly CP. A 76-year-old man with recurrent Clostridium difficile-associated diarrhea: review of C. difficile infection. JAMA 2009;301:954. [PMID: 19190304]

Crohn's Disease

- ■ Essentials of Diagnosis
  - Insidious onset, with intermittent bouts of diarrhea, low-grade fever, right lower quadrant pain
  - Complications include fistula formation, perianal disease with abscess, right lower quadrant mass and tenderness, obstruction
  - Anemia, leukocytosis, hypoalbuminemia, elevated erythrocyte sedimentation rate/C-reactive protein, positive fecal occult blood
  - Radiographic findings of thickened, stenotic bowel with ulceration, stricturing, or fistulas; characteristic skip areas
  - Endoscopic biopsy with histologic demonstration of acute or chronic submucosal inflammation with fibrosis and granulomatous lesions

- ■ Differential Diagnosis
  - Ulcerative colitis
  - Appendicitis
  - Diverticulitis
  - Intestinal tuberculosis
  - Infectious diarrhea
  - Lymphoma, other tumors of small intestine

- ■ Treatment
  - High protein, low-residue, and lactose-free diet during acute flares
  - Consider 5-ASA for mild colonic disease and budesonide for mild ileal and right colonic disease.
  - Corticosteroids can be used during acute flares, but if a patient requires steroids, then the treatment strategy should include a maintenance regimen (such as an immunomodulator, like 6-merpcatopurine/azathioprine or methotrexate). In the case of severe, refractory, or fistulous disease, consider a biologic agent (anti-tumor necrosis factor monoclonal antibodies)
  - Perianal abscess requires surgical drainage prior to treatment. For nonsuppurative fistulizing and perianal disease, consider antibiotics, immunomodulators, and infliximab.
  - Surgery for refractory obstruction, fistula, or abscess

- ■ Pearl

A disorder with a remarkable panoply of extraintestinal manifestations; mucosal ulcers, hypercoagulability states, and even systemic vasculitis may be associated.

Reference

Lichtenstein GR, Hanauer SB, Sandborn WJ; Practice Parameters Committee of American College of Gastroenterology. Management of Crohn's disease in adults. Am J Gastroenterol 2009;104:465. [PMID: 19174807]

Diffuse Esophageal Spasm

3

- **Essentials of Diagnosis**
  - Dysphagia, noncardiac chest pain, hypersalivation, reflux of recently ingested food
  - May be precipitated by ingestion of hot or cold foods
  - Endoscopic, radiographic, and manometric demonstration of non-propulsive hyperperistalsis; lower esophageal sphincter relaxes normally
  - "Nutcracker esophagus" variant with prolonged, high-pressure (> 175 mm Hg) propulsive contractions

- **Differential Diagnosis**
  - Angina pectoris
  - Esophageal or mediastinal tumors
  - Aperistalsis
  - Achalasia
  - Psychiatric disease

- **Treatment**
  - Trial of acid suppression.
  - Calcium channel blockers such as nifedipine or diltiazem in combination with nitrates often effective. For patient failing to respond, possible role for sildenafil, botulinum toxin.
  - Trazodone or tricyclic antidepressants for substernal pain

- **Pearl**

This condition may be indistinguishable from myocardial ischemia; exclude that possibility before investigating the esophagus.

Reference

Grübel C, Borovicka J, Schwizer W, Fox M, Hebbard G. Diffuse esophageal spasm. Am J Gastroenterol 2008;103:450. [PMID: 18005367]

Disaccharidase (Lactase) Deficiency

- ■ Essentials of Diagnosis
  - • Common in Asians and blacks, in whom lactase enzyme deficiency is nearly ubiquitous and begins in childhood; can also be acquired temporarily after gastroenteritis of other causes
  - • Symptoms vary from abdominal bloating, distention, cramps, and flatulence to explosive diarrhea in response to disaccharide ingestion
  - • Stool pH < 5.5; reducing substances present in stool
  - • Abnormal lactose hydrogen breath test, resolution of symptoms on lactose-free diet, or flat glucose response to disaccharide loading suggests the diagnosis

- ■ Differential Diagnosis
  - • Chronic mucosal malabsorptive disorders
  - • Irritable bowel syndrome
  - • Celiac sprue
  - • Small intestinal bacterial overgrowth
  - • Inflammatory bowel disease
  - • Pancreatic insufficiency
  - • Giardiasis
  - • Excess artificial sweetener use

- ■ Treatment
  - • Restriction of dietary lactose; usually happens by experience in affected minorities from early life
  - • Lactase enzyme supplementation
  - • Maintenance of adequate nutritional and calcium intake

- ■ Pearl

Consider this in undiagnosed diarrhea; the patient may not be aware of ingesting lactose-containing foods.

Reference

Lomer MC, Parkes GC, Sanderson JD. Review article: lactose intolerance in clinical practice—myths and realities. Aliment Pharmacol Ther 2008;27:93. [PMID: 17956597]

Duodenal Ulcer

- **Essentials of Diagnosis**
  - Epigastric pain 45–60 minutes following meals or nocturnal pain, both relieved by food or antacids, sometimes by vomiting; symptoms chronic and periodic; radiation to back common; patients may complain of weight gain
  - Iron deficiency anemia, positive fecal occult blood; amylase elevated with posterior penetration
  - Radiographic or endoscopic evaluation will demonstrate ulcer crater or deformity of duodenal bulb, and exclude other diagnoses such as malignancy
  - Caused by *Helicobacter pylori* in 70% of cases, NSAIDs in 20–30%, Zollinger-Ellison syndrome in < 1%; *H. pylori* infection may be diagnosed serologically, with biopsy or by breath test
  - Complications include hemorrhage, intractable pain, penetration, perforation, and obstruction

- **Differential Diagnosis**
  - Reflux esophagitis
  - Gastritis
  - Pancreatitis
  - Cholecystitis
  - Other peptic disease (eg, Zollinger-Ellison syndrome [1% of patients with peptic ulcer disease] or gastric ulcer)

- **Treatment**
  - Eradicate *H. pylori* when present
  - Avoid tobacco, alcohol, xanthines, and ulcerogenic drugs, especially NSAIDs
  - H_2 blockers, proton pump inhibitors, and sucralfate
  - Endoscopic therapy for actively bleeding ulcers
  - Surgery—now far less common—may be needed for ulcers refractory to medical management (rare) or for the management of complications (eg, perforation, uncontrolled bleeding); supraselective vagotomy preferred unless patient unstable or is obstructed

- **Pearl**

Once an ulcer, always an ulcer; patients who develop a peptic ulcer have a lifetime increase in risk for recurrence.

Reference

Ramakrishnan K, Salinas RC. Peptic ulcer disease. Am Fam Physician 2007;76:1005. [PMID: 17956071]

Emetogenic Esophageal Perforation (Boerhaave's Syndrome)

- ■ Essentials of Diagnosis
  - • History of alcoholic binge drinking, excessive and rapid food intake, or both; may also occur after esophageal medical procedures
  - • Violent vomiting or retching followed by sudden pain in chest or abdomen, odynophagia, dyspnea
  - • Fever, shock, profound systemic toxicity, subcutaneous emphysema, mediastinal crunching sounds, rigid abdomen, tachypnea
  - • Leukocytosis, salivary hyperamylasemia
  - • Chest x-ray shows mediastinal widening, mediastinal emphysema, pleural effusion (often delayed)
  - • Demonstration of rupture of lower esophagus by esophagogram with water-soluble opaque media or CT scan; no role for endoscopy

- ■ Differential Diagnosis
  - • Myocardial infarction, pericarditis
  - • Pulmonary embolism, pulmonary abscess
  - • Aortic dissection
  - • Ruptured viscus
  - • Acute pancreatitis
  - • Shock due to other causes
  - • Caustic ingestion, pill esophagitis
  - • Instrumental esophageal perforation

- ■ Treatment
  - • Aggressive supportive measures with broad-spectrum antibiotics covering mouth organisms, nasogastric tube suctioning, and total parenteral nutrition
  - • Surgical consultation with repair
  - • In patients who are poor surgical candidates and without signs of sepsis, can consider endoscopic treatment with self-expanding stents

- ■ Pearl

One of the few causes in medicine of hydrophobia.

Reference

de Schipper JP, Pull ter Gunne AF, Oostvogel HJ, van Laarhoven CJ. Spontaneous rupture of the oesophagus: Boerhaave's syndrome in 2008. Literature review and treatment algorithm. Dig Surg 2009;26:1. [PMID: 19145081]

Esophageal Web

- **Essentials of Diagnosis**
  - Dysphagia, particularly for solids more than liquids
  - Plummer-Vinson syndrome if associated with iron deficiency anemia, glossitis, and spooning of nails; may be higher incidence of hypopharyngeal carcinoma
  - Can be associated with dermatologic diseases such as bullous pemphigoid, pemphigus vulgaris, or epidermolysis bullosa
  - Barium swallow (lateral view often required), esophagoscopy diagnostic (but often misses cervical esophageal webs)

- **Differential Diagnosis**
  - Esophageal ring (at gastroesophageal junction, may be due to acid reflux)
  - Achalasia
  - Esophageal diverticulum
  - Aperistalsis
  - Esophageal or mediastinal tumor
  - Esophageal stricture

- **Treatment**
  - Treat the iron deficiency after finding its cause—the web may resolve spontaneously
  - Esophagoscopy with disruption of webs adequate in most cases
  - Bougienage or endoscopic dilation required on occasion

- **Pearl**

Webs do not cause iron deficiency; the iron deficiency causes webs.

Reference

Chung S, Roberts-Thomson IC. Gastrointestinal: upper oesophageal web. J Gastroenterol Hepatol 1999;14:611. [PMID: 10385074]

Foreign Bodies in the Esophagus

- ■ Essentials of Diagnosis
  - • Most common in children, edentulous older patients, and the severely mentally impaired
  - • Occurs at physiologic areas of narrowing (upper esophageal sphincter, the level of the aortic arch, or the diaphragmatic hiatus)
  - • Other predisposing factors favoring impaction include Zenker's diverticulum, webs, achalasia, peptic strictures, or malignancy
  - • Recent ingestion of food or foreign material (coins most commonly in children, meat bolus most common in adults), but the history may be missing
  - • Vague discomfort in chest or neck, dysphagia, inability to handle secretions, odynophagia, hypersalivation, and stridor or dyspnea in children
  - • Radiographic or endoscopic evidence of esophageal obstruction by foreign body

- ■ Differential Diagnosis
  - • Esophageal stricture
  - • Eosinophilic esophagitis
  - • Esophageal or mediastinal tumor
  - • Angina pectoris

- ■ Treatment
  - • Endoscopic removal with airway protection as needed and the use of an overtube if sharp objects are present
  - • Emergent endoscopy should be used for sharp objects, disk batteries (secondary to risk of perforation due to their caustic nature), or evidence of the inability to handle secretions; objects retained in the esophagus should be removed within 24 hours of ingestion
  - • Endoscopy is successful in > 90% of cases; avoid barium studies before endoscopy, as they impair visualization

- ■ Pearl

Treatment is ordinarily straightforward; diagnosis may not be, especially in the very young and very old.

Reference

Eisen GM, Baron TH, Dominitz JA, et al; American Society for Gastrointestinal Endoscopy. Guideline for the management of ingested foreign bodies. Gastrointest Endosc 2002;55:802. [PMID: 12024131]

Gastric Ulcer

■ Essentials of Diagnosis

- Epigastric pain unpredictably relieved by food or antacids; weight loss, anorexia, vomiting
- Iron deficiency anemia, fecal occult blood positive
- Ulcer demonstrated by barium study or endoscopy
- Caused by *Helicobacter pylori* (in 70% of cases), NSAIDs, gastric malignancy, or rarely, Zollinger-Ellison syndrome
- Endoscopic biopsy or documentation of complete healing necessary to exclude malignancy
- Complications include hemorrhage, perforation, and obstruction

■ Differential Diagnosis

- Other peptic ulcer disease
- Gastroesophageal reflux
- Gastric carcinoma
- Cholecystitis
- Esophagitis
- Gastritis
- Irritable or functional bowel disease such as nonulcer dyspepsia

■ Treatment

- Eradicate *H. pylori* when present
- Avoid tobacco, alcohol, xanthines, and ulcerogenic drugs, especially NSAIDs
- Proton pump inhibitors, sucralfate, H_2-receptor antagonists
- Endoscopic therapy for actively bleeding ulcers
- Surgery may be needed for ulcers refractory to medical management (rare, and must exclude cancer if ulcer not healing) or for the management of complications (eg, perforation, uncontrolled bleeding)

■ Pearl

Gastric ulcers lose weight; duodenal ulcers gain it.

Reference

Ramakrishnan K, Salinas RC. Peptic ulcer disease. Am Fam Physician 2007;76:1005. [PMID: 17956071]

Gastritis

- **Essentials of Diagnosis**
  - May be acute (erosive) or indolent (atrophic); multiple varied causes
  - Symptoms often vague and include nausea, vomiting, anorexia, nondescript upper abdominal distress
  - Mild epigastric tenderness to palpation; in some, physical signs absent
  - Iron deficiency anemia not unusual
  - Endoscopy with gastric biopsy for definitive diagnosis
  - Multiple associations include stress and diminished mucosal blood flow (burns, sepsis, critical illness), drugs (NSAIDs, salicylates), atrophic states (aging, pernicious anemia), previous surgery (gastrectomy, Billroth II), *H. pylori* infection, acute or chronic alcoholism

- **Differential Diagnosis**
  - Peptic ulcer
  - Hiatal hernia
  - Malignancy of stomach or pancreas
  - Cholecystitis
  - Ischemic cardiac disease

- **Treatment**
  - Avoidance of alcohol, caffeine, salicylates, tobacco, and NSAIDs
  - Investigate for presence of *H. pylori*; eradicate if present
  - Proton pump inhibitors in patients receiving oral feedings, H_2 inhibitors, or sucralfate
  - Prevention in high-risk patients (eg, intensive care setting) using these same agents

- **Pearl**

Ninety-five percent of gastroenterologists and a high proportion of other health care workers carry H. pylori.

Reference

El-Zimaity H. Gastritis and gastric atrophy. Curr Opin Gastroenterol 2008;24:682. [PMID: 19122515]

Gastroesophageal Reflux Disease (GERD)

■ **Essentials of Diagnosis**

- Substernal burning (pyrosis) or pressure, aggravated by recumbency and relieved with sitting; can cause dysphagia, odynophagia, atypical chest pain; proton pump inhibitor may be diagnostic and therapeutic; further testing when diagnosis unclear, symptoms refractory
- Reflux, hiatal hernia may be found at barium study
- Incompetent lower esophageal sphincter (LES); endoscopy with biopsy may be necessary to exclude other diagnoses
- Esophageal pH helpful during symptoms
- Diminished LES tone also seen in obesity, pregnancy, hiatal hernia, nasogastric tube

■ **Differential Diagnosis**

- Peptic ulcer disease
- Angina pectoris
- Achalasia, esophageal spasm, pill esophagitis

■ **Treatment**

- Weight loss, avoidance of late-night meals, elevation of head of bed
- Avoid chocolate, caffeine, tobacco, alcohol
- High-dose H_2 blockers or proton pump inhibitors
- Surgical fundoplication for patients intolerant or allergic to medical therapy or refractory cases with predominantly regurgitation or nonacid reflux; use caution in patients whose primary complaint is heartburn and who are found to have nonerosive GER, as these patients likely have a component of visceral hypersensitivity that may be exacerbated by surgery.

■ **Pearl**

Eradication of H. pylori *may actually worsen GERD; the gastric acid secretion increases upon eradication of the bacterium.*

Reference

Fass R. Proton pump inhibitor failure: what are the therapeutic options? Am J Gastroenterol 2009;104(suppl):S33. [PMID: 19262545]

Intestinal Tuberculosis

- ■ Essentials of Diagnosis
  - • Chronic abdominal pain, anorexia, bloating; weight loss, fever, diarrhea, new-onset ascites in many
  - • Mild right lower quadrant tenderness, as ileocecal area is the most commonly involved intestinal site; fistula-in-ano sometimes seen
  - • Barium study may reveal mucosal ulcerations or scarring and fibrosis with narrowing of the small or large intestine
  - • In peritonitis, ascitic fluid has high protein and mononuclear pleocytosis; peritoneal biopsy with granulomas is more sensitive than ascites AFB culture; high adenosine deaminase levels in ascitic fluid may suggest the diagnosis; TB peritonitis more common in those with immune compromise
  - • Complications include intestinal obstruction, hemorrhage, fistula formation, and bacterial overgrowth with malabsorption

- ■ Differential Diagnosis
  - • Carcinoma of the colon or small bowel
  - • Inflammatory bowel disease: Crohn's disease
  - • Ameboma or *Yersinia* infection
  - • Intestinal lymphoma or amyloidosis
  - • Ovarian or peritoneal carcinomatosis
  - • *Mycobacterium avium-intracellulare* infection

- ■ Treatment
  - • Standard therapy for tuberculosis; as infection heals, the affected bowel may develop stricture

- ■ Pearl

Seen uncommonly in the developed world, but experienced clinicians have long noted that exploratory laparotomy for suspected small bowel obstruction relieves symptoms without antituberculous therapy.

Reference

Donoghue HD, Holton J. Intestinal tuberculosis. Curr Opin Infect Dis 2009;22:490. [PMID: 19623062]

Irritable Bowel Syndrome (IBS)

- ■ Essentials of Diagnosis
  - Chronic functional disorder characterized by abdominal pain or discomfort associated with altered bowel habits, occurring for at least 3 months
  - Variable abdominal tenderness
  - More common in women and if a history of physical abuse
  - Evaluation: History and physical exam, colonoscopy in patients over age 50; further testing as indicated for alarm symptoms or physical exam findings
  - Studies (such as complete blood count, ova and parasite, thyroid-stimulating hormone) are normal

- ■ Differential Diagnosis
  - Inflammatory bowel disease
  - Celiac sprue
  - Lactose intolerance
  - Diverticular disease
  - Peptic ulcer disease

- ■ Treatment
  - Rule out celiac disease in patients with diarrhea-predominant IBS or mixed (alternating diarrhea/constipation) IBS
  - Endoscopic evaluations in patients with alarm features or > 50 years of age
  - Reassurance and explanation
  - High-fiber (avoid insoluble fiber) diet with or without fiber supplements; restricting dairy products may be helpful
  - Antispasmodic agents (eg, dicyclomine, hyoscyamine, peppermint oil); antidiarrheal or anticonstipation agents
  - Tricyclic antidepressants, selective serotonin reuptake inhibitors, and behavioral modification with relaxation techniques helpful for some patients
  - Alosetron for women with severe diarrhea-predominant IBS that has not responded to conventional therapies (rare but serious increased risk for ischemic colitis); lubiprostone for women with constipation-predominant IBS (pregnancy category C).

- ■ Pearl

IBS is high on the list of causes of visits to gastroenterologists.

Reference

American College of Gastroenterology Task Force on Irritable Bowel Syndrome, Brandt LJ, Chey WD, et al. An evidence-based position statement on the management of irritable bowel syndrome. Am J Gastroenterol 2009;104(suppl 1): S1. [PMID: 19521341]

Mallory-Weiss Syndrome (Mucosal Laceration of the Gastroesophageal Junction)

3

- ■ Essentials of Diagnosis
  - Hematemesis of bright red blood, often after prolonged or forceful vomiting or retching; majority lack this history
  - Because many patients are hypovolemic, portal pressure is low and bleeding unimpressive
  - More impressive in alcoholics with brisk bleeding because of associated coagulopathy and may involve esophageal varices
  - Endoscopic demonstration of vertical mucosal tear at cardioesophageal junction or proximal stomach
  - Hiatal hernia often associated

- ■ Differential Diagnosis
  - Peptic ulcer
  - Esophageal varices
  - Gastritis
  - Reflux, infectious, or pill esophagitis

- ■ Treatment
  - Usually none required; spontaneous resolution of bleeding unless concomitant varices present
  - Endoscopic hemostatic intervention with epinephrine injection, thermal coaptation, banding or endoscopic clipping for active bleeding; rarely, balloon tamponade, embolization, or surgery is required for uncontrolled bleeding

- ■ Pearl

Hyperemesis gravidarum is likely the most common cause, although bleeding is scant because of low portal pressures attendant to vomiting-induced dehydration.

Reference

Cho YS, Chae HS, Kim HK, et al. Endoscopic band ligation and endoscopic hemoclip placement for patients with Mallory-Weiss syndrome and active bleeding. World J Gastroenterol 2008;14:2080. [PMID: 18395910]

Polyps of the Colon & Rectum

- ■ Essentials of Diagnosis
  - • Discrete mass lesions arising from colonic epithelium and protruding into the intestinal lumen; polyps may be pedunculated, sessile, or flat
  - • Most patients asymptomatic; can be associated with chronic occult blood loss
  - • Family history may be present
  - • Diagnosed by sigmoidoscopy, colonoscopy, or virtual colonoscopy
  - • Removing polyps decreases the incidence of adenocarcinoma

- ■ Differential Diagnosis
  - • Adenocarcinoma
  - • Radiographic artifact
  - • Other luminal findings: Nonadenomatous (hyperplastic) polyps, lipomas, inverted diverticula

- ■ Treatment
  - • Surgical or endoscopic polypectomy in all cases with histologic review
  - • Colectomy for familial polyposis or Gardner's syndrome
  - • Surveillance colonoscopy every 3–5 years depending on number and histology of the polyps

- ■ Pearl

Rigorous screening programs in delivery systems such as the VAMC have markedly reduced the incidence of malignant deterioration; a real success story for appropriate screening.

Reference

Lieberman DA. Clinical practice. Screening for colorectal cancer. N Engl J Med 2009;361:1179. [PMID: 19759380]

Ulcerative Colitis (UC)

- ■ Essentials of Diagnosis
  - Low-volume diarrhea, often bloody; urgency, tenesmus, and cramping lower abdominal pain; associated with fever, weight loss
  - Mild abdominal tenderness, mucocutaneous lesions, erythema nodosum or pyoderma gangrenosum
  - Anemia, accelerated sedimentation rate, hypoproteinemia, absent stool pathogens
  - Colon involved contiguously from rectum
  - Mucosal biopsy with chronic active inflammation, crypt abscesses
  - Increased incidence of colonic adenocarcinoma with young age at onset, long-standing active disease, and pancolitis

- ■ Differential Diagnosis
  - Bacterial, amebic, or ischemic colitis
  - Adenocarcinoma of the colon
  - Pseudomembranous colitis
  - Granulomatous colitis or Crohn's disease
  - Antibiotic-associated diarrhea
  - Radiation colitis or collagenous colitis

- ■ Treatment
  - High-protein, low-residue, lactose-free diet during flares
  - Mild or moderate UC can be treated with oral 5-ASA or topical mesalamine (by enema or suppository) to induce and maintain a remission; can add corticosteroid enemas or suppositories for additional symptomatic relief
  - Corticosteroids for acute flare refractory to maximal dose oral/rectal 5-ASA; consider addition of 6-mercaptopurine (6-MP) or azathioprine in patients who cannot achieve steroid-free remission.
  - Consider infliximab in patients who are steroid refractory or steroid dependent despite therapy with 6-MP or azathioprine
  - For a severe flare requiring hospitalization, IV corticosteroids should be given; patients failing to respond within 3–5 days should be considered for colectomy versus a trial of cyclosporine or infliximab.
  - Colectomy for toxic megacolon unresponsive to medical therapy
  - Yearly colonoscopy after 8 years of pancolitis for dysplasia surveillance

- ■ Pearl

The four hepatobiliary complications are pericholangitis, chronic active hepatitis, sclerosing cholangitis, and cholangiocarcinoma; the first two parallel activity of colitis, the last two do not.

Reference

Kornbluth A, Sachar DB. Ulcerative Colitis Practice Guidelines in Adults: American College of Gastroenterology, Practice Parameters Committee. Am J Gastroenterol 2010;105:501. [PMID: 20068560]

Whipple's Disease

■ Essentials of Diagnosis

- Caused by infection with the bacillus *Tropheryma whippelii*
- Rare disease, even more so in women and blacks
- Insidious onset of fever, abdominal pain, malabsorption, arthralgias, weight loss, symptoms of steatorrhea, polyarthritis
- Lymphadenopathy, arthritis, macular skin rash, various neurologic findings
- Anemia, hypoalbuminemia, hypocarotenemia
- Small bowel mucosal biopsy reveals characteristic foamy mononuclear cells filled with periodic acid-Schiff staining material; electron microscopy shows bacilli in multiple affected organs

■ Differential Diagnosis

- Celiac or tropical sprue
- Inflammatory bowel disease, Crohn's disease
- Ulcerative colitis
- Intestinal lymphoma
- Rheumatoid arthritis or HLA-B27 spondyloarthropathy
- Hyperthyroidism
- HIV infection

■ Treatment

- Penicillin and streptomycin intravenously (ceftriaxone and streptomycin for central nervous system disease) for 10–14 days followed by trimethoprim-sulfamethoxazole (cefixime or doxycycline in sulfonamide-allergic patients)
- Treatment for at least 1 year

■ Pearl

Oculomasticatory myorhythmia (rhythmic motion of the eye muscles with chewing) is unique to Whipple's; it is harder to pronounce than diagnose.

Reference

Marth T. New insights into Whipple's disease: a rare intestinal inflammatory disorder. Dig Dis 2009;27:494. [PMID: 19897965]

Zollinger-Ellison Syndrome (Gastrinoma)

■ Essentials of Diagnosis

- Severe, recurrent, intractable peptic ulcer disease, often associated with concomitant esophagitis; ulcers may be in atypical locations, like jejunum, but most occur in usual sites
- Eighty percent of cases are sporadic; the rest are associated with multiple endocrine neoplasia type 1 (MEN1)
- Fasting serum gastrin > 150 pg/mL (often much higher) in the setting of a low gastric pH; elevated serum chromogranin A; renal insufficiency; proton pump inhibitors can also raise serum gastrin
- Diarrhea common, caused by inactivation of pancreatic enzymes; relieved by nasogastric tube suctioning immediately
- Gastrinomas may arise in pancreas, duodenum, or lymph nodes; > 50% are malignant but not usually aggressive
- Localization techniques include somatostatin receptor scintigraphy, thin-cut CT, MRI, endoscopic ultrasound, or intraoperative localization

■ Differential Diagnosis

- Peptic ulcer disease of other cause
- Esophagitis
- Gastritis
- Pancreatitis
- Cholecystitis
- Diarrhea or malabsorption from other causes

■ Treatment

- High-dose proton pump inhibitor (with goal of < 10 mEq/h of gastric acid secretion)
- Exploratory laparotomy for patients without preoperative evidence of unresectable metastatic disease; not recommended for patients with MEN1
- Chemotherapy ineffective; interferon, octreotide, and hepatic artery embolization for metastatic disease
- Resection for localized disease
- Family counseling
- MEN1-associated gastrinoma appears to have a lower incidence of hepatic metastases and a better long-term prognosis

■ Pearl

In Zollinger-Ellison syndrome, isolated gastric ulcer is never encountered.

Reference

Murugesan SV, Varro A, Pritchard DM. Review article: strategies to determine whether hypergastrinaemia is due to Zollinger-Ellison syndrome rather than a more common benign cause. Aliment Pharmacol Ther 2009;29:1055. [PMID: 19226290]

4

Hepatobiliary Disorders

Acute Liver Failure

- ### Essentials of Diagnosis
  - Severe liver injury in a person with previously normal liver function, associated with development of hepatic encephalopathy and evidence of hepatic synthetic dysfunction
  - Patients often present with new-onset jaundice, anorexia, nausea, vomiting, flulike symptoms, or altered mental status
  - Etiologies include acetaminophen overdose, idiosyncratic drug reaction, acute viral hepatitis, exposure to hepatotoxins, autoimmune hepatitis, Wilson's disease, complications of pregnancy, and vascular disorders
  - Markedly abnormal liver function tests: Elevated bilirubin, AST/ALT > 1000, elevated international normalized ratio.
  - Prognosis depends on etiology, rapidity of onset and degree of encephalopathy, and development of complications

- ### Differential Diagnosis
  - Acute decompensation of chronic liver disease
  - Acute viral hepatitis; alcoholic hepatitis; sepsis
  - Idiopathic drug reaction

- ### Treatment
  - Prompt recognition of acute liver failure key
  - Consider giving N-acetylcysteine to all cases of acute liver failure, not just patients with acetaminophen overdose
  - After resuscitation and stabilization, transfer to a transplant center
  - Surveillance for infection; consider prophylactic antibiotics in patients with advanced encephalopathy, systemic inflammatory response syndrome, or awaiting liver transplantation
  - Management of complications: hepatic encephalopathy, cerebral edema, acute renal failure, acute respiratory distress syndrome, cardiovascular compromise, metabolic disturbances, bleeding
  - Liver transplantation in select patients

- ### Pearl

In pregnant patients presenting with acute fatty liver of pregnancy or HELLP syndrome, treatment is early delivery.

Reference

Stravitz RT, Kramer DJ; Medscape. Management of acute liver failure. Nat Rev Gastroenterol Hepatol 2009;6:542. [PMID: 19652652]

Acute Viral Hepatitis

■ Essentials of Diagnosis

- Jaundice, fever, chills; enlarged, tender liver
- Anorexia, nausea, vomiting, malaise, symptoms of flulike syndrome, arthralgias, and aversion to smoking
- Normal to low white cell count; abnormal liver function studies (ALT > AST); serologic tests for hepatitis A (HAV IgM), hepatitis B (HBsAg, HB core ab IGM), or hepatitis C (HCV RNA) may be positive
- Liver biopsy shows characteristic hepatocellular necrosis and mononuclear infiltrates
- Hepatitis A: Fecal-oral transmission, short incubation period; good prognosis, but rare cases of fulminant hepatic failure
- Hepatitis B and hepatitis C: Parenteral transmission, longer incubation period, progression to chronic disease more likely
- Hepatitis E: Fecal-oral transmission, usually by contaminated water in endemic regions, although other transmission routes probable; during pregnancy, infection can lead to fulminant hepatitis with mortality rates of 15–25%

■ Differential Diagnosis

- Alcoholic hepatitis
- Cholestatic jaundice secondary to medications or herbals
- Acetaminophen toxicity
- Leptospirosis
- Secondary syphilis
- Q fever
- Choledocholithiasis
- Carcinoma of the pancreas
- Hepatic vein thrombosis

■ Treatment

- Supportive care
- Avoidance of hepatotoxins: alcohol, acetaminophen
- Treatment of acute hepatitis C (if spontaneous clearance has not occurred by 8–12 weeks) with pegylated interferon

■ Pearl

Hepatitis A is the only viral hepatitis causing spiking fevers; if you believe a patient has hepatitis but serology is negative, remember ascending cholangitis however.

Reference

Degertekin B, Lok AS. Update on viral hepatitis: 2008. Curr Opin Gastroenterol 2009;25:180. [PMID: 19387254]

Alcoholic Hepatitis

- **Essentials of Diagnosis**
  - Onset usually after years of alcohol intake; anorexia, nausea, abdominal pain
  - Fever, jaundice, tender hepatomegaly, ascites, encephalopathy
  - Macrocytic anemia, leukocytosis with left shift, thrombocytopenia, abnormal liver function tests (AST about double ALT, increased bilirubin, prolonged prothrombin time), hypergamma globulinemia; AST rarely exceeds 300 U/L despite severity of illness
  - Liver biopsy if diagnosis is in doubt

- **Differential Diagnosis**
  - Cholelithiasis, cholecystitis, cholangitis
  - Cirrhosis due to other causes
  - Nonalcoholic fatty liver
  - Viral hepatitis
  - Drug-induced hepatitis
  - Autoimmune liver disease

- **Treatment**
  - General supportive measures including nutritional support, withdrawal of alcohol, avoidance of hepatotoxins (especially acetaminophen)
  - Treat any ascites, hepatic encephalopathy
  - Screen for bacterial infections (CBC, blood and urine cultures, ascites fluid cell count and culture if present, chest x-ray)
  - Methylprednisolone (32 mg/d for 4 weeks) or pentoxifylline (400 mg three times a day for 4 weeks) may be beneficial in severe acute disease when discriminant function (4.6 [PT − control] + bilirubin [mg/dL]) is > 32 (study exclusion criteria: active GI bleeding, infection)

- **Pearl**

  Transaminase is paradoxically only mildly elevated even in severe cases; if the AST exceeds 300, make another diagnosis.

Reference

Lucey MR, Mathurin P, Morgan TR. Alcoholic hepatitis. N Engl J Med 2009;360:2758. [PMID: 19553649]

Amebic Hepatic Abscess

- **Essentials of Diagnosis**
  - Fever, right-sided abdominal pain, right pleuritic chest pain; preceding or concurrent diarrheal illness in minority
  - History of travel to or recent immigration from endemic region
  - Tender palpable liver ("punch" tenderness), localized intercostal tenderness
  - Anemia, leukocytosis with left shift, nonspecific liver test abnormalities
  - Positive serologic tests for *Entamoeba histolytica* in > 95% of patients, though may be negative early in infection
  - Increased right hemidiaphragm by radiography; ultrasound, CT scan, or liver scan demonstrates location and number of lesions

- **Differential Diagnosis**
  - Pyogenic abscess
  - Echinococcal cyst
  - Primary or metastatic tumor
  - Acute hepatitis
  - Right lower lobe pneumonia
  - Cholelithiasis, cholecystitis

- **Treatment**
  - Metronidazole drug of choice; repeated courses occasionally necessary
  - Percutaneous needle aspiration for toxic patient failing to respond to therapy or with suspected imminent rupture or possible bacterial superinfection
  - Oral course of luminal amebicides (iodoquinol, paromomycin sulfate) after acute therapy to eradicate intestinal cyst phase

- **Pearl**

More a cyst than an abscess; the "anchovy paste" within the lesion is free of neutrophils.

Reference

Pritt BS, Clark CG. Amebiasis. Mayo Clin Proc 2008;83:1154. [PMID: 18828976]

Ascites

4

■ Essentials of Diagnosis

- Usually associated with cirrhosis, but heart or kidney disease also causative
- Evidence of shifting dullness, bulging flanks
- Paracentesis for new-onset ascites or symptoms suggestive of spontaneous bacterial peritonitis
- Fluid sent for cell count, protein, bacterial culture; amylase, cytology, and triglycerides as indicated
- Serum–ascites albumin gradient ≥ 1.1 g/dL is virtually diagnostic of portal hypertension
- > 250 neutrophils/μL characteristic of infection

■ Differential Diagnosis

Due to portal hypertension:
- Chronic liver disease (80–85% of all cases)
- Cardiac failure (3%)

Not due to portal hypertension:
- Malignancy-related (10%), TB, pancreatic, chylous ascites

■ Treatment

Treat as follows for ascites due to portal hypertension:
- Sodium restriction (< 2 g/d)
- Fluid restriction if serum sodium < 120 mmol/L
- Diuretics: Usually spironolactone and furosemide in 100-mg to 40-mg ratio to address potassium balance
- Large-volume paracentesis (4–6 L) for tense or refractory ascites with albumin replacement (6–10 g/L)
- Transjugular intrahepatic portosystemic shunt (TIPS) or surgical shunting in refractory cases
- Patients with spontaneous bacterial peritonitis are treated for 5 days with a third-generation cephalosporin (eg, cefotaxime); should also receive IV albumin (dose is 1.5 g/kg on day 1 and 1 g/kg on day 3)
- Spontaneous bacterial peritonitis prophylaxis for patients with spontaneous bacterial peritonitis, gastrointestinal hemorrhage, or low-protein ascites (< 1.5 g/dL)

■ Pearl

Once spontaneous bacterial peritonitis occurs, liver transplantation is the only intervention that will prolong life.

Reference

Kuiper JJ, de Man RA, van Buuren HR. Review article: management of ascites and associated complications in patients with cirrhosis. Aliment Pharmacol Ther 2007;26(suppl 2):183. [PMID: 18081661]

Autoimmune Hepatitis

- ■ Essentials of Diagnosis
  - Insidious onset; usually affects young women
  - Fatigue, anorexia, arthralgias; dark urine; light stools in some
  - Jaundice, spider angiomas, hepatomegaly, acne, hirsutism
  - Abnormal liver function tests, most notably increased amino-transferases, polyclonal gammopathy
  - Associated with arthritis, thyroiditis, nephritis, Coombs-positive hemolytic anemia
  - Type 1: Antinuclear antibody (ANA) or anti–smooth muscle antibody–positive; type 2: anti–liver/kidney microsomal antibody–positive
  - Patients may develop cirrhosis, predicted by biopsy features of chronic active hepatitis

- ■ Differential Diagnosis
  - Chronic viral hepatitis
  - Nonalcoholic steatohepatitis
  - Sclerosing cholangitis
  - Primary biliary cirrhosis
  - Wilson's disease
  - Hemochromatosis

- ■ Treatment
  - General supportive measures (including exercise, calcium, and hormonal therapy to prevent osteoporosis)
  - In patients with elevated aminotransferases or gammaglobulins or for individualized reasons: Prednisone for induction of remission and azathioprine for maintenance of remission
  - Liver transplantation for cirrhosis; cirrhotic patients should also be screened for hepatocellular carcinoma

- ■ Pearl

If you think you see a spider angioma below the waist, think again; this practically never happens in all types of liver disease.

Reference

Yeoman AD, Longhi MS, Heneghan MA. Review article: the modern management of autoimmune hepatitis. Aliment Pharmacol Ther 2010;31:771. [PMID: 20096018]

Choledocholithiasis/Cholangitis

- ■ Essentials of Diagnosis
  - • Often a history of biliary tract disease; episodic attacks of right abdominal or epigastric pain that may radiate to the right scapula or shoulder; occasionally painless jaundice
  - • Pain, fever, and jaundice (Charcot's triad), associated with nausea, vomiting, hypothermia, shock, and leukocytosis with a left shift
  - • Elevated liver function tests, especially bilirubin and alkaline phosphatase; during acute impaction, there may be a rapid rise of serum AST/ALT due to hepatocellular injury
  - • Abdominal imaging studies may reveal gallstones. Ultrasound or CT scan shows dilated biliary tree and can sometimes identify stones within the bile duct.
  - • Endoscopic ultrasound (EUS), endoscopic retrograde cholangiopancreatography (ERCP), or magnetic resonance cholangiopancreatography (MRCP) localizes the degree and location of obstruction

- ■ Differential Diagnosis
  - • Carcinoma of the pancreas, ampulla of Vater, or common duct
  - • Acute hepatitis
  - • Acute cholecystitis or Mirizzi's syndrome
  - • Biliary stricture
  - • Drug-induced cholestatic jaundice
  - • Pancreatitis
  - • Other septic syndromes

- ■ Treatment
  - • Intravenous broad-spectrum antibiotics
  - • Endoscopic papillotomy and stone extraction for retained stones, followed by laparoscopic or open cholecystectomy
  - • Percutaneous biliary drainage in patients too hemodynamically unstable to tolerate sedation for ERCP or if endoscopic expertise not available

- ■ Pearl

  Although choledocholithiasis is often asymptomatic, septic shock due to cholangitis may occur with stunning rapidity; the sun should never set on this diagnosis.

Reference

Lee JG. Diagnosis and management of acute cholangitis. Nat Rev Gastroenterol Hepatol 2009;6:533. [PMID: 19652653]

Cholelithiasis (Gallstones)

- **Essentials of Diagnosis**
  - Frequently asymptomatic but may be associated with recurrent bouts of right-sided or midepigastric pain and nausea or vomiting after eating
  - Ultrasound, CT scan, and plain films demonstrate stones within the gallbladder
  - Increased incidence with female gender, chronic hemolysis, obesity, Native American origin, inflammatory bowel disease, diabetes mellitus, pregnancy, hypercholesterolemia

- **Differential Diagnosis**
  - Acute cholecystitis
  - Acute pancreatitis
  - Peptic ulcer disease
  - Acute appendicitis
  - Acute hepatitis
  - Right lower lobe pneumonia
  - Myocardial infarction
  - Radicular pain in T6–T10 dermatome

- **Treatment**
  - Laparoscopic or open cholecystectomy for symptomatic patients only
  - Bile salts (ursodeoxycholic acid) may cause dissolution of cholesterol stones, but should only be considered for patients who are not surgical candidates

- **Pearl**

In a patient with right upper quadrant densities on an abdominal plain film and an increased MCHC with low mean corpuscular volume, hereditary spherocytosis is the diagnosis.

Reference

Bellows CF, Berger DH, Crass RA. Management of gallstones. Am Fam Physician 2005;72:637. [PMID: 16127953]

Chronic Viral Hepatitis

- **Essentials of Diagnosis**
  - Fatigue, right upper quadrant discomfort, arthralgias, depression, nausea, anorexia
  - In advanced cases (cirrhosis): Jaundice, variceal bleeding, encephalopathy, ascites, spontaneous bacterial peritonitis, and hepatocellular carcinoma
  - Persistent elevation in ALT (> 6 months)
  - In hepatitis B, positive hepatitis B DNA with HBsAg present
  - In hepatitis C, positive hepatitis C RNA

- **Differential Diagnosis**
  - Alcoholic cirrhosis
  - Metabolic liver disorders (eg, nonalcoholic steatohepatitis), Wilson's disease, hemochromatosis
  - Autoimmune hepatitis
  - Cholestatic jaundice secondary to drugs

- **Treatment**
  - Avoidance of alcohol
  - For chronic active hepatitis B, treatment with nucleoside analogs (lamivudine, telbivudine, entecavir) or nucleotide analogs (adefovir, tenofovir); tenofovir and entecavir are considered first-line therapies due to their high-potency, low-resistance profiles, and overall tolerability; consider interferon in select patients.
  - Pegylated interferon alfa and ribavirin for chronic hepatitis C; specifically targeted antiviral therapy for HCV (STAT-C) in development
  - Screening for hepatocellular cancer in all patients with chronic hepatitis B or hepatitis C with cirrhosis
  - Vaccination against hepatitis A (and hepatitis B in patients with hepatitis C)
  - Liver transplantation for advanced disease or hepatocellular carcinoma

- **Pearl**

Hepatitis B and C are the most common causes worldwide of hepatocellular carcinoma.

Reference

Dakhil N, Junaidi O, Befeler AS. Chronic viral hepatitis. Mo Med 2009;106:361. [PMID: 19902718]

Cirrhosis

■ Essentials of Diagnosis

- The outcome of many types of chronic hepatitis—viral, toxic, immune, and metabolic
- Insidious onset of malaise, weight loss, increasing abdominal girth
- Spider angiomas, hepatosplenomegaly, palmar erythema, Dupuytren's contractures, gynecomastia, ascites, edema, asterixis
- Macrocytic anemia, thrombocytopenia, impaired synthetic function
- Biopsy diagnostic with micro- or macronodular fibrosis
- Complications include gastrointestinal bleeding from esophageal or gastric varices, ascites and spontaneous bacterial peritonitis, hepatorenal syndrome, encephalopathy

■ Differential Diagnosis

- Congestive heart failure
- Constrictive pericarditis
- Schistosomiasis
- Nephrotic syndrome
- Hypothyroidism
- Budd-Chiari syndrome

■ Treatment

- Supportive care, abstinence from alcohol
- Beta-blockers or endoscopic eradication in patients with established varices
- Diuretics or large-volume paracenteses for ascites and edema
- Antibiotic treatment and secondary prophylaxis for spontaneous bacterial peritonitis; debatably, primary prophylaxis if ascites total protein is < 1.5 g/dL
- Lactulose for encephalopathy
- Transjugular intrahepatic portosystemic shunt for bleeding gastric varices, bleeding esophageal varices not controlled by endoscopic therapy, or refractory ascites (encephalopathy is a contraindication)
- Liver transplantation in selected cases

■ Pearl

Comes from the Greek word kirrhos, *meaning orange-colored; see one in the pathology lab and you'll understand.*

Reference

Kuiper JJ, de Man RA, van Buuren HR. Review article: management of ascites and associated complications in patients with cirrhosis. Aliment Pharmacol Ther 2007;26(suppl 2):183. [PMID: 18081661]

Hepatic Encephalopathy

- ■ Essentials of Diagnosis
  - • Neurologic and psychiatric abnormalities resulting from liver dysfunction due to acute liver failure, cirrhosis, or major noncirrhotic portosystemic shunting
  - • Diagnosis requires history and physical examination suggestive of liver disease or portosystemic shunting
  - • Clinical manifestations range from mild confusion, personality changes, and sleep disturbances (stage I) to coma (stage IV)
  - • Asterixis, hyperreflexia, muscular rigidity, extensor plantar response, parkinsonian features, immobile facies, slow and monotonous speech
  - • Often triggered by gastrointestinal bleeding, infection, lactulose noncompliance, dietary protein overload, hypokalemia, dehydration, or medications such as sedatives or narcotics

- ■ Differential Diagnosis
  - • Systemic or central nervous system sepsis
  - • Hypoxia or hypercapnia
  - • Acidosis
  - • Uremia
  - • Use of sedatives or narcotics
  - • Postictal confusion
  - • Wernicke-Korsakoff syndrome
  - • Acute liver failure (cerebral edema or hypoglycemia)
  - • Delirium tremens
  - • Hyponatremia

- ■ Treatment
  - • Identify and treat precipitating factors listed above
  - • Lactulose 30–60 mL by mouth or nasogastric tube (or rectally) every 2 hours until bowel movements occur; in resolving or chronic encephalopathy, titrate to maintain two or three loose stools per day; if patients become hypernatremic, reduce lactulose dose
  - • Newer medical therapies include rifaximin, a nonabsorbable antibiotic
  - • Dietary protein restriction (< 70 g/d but > 40 g/d)
  - • Liver transplantation for chronic hepatic encephalopathy

- ■ Pearl

In a patient with cirrhosis and a normal hematocrit, be wary of hepatocellular carcinoma; it is the second most likely tumor to elaborate erythropoietin.

Reference

Bajaj J. Review article: modern management of hepatic encephalopathy. Aliment Pharmacol Ther 2010;31:537. [PMID: 20002027]

Hepatic Vein Obstruction (Budd-Chiari Syndrome)

- ■ Essentials of Diagnosis
  - Spectrum of disorders characterized by occlusion of the hepatic veins from a variety of causes; more common in women
  - Acute or chronic onset of tender, painful hepatic enlargement, jaundice, splenomegaly, and ascites
  - Doppler ultrasound or venography demonstrates occlusion of the hepatic veins; CT and MRI can also be helpful
  - Liver scintigraphy may show a prominent caudate lobe because its venous drainage may not be occluded; liver biopsy reveals characteristic central lobular congestion
  - Underlying causes include hypercoagulable states (both inherited and acquired), caval webs, polycythemia, right-sided heart failure, malignancy, "bush teas" (pyrrolizidine alkaloids), paroxysmal nocturnal hemoglobinuria, birth control pills, pregnancy, Behçet's disease

- ■ Differential Diagnosis
  - Cirrhosis
  - Constrictive pericarditis
  - Restrictive or dilated cardiomyopathy
  - Metastatic disease involving the liver
  - Granulomatous liver disease

- ■ Treatment
  - Treatment of complications (eg, ascites, encephalopathy)
  - Lifelong anticoagulation or treatment of underlying disease
  - Local thrombolysis in acute form of the disease
  - Transvenous intravascular portosystemic shunt may be considered in noncirrhotic patients
  - Liver transplantation for severe hepatocellular dysfunction

- ■ Pearl

Most hepatic vein obstructions involve a branch of that vessel; abrupt elevation of AST to exceptionally high levels gives a clue to the diagnosis in susceptible patients.

Reference

Valla DC. Primary Budd-Chiari syndrome. J Hepatol 2009;50:195. [PMID: 19012988]

Hepatocellular Carcinoma

■ Essentials of Diagnosis

- One of the world's most common visceral tumors
- Hepatitis B (with and without cirrhosis), hepatitis C cirrhosis, alcoholic cirrhosis, hemochromatosis among the important risk factors
- Symptoms and physical exam findings may not help, as they are similar to those of underlying liver disease
- Decompensation (new ascites, hepatic encephalopathy, or jaundice) of previously stable cirrhosis may be the presenting symptom
- Elevated (sometimes markedly) alpha-fetoprotein in some but not all; characteristic arterial phase enhancement with venous phase washout on helical CT scan

■ Differential Diagnosis

- Metastatic primary of other source
- Regenerating nodule

■ Treatment

- Surgical resection if adequate hepatic function and if tumor factors favorable (only one lobe involved and no extrahepatic spread)
- Transplant in highly selected patients
- If not transplant or resection candidates: Radiofrequency or alcohol ablation
- For patients with large or multifocal tumors not amenable to ablation, consider transarterial chemoembolization for palliation; systemic chemotherapy for patients with advanced disease (extrahepatic disease or evidence of vascular invasion)

■ Pearl

Remember, a normal AFP does not exclude HCC.

Reference

Cabrera R, Nelson DR. Review article: the management of hepatocellular carcinoma. Aliment Pharmacol Ther 2010;31:461. [PMID: 19925500]

Primary Biliary Cirrhosis

- ■ Essentials of Diagnosis
  - Usually affects women aged 40–60 years with the insidious onset of pruritus, jaundice, fatigue, and hepatomegaly
  - Malabsorption, xanthomas, xanthomatous neuropathy, osteomalacia, and portal hypertension may be complications
  - Increased alkaline phosphatase and gamma glutamyl transpeptidase, cholesterol, bilirubin; positive antimitochondrial antibody in 95%
  - Liver biopsy reveals dense inflammatory infiltrate centered on bile duct

- ■ Differential Diagnosis
  - Chronic biliary tract obstruction (ie, cholelithiasis-related stricture)
  - Bile duct carcinoma
  - Inflammatory bowel disease complicated by cholestatic liver disease
  - Sarcoidosis
  - Sclerosing cholangitis
  - Drug-induced cholestasis

- ■ Treatment
  - Cholestyramine, colestipol, or rifampin for pruritus
  - Calcium (high risk of osteoporosis, osteomalacia) and supplementation with vitamins A, D, E, and K
  - Ursodeoxycholic acid delays progression and extends survival
  - Liver transplant for refractory cirrhosis or hepatocellular cancer

- ■ Pearl

The perfect disease for cure by transplantation; no virus, no autoimmunity, no malignancy in explant.

Reference

Hohenester S, Oude-Elferink RP, Beuers U. Primary biliary cirrhosis. Semin Immunopathol 2009;31:283. [PMID: 19603170]

Pyogenic Hepatic Abscess

■ Essentials of Diagnosis

- Fever, jaundice, right upper quadrant tenderness, weight loss, pleuritic chest pain, cough, anorexia or nausea
- Usually due to hematogenous or local spread of an intra-abdominal infection
- Leukocytosis with left shift; nonspecific abnormalities of liver function studies
- Most common organisms are *Escherichia coli, Proteus vulgaris, Enterobacter aerogenes,* and anaerobic species
- Elevated right hemidiaphragm by radiography; ultrasound, CT scan, or liver scan demonstrates intrahepatic defect
- Predisposing factors: Malignancy, recent endoscopy or surgery, diabetes, Crohn's disease, diverticulitis, appendicitis, recent trauma

■ Differential Diagnosis

- Amebic hepatic abscess
- Acute hepatitis
- Right lower lobe pneumonia
- Cholelithiasis, cholecystitis
- Appendicitis

■ Treatment

- Antibiotics with coverage of gram-negative organisms and anaerobes, antibiotics narrowed if specific organisms identified
- Percutaneous or surgical drainage for cases refractory to medical management

■ Pearl

The classic triad of fever, jaundice, and hepatomegaly is not so classic; it is found in less than 10% of cases.

Reference

Johannsen EC, Sifri CD, Madoff LC: Pyogenic liver abscesses. Infect Dis Clin North Am 2000;14:547, vii. [PMID: 10987109]

Sclerosing Cholangitis

■ Essentials of Diagnosis

- Progressively obstructive jaundice, pruritus, malaise, and anorexia; most common in young men aged 20–40 years
- 60–80% of cases have associated IBD, predominantly ulcerative colitis; some may be asymptomatic
- Positive antineutrophil cytoplasmic antibody found in 70%; elevated total bilirubin and alkaline phosphatase common
- Imaging by MRCP or ERCP; MRCP demonstrates multifocal strictures and segmental dilations ("beading") and is the diagnostic modality of choice for suspected primary sclerosing cholangitis (PSC); ERCP is more invasive, results in hospitalizations due to complications in 10% of PSC patients; reserved for endoscopic therapy

■ Differential Diagnosis

- Choledocholithiasis
- Drug-induced cholestasis
- Carcinoma of pancreas or biliary tree
- Hepatitis due to any cause
- *Clonorchis sinensis* infection
- AIDS cholangiopathy

■ Treatment

- At present, no specific medical therapy has been shown to have a major impact on the prevention of complications (cholangitis, obstruction, cholangiocarcinoma and hepatic failure) or survival
- Ursodeoxycholic acid may improve liver function tests but does not alter symptoms or natural history
- Fat-soluble vitamin and calcium supplementation
- Stenting or balloon dilation of symptomatic obstruction due to dominant strictures by ERCP
- At diagnosis, all patients with PSC should be evaluated for IBD with colonoscopy and biopsy; these patients are at significantly increased risk of IBD-associated colorectal cancer, and surveillance colonoscopy is recommended at 1–2-year intervals from time of diagnosis
- Liver transplantation for decompensated disease

■ Pearl

Most sclerosing cholangitis is seen in inflammatory bowel disease, but most inflammatory bowel disease is not complicated by sclerosing cholangitis.

Reference

Chapman R, Fevery J, Kalloo A, Nagorney DM, Boberg KM, Shneider B, Gores GJ. Diagnosis and management of primary sclerosing cholangitis. Hepatology 2010;51:660. [PMID: 20101749]

Variceal Bleeding

- **Essentials of Diagnosis**
  - Sudden, painless large-volume episode of hematemesis with melena or hematochezia typical
  - Antecedent history of liver disease and stigmata of liver disease or portal hypertension on physical examination
  - Hepatic portal venous pressure gradient of ≥ 12 mm Hg is generally necessary for variceal bleeding
  - Fifty percent of patients with alcoholic cirrhosis will present with esophageal varices within 2 years of diagnosis
  - A 30–50% risk of death with each episode

- **Differential Diagnosis**
  - Peptic ulcer disease
  - Mallory-Weiss tear
  - Gastric varices
  - Alcoholic gastritis
  - Esophagitis
  - Bleeding from portal hypertensive gastropathy
  - Other less common sources: Dieulafoy's lesion, hemosuccus pancreaticus, aortoenteric fistulas

- **Treatment**
  - Appropriate resuscitation (intravenous resuscitation, correction of coagulopathy, blood transfusions, airway protection)
  - Intravenous octreotide (100-μg bolus, 50-μg/h drip)
  - Antibiotic prophylaxis (reduces rebleed rate and mortality)
  - Urgent endoscopic evaluation and treatment with band ligation; less successful in gastric varices
  - Balloon tamponade (Minnesota-Sengstaken-Blakemore) as a temporizing measure or for endoscopic failures
  - Transjugular intrahepatic portosystemic shunt (TIPS) or shunt surgery for gastric varices or refractory cases of esophageal varices
  - Liver transplantation for appropriate candidates with recurrent bleeding episodes
  - Prophylaxis of recurrent bleeding with endoscopic (band ligation) and pharmacologic therapy (propranolol, nadolol)

- **Pearl**

Splenic vein thrombosis may be due to pancreatitis, resulting in a cause of varices which is curable by splenectomy.

Reference

Bosch J, Abraldes JG, Berzigotti A, Garcia-Pagan JC. Portal hypertension and gastrointestinal bleeding. Semin Liver Dis 2008;28:3. [PMID: 18293274]

5

Hematologic Diseases

Acute Leukemia

- **Essentials of Diagnosis**
  - Rapid onset of fever, weakness, malaise, bleeding, bone or joint pain, infection
  - Pallor, fever, petechiae; lymphadenopathy, generally unimpressive; splenomegaly unusual
  - Pancytopenia with circulating leukemic blasts (rarely pancytopenia alone)
  - > 20% immature blasts in bone marrow and/or peripheral blood
  - Abnormal cells either lymphoblasts (ALL) or myeloblasts (AML), and immunohistochemistry immunohistochemistry and flow cytometry can help distinguish; Auer rods (eosinophilic cytoplasmic inclusions) in blasts are diagnostic of myeloid origin

- **Differential Diagnosis**
  - Aplastic anemia
  - Severe B_{12} or folate deficiency
  - Severe infection, pertussis in particular
  - Chronic myelogenous leukemia/myeloproliferative disorders
  - Chronic lymphocytic leukemia
  - Infectious mononucleosis
  - Hodgkin's or non-Hodgkin's lymphoma
  - Metastatic malignancy to bone marrow
  - Miliary tuberculosis
  - Paroxysmal nocturnal hemoglobinuria

- **Treatment**
  - Aggressive combination chemotherapy with specific drugs dictated by cell type
  - Conventional-dose chemotherapy curative in minority of adults with acute leukemia; allogeneic and autologous bone marrow transplantation considered for appropriate patients

- **Pearl**

Pain in expansile bone marrow can simulate mechanical back pain with bilateral leg radiation.

Reference

Ribera JM, Oriol A. Acute lymphoblastic leukemia in adolescents and young adults. Hematol Oncol Clin North Am 2009;23:1033, vi. [PMID: 19825451]

Agranulocytosis

- **Essentials of Diagnosis**
  - Malaise of abrupt onset, chills, fever, sore throat
  - Mucosal ulceration
  - History of drug ingestion common (eg, trimethoprim-sulfamethoxazole, ganciclovir, propylthiouracil)
  - Profound granulocytopenia with relative lymphocytosis

5

- **Differential Diagnosis**
  - Aplastic anemia
  - Myelodysplasia
  - Systemic lupus erythematosus (SLE)
  - Viral infection (HIV, cytomegalovirus, hepatitis)
  - Acute leukemia
  - Felty's syndrome

- **Treatment**
  - Stop offending drugs
  - Broad-spectrum antibiotics for fever
  - Trial of filgrastim (granulocyte colony-stimulating factor) for severe neutropenia
  - Allogeneic bone marrow transplant for appropriate refractory patients

- **Pearl**

Sequential neutrophil counts are valueless in diagnosis, as a normal neutrophil count today may be agranulocytosis tomorrow; depend on symptoms, especially sore throat, to make the diagnosis.

Reference

Repetto L; CIPOMO investigators. Incidence and clinical impact of chemotherapy induced myelotoxicity in cancer patients: an observational retrospective survey. Crit Rev Oncol Hematol 2009;72:170. [PMID: 19406660]

Alpha-Thalassemia Trait

■ Essentials of Diagnosis

- Commonly comes to attention because of CBC done for other reasons
- Increased frequency in persons of African, Mediterranean, or southern Chinese ancestry
- Microcytosis out of proportion to anemia; occasional target cells and acanthocytes on smear, but far less so than with beta-thalassemia; normal iron studies
- Mentzer's index (mean corpuscular volume [MCV]/RBC) < 13
- Results from two-gene deletion among the possible four copies of the α-globin gene
- No increase in hemoglobin A_2 or hemoglobin F
- Diagnosis of exclusion in patient with modest anemia (definitive diagnosis depends on hemoglobin gene mapping)

■ Differential Diagnosis

- Iron deficiency anemia
- Other hemoglobinopathies
- Sideroblastic anemia
- Beta-thalassemia minor

■ Treatment

- Oral folic acid supplementation
- Avoidance of medicinal iron or oxidative agents
- Red blood cell transfusions during pregnancy or stress (intercurrent illness) if hemoglobin falls below 9 g/dL

■ Pearl

Microcytosis without anemia, hyperchromia, or target cells is with few exceptions this condition.

Reference

Sirichotiyakul S, Wanapirak C, Srisupundit K, Luewan S, Tongsong T. A comparison of the accuracy of the corpuscular fragility and mean corpuscular volume tests for the alpha-thalassemia 1 and beta-thalassemia traits. Int J Gynaecol Obstet 2009;107:26. [PMID: 19591999]

Anemia of Chronic Disease

- **Essentials of Diagnosis**
  - Known chronic disease, particularly inflammatory; symptoms and signs usually those of responsible disease
  - Modest anemia (hematocrit [Hct] ≥ 25%); red cells normal morphologically but may be slightly microcytic
  - Low serum iron with normal or low total iron-binding capacity, normal or high serum ferritin, normal or increased bone marrow iron stores, low soluble transferrin receptor and soluble transferrin receptor:log ferritin ratio

- **Differential Diagnosis**
  - Iron deficiency anemia
  - Myelodysplasia
  - Sideroblastic anemia
  - Thalassemia

- **Treatment**
  - None usually necessary; treat underlying illness
  - Red blood cell transfusions for symptomatic anemia
  - Recombinant erythropoietin (epoetin alfa or darbepoetin alfa); supplemental iron often needed to maintain iron stores while on erythropoiesis-stimulating agent

- **Pearl**

In anemia of chronic disease, the hemoglobin and hematocrit do not fall below 60% of baseline; if they do, there is another cause, most often kidney failure.

Reference

Dharmarajan TS, Widjaja D. Erythropoiesis-stimulating agents in anemia: use and misuse. J Am Med Dir Assoc 2009;10:607. [PMID: 19883882]

Aplastic Anemia

- ■ Essentials of Diagnosis
  - • Lassitude, fatigue, malaise, other nonspecific symptoms
  - • Pallor, purpura, mucosal bleeding, petechiae, signs of infection
  - • Pancytopenia with normal cellular morphology; hypocellular bone marrow with fatty infiltration
  - • Occasional history of exposure to an offending drug or radiation

- ■ Differential Diagnosis
  - • Bone marrow infiltrative process (tumor, some infections, granulomatous diseases)
  - • Myelofibrosis
  - • Myelodysplasia (hypocellular in 20% of cases)
  - • Acute leukemia
  - • Hypersplenism
  - • Viral infections including HIV, hepatitis
  - • SLE
  - • Hairy cell leukemia
  - • Large granular lymphocyte disease

- ■ Treatment
  - • Allogeneic bone marrow transplantation for patients under age 30
  - • Intensive immunosuppression with antithymocyte globulin, cyclosporine if transplantation not feasible
  - • Oral androgens may be of benefit
  - • If SLE-associated, plasmapheresis and corticosteroids effective
  - • Avoid transfusions if possible in patients who may be transplant candidates; otherwise, red blood cells and platelet transfusions, filgrastim (granulocyte colony-stimulating factor), or sargramostim (granulocyte-macrophage colony-stimulating factor) as necessary

- ■ Pearl

The risk of aplastic anemia has resulted in the virtual absence of chloramphenicol from formularies, yet it requires one prescription per day for more than 100 years to produce a single case.

Reference

Marsh J. Making therapeutic decisions in adults with aplastic anemia. Hematol Am Soc Hematol Educ Program 2006:78. [PMID: 17124044]

Autoimmune Hemolytic Anemia

- ■ Essentials of Diagnosis
  - • Acquired anemia caused by immunoglobulin (Ig) G (warm) or IgM (cold) autoantibody
  - • Fatigue, malaise in many; occasional abdominal or back pain
  - • Pallor, jaundice, but palpable spleen uncommon
  - • Persistent anemia with microspherocytes and reticulocytosis; elevated indirect bilirubin and serum lactate dehydrogenase (LDH)
  - • Positive Coombs (direct antiglobulin) test
  - • Various drugs, underlying autoimmune or lymphoproliferative disorder may be causative

- ■ Differential Diagnosis
  - • Disseminated intravascular coagulation
  - • Hemoglobinopathy
  - • Hereditary spherocytosis
  - • Nonspherocytic hemolytic anemia
  - • Sideroblastic anemia
  - • Megaloblastic anemia

- ■ Treatment
  - • High-dosage steroids (warm antibody)
  - • Intravenous immune globulin (warm antibody)
  - • Plasmapheresis in severe cases (warm or cold antibody)
  - • Avoid cold; administer warmed blood/fluids (cold antibody)
  - • Splenectomy for refractory or recurrent cases (warm antibody)
  - • Immunosuppression (both warm and cold antibody)
  - • Cross-match difficult because of autoantibodies, so least incompatible blood used
  - • Splenectomy for refractory or recurrent cases
  - • More intensive immunosuppressive regimens available for refractory cases after splenectomy

- ■ Pearl

As in all cases of extravascular hemolysis, iron is recycled; multiple transfusions thus lead to iron overload.

Reference

Valent P, Lechner K. Diagnosis and treatment of autoimmune haemolytic anaemias in adults: a clinical review. Wien Klin Wochenschr 2008;120:136. [PMID: 18365153]

Beta-Thalassemia Minor

- ■ Essentials of Diagnosis
  - • Symptoms variable depending on degree of anemia; no specific physical findings
  - • Mild and persistent anemia, hypochromia with microcytosis and target cells; red blood cell count normal or elevated
  - • Similar findings in one of patient's parents
  - • Patient often of Mediterranean, African, or southern Chinese ancestry
  - • Elevated hemoglobin A_2 and hemoglobin F
  - • Mentzer's index (MCV/RBC) < 13

- ■ Differential Diagnosis
  - • Iron deficiency anemia
  - • Other hemoglobinopathies, especially hemoglobin C disorders
  - • Sideroblastic anemia
  - • Alpha-thalassemia
  - • Anemia of chronic disease

- ■ Treatment
  - • Oral folic acid supplementation
  - • Avoidance of medicinal iron or oxidative agents
  - • Red blood cell transfusions during pregnancy or stress (intercurrent illness) if hemoglobin falls below 9 g/dL

- ■ Pearl

The hemoglobinopathies exhibit central red cell targeting; liver disease targeting tends to be eccentric.

Reference

Ceylan C, Miskioğlu M, Colak H, Kiliççioğlu B, Ozdemir E. Evaluation of reticulocyte parameters in iron deficiency, vitamin B(12) deficiency and beta-thalassemia minor patients. Int J Lab Hematol 2007;29:327. [PMID: 17824912]

Chronic Lymphocytic Leukemia (CLL)

- **Essentials of Diagnosis**
  - Fatigue in some; most asymptomatic; often discovered incidentally
  - Pallor, lymphadenopathy, splenomegaly common
  - Sustained lymphocytosis > 5000/μL or higher, with some counts up to 1,000,000/μL; morphologically mature cells in most cases
  - Coombs-positive hemolytic anemia, immune thrombocytopenia, hypogammaglobulinemia late in course
  - Anemia, thrombocytopenia, bulky lymphadenopathy associated with poorer prognosis
  - Flow cytometry separates CLL from reactive lymphocytosis
  - May transform into high-grade lymphoid neoplasm (Richter's transformation)
  - Poor prognostic markers, including ZAP 70, CD 38, and del 17p, predict for more rapid progression and poorer survival

- **Differential Diagnosis**
  - Infectious mononucleosis
  - Prolymphocytic leukemia
  - Pertussis
  - Mantle cell lymphoma
  - Hairy cell leukemia
  - Adult T-cell leukemia/lymphoma
  - Other lymphoma with leukemic phase

- **Treatment**
  - Given the chronic, frequently indolent nature of the disease, chemotherapy is reserved for symptomatic patients, end organ disease, progressive lymphadenopathy, or young patients with advanced disease
  - Treatment involves purine analogs (fludarabine), alkylating agents (cyclophosphamide), or monoclonal antibodies, such as rituximab (antibody to CD20) or alemtuzumab (antibody to CD52)
  - Combination therapy, such as fludarabine, cyclophosphamide, and/or rituximab, has resulted in improved response rates and failure-free survival rates, but increased toxicity
  - Allogeneic bone marrow transplantation potentially curative in selected patients
  - Steroids, immunoglobulin may help associated immune cytopenias

- **Pearl**

Smudge cells result from crushing of fragile leukemic cells during preparation of the blood smear, not from any intrinsic abnormality in the cell.

Reference

Delgado J, Briones J, Sierra J. Emerging therapies for patients with advanced chronic lymphocytic leukaemia. Blood Rev 2009;23:217. [PMID: 19643519]

Chronic Myelogenous Leukemia (CML)

- ■ Essentials of Diagnosis
  - Symptoms variable; often diagnosed by examination or blood count done for unrelated reasons
  - Splenomegaly in all cases; sternal tenderness in some
  - Leukocytosis, typically striking; immature white cells in peripheral blood and bone marrow; thrombocytosis, eosinophilia, basophilia common
  - Diagnosis relies on demonstration of Philadelphia chromosome t(9:22) (bcr-abl fusion gene) by conventional cytogenetics, reverse transcriptase polymerase chain reaction of peripheral blood or bone marrow, or fluorescent in situ hybridization
  - Low leukocyte alkaline phosphatase level, markedly elevated serum vitamin B_{12} due to high B_{12} binding transcobalamins
  - Results in acute leukemia in 3–5 years without treatment

- ■ Differential Diagnosis
  - Leukemoid reactions associated with infection, inflammation, or cancer
  - Other myeloproliferative disorders

- ■ Treatment
  - Tyrosine kinase inhibitor (imatinib mesylate [Gleevec]) targeting specific molecular defect in CML cells (bcr-abl fusion gene) is first-line therapy; imatinib-resistant patients who are not transplantation candidates can be treated with other tyrosine kinase inhibitors (dasatinib, nilotinib)
  - Combination of cytarabine and interferon leads to cytogenetically complete remissions in a small minority of patients
  - Due to its significant toxicity, allogeneic bone marrow transplantation is often reserved for imatinib-resistant disease, but can be applied earlier for younger patients with matched sibling donors because it remains the only curative modality

- ■ Pearl

Pseudohypoglycemia is an in vitro artifact resulting from continuing white cell metabolism of glucose after phlebotomy; an asymptomatic patient with a blood glucose of zero should suggest this artifact.

Reference

Champlin R, de Lima M, Kebriaei P, et al. Nonmyeloablative allogeneic stem cell transplantation for chronic myelogenous leukemia in the imatinib era. Clin Lymphoma Myeloma 2009;9(suppl 3):S261. [PMID: 19778850]

Disseminated Intravascular Coagulation (DIC)

- ■ Essentials of Diagnosis
  - Evidence of abnormal bleeding or clotting, usually in a critically ill patient
  - Occurs as a result of activation and consumption of clotting and antithrombotic factors due to severe stressors such as sepsis, burns, massive hemorrhage
  - May occur in chronic, indolent form, usually associated with malignancy
  - Anemia, thrombocytopenia, elevated prothrombin time, and later, partial thromboplastin time, low fibrinogen, elevated fibrin degradation products and fibrin D-dimers

- ■ Differential Diagnosis
  - Severe liver disease
  - Thrombotic thrombocytopenic purpura
  - Hemolytic-uremic syndrome
  - Vitamin K deficiency
  - Other microangiopathic hemolytic anemias (eg, prosthetic heart valve)
  - Sepsis-induced thrombocytopenia or anemia
  - Heparin-induced thrombocytopenia

- ■ Treatment
  - Treat underlying disorder
  - Replacement of consumed blood factors with fresh-frozen plasma, cryoprecipitate, and potentially antithrombin III, as well as platelet transfusions only if active bleeding and/or severe thrombocytopenia in trauma patient
  - Low-dose heparin infusion is limited to cases of acute promyelocytic leukemia or chronic low-grade DIC with predominant thrombotic picture; confirm normal or near-normal antithrombin levels before administration
  - Antifibrinolytic therapy (aminocaproic acid or tranexamic acid) is generally contraindicated because it can increase risk for thrombosis, but if used for severe refractory bleeding, must be used only in the presence of heparin therapy

- ■ Pearl
  If DIC is chronic, increased synthesis of fibrinogen and increased production of platelet counts may normalize those determinations.

Reference

Gando S, Saitoh D, Ogura H, et al. Natural history of disseminated intravascular coagulation diagnosed based on the newly established diagnostic criteria for critically ill patients: results of a multicenter, prospective survey. Crit Care Med 2008;36:145. [PMID: 18090367]

Drug-Induced Hemolytic Anemia

- ■ Essentials of Diagnosis
  - • Immune hemolytic anemia due to host antibody recognition of drug and red blood cell membrane
  - • Acute to subacute onset; elevated LDH, hyperbilirubinemia, reticulocytosis
  - • Rarely, fulminant presentation with laboratory abnormalities as noted plus hemoglobinemia-hemoglobinuria, renal failure, and hemodynamic instability
  - • Positive Coombs test with patient's blood; Coombs test using reagent red blood cells positive only in presence of offending drug

- ■ Differential Diagnosis
  - • Autoimmune hemolytic anemia
  - • Microangiopathic hemolytic anemia (eg, DIC, thrombotic thrombocytopenic purpura)
  - • Delayed transfusion-related hemolysis
  - • Blood loss

- ■ Treatment
  - • Discontinue offending drug
  - • Plasmapheresis for severe cases, especially if drug has long serum half-life
  - • Intravenous immune globulin, steroids potentially of benefit

- ■ Pearl

An annoying prospect in primary care: because many drugs can cause it and many patients take many drugs, the only way to be sure is to stop them one at a time.

Reference

Johnson ST, Fueger JT, Gottschall JL. One center's experience: the serology and drugs associated with drug-induced immune hemolytic anemia—a new paradigm. Transfusion 2007;47:697. [PMID: 17381629]

Essential Thrombocytosis

- ■ Essentials of Diagnosis
  - • Sustained elevated platelet count without other cause
  - • Painful burning of palms and soles (erythromelalgia) promptly and typically relieved with low-dose aspirin
  - • Arterial > venous thromboses
  - • Approximately 60% of cases have JAK2V617F mutation, resulting in constitutive activation of tyrosine kinase–dependent cellular signaling pathways and ultimately cytokine-independent growth of hematopoietic cells.
  - • Bone marrow proliferation mainly of megakaryocytic lineage, with no significant increase in granulopoiesis or erythropoiesis
  - • Can progress to post-thrombocythemic myelofibrosis ("spent" stage) or acute leukemia late in course
  - • May have mild elevations in white blood cell count and hematocrit; basophilia, eosinophilia, hypervitaminosis B_{12}

- ■ Differential Diagnosis
  - • Other myeloproliferative disorders; if JAK2 mutation–positive, use other constellation of signs and/or symptoms to distinguish polycythemia vera versus essential thrombocytosis versus primary myelofibrosis
  - • Chronic infection or autoimmune disease, visceral malignancy (reactive thrombocytosis)
  - • Iron deficiency

- ■ Treatment
  - • Platelet-lowering therapy for those with high risk of clotting (history of prior clotting, age > 60 years, established arterial vascular disease)
  - • Hydroxyurea and anagrelide most commonly used agents; interferon alfa for younger or pregnant patients
  - • Low-dose aspirin for vasomotor symptoms

- ■ Pearl

Platelet counts of over 1 million in reactive thrombocytosis; essential thrombocytosis clots and bleeds because of qualitative, not quantitative, abnormalities.

Reference

Brière JB. Essential thrombocythemia. Orphanet J Rare Dis 2007;2:3. [PMID: 17210076]

Folic Acid Deficiency

- ■ Essentials of Diagnosis
  - Nonspecific gastrointestinal symptoms, fatigue, dyspnea without neurologic complaints in a patient with malnutrition, often related to alcoholism
  - Pallor, mild jaundice
  - Pancytopenia, but counts not as low as in vitamin B_{12} deficiency; oval macrocytosis and hypersegmented neutrophils; megaloblastic marrow; normal vitamin B_{12} levels
  - Red blood cell folate < 150 ng/mL diagnostic
  - Homocysteine levels elevated while methylmalonic acid remains normal; both are usually elevated in vitamin B_{12} deficiency

- ■ Differential Diagnosis
  - Vitamin B_{12} deficiency
  - Myelodysplastic syndromes
  - Infiltrative granulomatous or neoplastic bone marrow process
  - Hypersplenism
  - Paroxysmal nocturnal hemoglobinuria
  - Acute leukemia

- ■ Treatment
  - Exclude vitamin B_{12} deficiency before therapy
  - Oral folic acid supplementation
  - If diet is adequate, a gastrointestinal evaluation is warranted; most cases of folate deficiency are preventable or treatable

- ■ Pearl

Like any megaloblastic anemia, this is hemolytic; however, hemolysis takes place in the bone marrow, causing sensational elevations of marrow serum LDH.

Reference

McLean E, de Benoist B, Allen LH. Review of the magnitude of folate and vitamin B12 deficiencies worldwide. Food Nutr Bull 2008;29(suppl):S38. [PMID: 18709880]

Hairy Cell Leukemia

- **Essentials of Diagnosis**
  - Fatigue, abdominal pain, but often asymptomatic; susceptibility to bacterial infections
  - Pallor, prominent splenomegaly, rare lymphadenopathy
  - Bruising and bleeding due to severe thrombocytopenia
  - Pancytopenia, "hairy cell" morphology of leukocytes in periphery and marrow at high magnification
  - "Dry tap" on bone marrow aspiration; diagnosis confirmed by flow cytometry; tartrate-resistant acid phosphatase stain also positive

- **Differential Diagnosis**
  - Myelofibrosis
  - Chronic lymphocytic leukemia
  - Waldenström's macroglobulinemia
  - Non-Hodgkin's lymphoma
  - Aplastic anemia
  - Acute leukemia
  - Infiltration of marrow by tumor or granuloma
  - Paroxysmal nocturnal hemoglobinuria

- **Treatment**
  - Treat when significant cytopenias, constitutional symptoms, or symptomatic splenomegaly or lymphadenopathy
  - Purine analogs (cladribine, pentostatin) give durable remissions in > 80% of patients
  - Splenectomy for severe cytopenias or chemotherapy-resistant disease
  - Interferon alfa can be used for purine-resistant cases to help normalize counts, but does not result in complete remission

- **Pearl**

The splenomegaly tells the clinician this is not acute leukemia; visceromegaly is uncommon in that disorder.

Reference

Ravandi F. Hairy cell leukemia. Clin Lymphoma Myeloma 2009;9(suppl 3):S254. [PMID: 19778849]

Hemoglobin SC Disease

- ▪ Essentials of Diagnosis
  - Recurrent attacks of abdominal, joint, or bone pain
  - Splenomegaly, retinopathy (similar to diabetes)
  - Mild anemia, reticulocytosis, and few sickle cells on smear but many targets; 50% hemoglobin C, 50% hemoglobin S on electrophoresis
  - Functional asplenia occurs later than in SS disease
  - In situ thrombi of pulmonary artery or venous sinus of brain may simulate pulmonary emboli or may cause stroke, respectively, especially in pregnancy

- ▪ Differential Diagnosis
  - Sickle cell anemia
  - Sickle thalassemia
  - Hemoglobin C disease
  - Cirrhosis
  - Pulmonary embolism
  - Beta thalassemia

- ▪ Treatment
  - No specific therapy for most patients
  - Otherwise treat as for SS hemoglobin

- ▪ Pearl

Normally fairly well tolerated, it is to be recalled that anything sickle cell disease can do, then so can any one of the sickle traits.

Reference

Subbannan K, Ustun C, Natarajan K, et al. Acute splenic complications and implications of splenectomy in hemoglobin SC disease. Eur J Haematol 2009;83:258. [PMID: 19459924]

Hemoglobin S–Thalassemia Disease

- ■ Essentials of Diagnosis
  - • Recurrent attacks of abdominal, joint, or bone pain
  - • Splenomegaly, retinopathy
  - • Mild to moderate anemia with low MCV; reticulocytosis; few sickle cells on smear with many target cells; increased hemoglobin A_2 by electrophoresis distinguishes from sickle cell disease, hemoglobin C

- ■ Differential Diagnosis
  - • Sickle cell anemia
  - • Hemoglobin C disease
  - • Hemoglobin SC disease
  - • Cirrhosis

- ■ Treatment
  - • Chronic oral folic acid supplementation
  - • Acute therapy as in sickle cell anemia

- ■ Pearl

The low MCV and target cells in the face of microvascular ischemic disease should suggest this diagnosis.

Reference

Thein SL, Menzel S. Discovering the genetics underlying foetal haemoglobin production in adults. Br J Haematol 2009;145:455. [PMID: 19344402]

Hemolytic Transfusion Reaction

- ■ Essentials of Diagnosis
  - Chills and fever during blood transfusion
  - Back, chest pain; dark urine
  - Associated with vascular collapse, renal failure, and disseminated intravascular coagulation
  - Hemolysis, hemoglobinuria, and severe anemia

- ■ Differential Diagnosis
  - Leukoagglutination reaction
  - IgA deficiency with anaphylactic transfusion reaction
  - Myocardial infarction
  - Acute abdomen due to other causes
  - Pyelonephritis
  - Bacteremia due to contaminated blood product

- ■ Treatment
  - Stop transfusion immediately
  - Hydration and intravenous mannitol to prevent renal failure

- ■ Pearl

Although all adverse clinical events during transfusion raise this possibility, modern blood banking has resulted in a much lower incidence; transfusion-related acute lung injury is far more common.

Reference

Sigler E, Shvidel L, Yahalom V, Berrebi A, Shtalrid M. Clinical significance of serologic markers related to red blood cell autoantibodies production after red blood cell transfusion-severe autoimmune hemolytic anemia occurring after transfusion and alloimmunization: successful treatment with rituximab. Transfusion 2009;49:1370. [PMID: 19374728]

Hemolytic-Uremic Syndrome

■ Essentials of Diagnosis

- Petechial rash, hypertension, acute-to-subacute renal failure
- Often preceded by gastroenteritis or exposure to offending medication
- Frequently associated with antecedent *Campylobacter* infection (may be very mild to occult)
- Laboratory reports notable for thrombocytopenia, anemia, renal failure, elevated LDH, normal prothrombin time and partial thromboplastin time as well as fibrin and fibrinogen degeneration products

■ Differential Diagnosis

- Disseminated intravascular coagulation
- Thrombotic thrombocytopenic purpura (TTP)
- Catastrophic antiphospholipid antibody syndrome
- Pre-eclampsia–eclampsia
- Other microangiopathic hemolytic anemias

■ Treatment

- In children, disease is most often self-limited and managed with supportive care
- In adults, stop potentially offending drugs
- Plasmapheresis for refractory cases

■ Pearl

So similar to TTP that it may be impossible to tell them apart; this is an academic point because treatment is virtually identical for both.

Reference

Fakhouri F, Frémeaux-Bacchi V. Does hemolytic uremic syndrome differ from thrombotic thrombocytopenic purpura? Nat Clin Pract Nephrol 2007;3:679. [PMID: 18033227]

Hemophilia A & B

- ■ Essentials of Diagnosis
  - Lifelong history of bleeding in a male
  - Slow, prolonged bleeding after minor injury or surgery; spontaneous hemarthroses common
  - Prolonged partial thromboplastin time corrected by mixing patient's plasma with a normal specimen
  - Low factor VIII coagulant activity (hemophilia A) or factor IX coagulant activity (hemophilia B)

- ■ Differential Diagnosis
  - von Willebrand's disease
  - Disseminated intravascular coagulation
  - Afibrinogenemia and dysfibrinogenemia
  - Heparin administration
  - Acquired factor deficiencies or inhibitors (eg, paraproteins with anti-VIII or anti-IX activity)

- ■ Treatment
  - Avoidance of aspirin
  - Factor replacement for any bleeding with factor VIII concentrates (hemophilia A) or factor IX complex (hemophilia B) or during invasive procedures
  - Increased factor dosing, steroids, or immunosuppressants if factor inhibitor develops
  - Desmopressin acetate before surgical procedures for hemophilia A may benefit selected patients

- ■ Pearl

Factor IX deficiency is called Christmas disease, not because of the holiday, but because of the index patient's name.

Reference

Mannucci PM, Schutgens RE, Santagostino E, Mauser-Bunschoten EP. How I treat age-related morbidities in elderly persons with hemophilia. Blood 2009;114:5256. [PMID: 19837978]

Heparin-Induced Thrombocytopenia (HIT)

- ■ Essentials of Diagnosis
  - • Moderate thrombocytopenia developing 4–14 days after institution of heparin (type 2); may be sooner if previously exposed to heparin
  - • Venous and arterial thromboses, skin necrosis rarely
  - • Positive serotonin release assay, heparin-induced platelet aggregation, or enzyme-linked immunosorbent assay for antiheparin-platelet factor 4 antibodies
  - • Rapid recovery of platelet count after discontinuation of heparin

- ■ Differential Diagnosis
  - • DIC
  - • Drug-induced thrombocytopenia
  - • Sepsis
  - • Idiopathic thrombocytopenic purpura

- ■ Treatment
  - • Immediate discontinuation of all exposure to heparin (including IV heparin flushes)
  - • Anticoagulation with direct thrombin inhibitors (lepirudin or argatroban) or danaparoid

- ■ Pearl

Given the expanding use of heparin for prophylaxis, this condition is extremely common—and under-recognized.

Reference

Arepally GM, Ortel TL. Clinical practice. Heparin-induced thrombocytopenia. N Engl J Med 2006;355:809. [PMID: 16928996]

Hereditary Spherocytosis

- ## Essentials of Diagnosis
  - Chronic hemolytic anemia of variable severity, often with exacerbations during coincident illnesses
  - Malaise, abdominal discomfort in symptomatic patients
  - Jaundice, splenomegaly in severely affected patients
  - Variable anemia with spherocytosis and reticulocytosis; elevated mean corpuscular hemoglobin concentration; increased osmotic fragility test and increased red cell fragility as measured with ektacytometry (ie, measurement of the shear stress a red blood cell can withstand before lysing)
  - Negative Coombs test
  - Family history of anemia, jaundice, splenectomy

- ## Differential Diagnosis
  - Autoimmune hemolytic anemia
  - Hemoglobin C disease
  - Iron deficiency anemia
  - Alcoholism
  - Burns

- ## Treatment
  - Oral folic acid supplementation
  - Pneumococcal vaccination if splenectomy contemplated
  - Splenectomy for symptomatic patients

- ## Pearl

The only condition in medicine causing a hyperchromic, microcytic anemia.

Reference

Schilling RF, Gangnon RE, Traver MI. Delayed adverse vascular events after splenectomy in hereditary spherocytosis. J Thromb Haemost 2008;6:1289. [PMID: 18485083]

Hodgkin's Disease

5

- ## Essentials of Diagnosis
  - In most cases the disorder starts in one node group and spreads in an orderly, contiguous fashion
  - Regionally enlarged, rubbery, painless lymphadenopathy (often cervical); hepatosplenomegaly variable
  - Reed-Sternberg cells (or variants) in lymph node or bone marrow biopsy diagnostic
  - Diagnosis often requires excisional lymph node biopsy, fine-needle aspirates often nondiagnostic; patients considered stage A if no constitutional symptoms are present and stage B if they have fevers, night sweats, or significant weight loss
  - Younger patients tend to have supradiaphragmatic disease with favorable histology; older individuals tend toward more aggressive pathology, infradiaphragmatic involvement

- ## Differential Diagnosis
  - Non-Hodgkin's lymphoma
  - Lymphadenitis secondary to infections (tuberculosis and cat-scratch disease)
  - Pseudolymphoma caused by phenytoin
  - Lymphomatoid granulomatosis
  - Sarcoidosis
  - HIV disease
  - SLE

- ## Treatment
  - Staging (I–IV) with chest x-ray, CT scans of chest, abdomen, and pelvis, PET-CT scan, and bone marrow biopsy
  - Radiation therapy for localized disease or short course of combination chemotherapy with less extensive radiation
  - Combination chemotherapy for disseminated disease with or without radiation to bulky areas of disease

- ## Pearl

Now a minority of lymphomas, remember it if a patient develops pain in a lymph node soon after drinking alcohol; indeed, mediastinal or hilar lymphadenopathy may result in the cardiologist being consulted for chest pain.

Reference

Mani H, Jaffe ES. Hodgkin lymphoma: an update on its biology with new insights into classification. Clin Lymphoma Myeloma 2009;9:206. [PMID: 19525189]

Idiopathic Thrombocytopenic Purpura

- ■ Essentials of Diagnosis
  - • Mucosal bleeding, easy bruising and bleeding
  - • Petechiae, ecchymoses; splenomegaly rare
  - • Severe thrombocytopenia, prolonged bleeding time; elevated platelet-associated IgG in 95%, though nonspecific; bone marrow with normal to increased megakaryocytes
  - • May be associated with autoimmune diseases (eg, SLE), HIV infection, lymphoproliferative disorders, or with Coombs-positive hemolytic anemia (Evans' syndrome)

- ■ Differential Diagnosis
  - • Acute leukemia
  - • Myelodysplastic syndrome
  - • Thrombotic thrombocytopenic purpura
  - • Disseminated intravascular coagulation
  - • Chronic lymphocytic leukemia
  - • Aplastic anemia
  - • Alcohol abuse
  - • Drug toxicity (eg, quinidine, digoxin)
  - • AIDS
  - • SLE

- ■ Treatment
  - • Prednisone, intravenous immune globulin, and anti Rh-D immune globulin (WinRho) in Rh-positive patients all have high rates of success acutely
  - • Splenectomy if no response to initial therapy, for relapsed disease, or for patients requiring high doses of steroids to maintain an acceptable platelet count
  - • Danazol, vincristine, vinblastine, azathioprine, cyclophosphamide, cyclosporine, and rituximab for refractory cases; plasma immunoadsorption may also be successful in some refractory cases
  - • Reserve platelet transfusion for life-threatening hemorrhages; bleeding sometimes stops even as the platelet count rises slightly if at all
  - • Novel therapies, including thrombopoiesis-stimulating agents (romiplostim, eltrombopag), can be used in refractory cases

- ■ Pearl

The order of platelet bleeding as the count falls: first skin, then mucous membrane, finally viscera; thus absence of cutaneous petechiae means a low likelihood of intracranial hemorrhage.

Reference

Stasi R. Immune thrombocytopenic purpura: the treatment paradigm. Eur J Haematol Suppl 2009:13. [PMID: 19200303]

Iron Deficiency Anemia

- Essentials of Diagnosis
  - Lassitude; in children under age 2, poor muscle tone, delayed motor development
  - Pallor, cheilosis, and koilonychia
  - Hypochromic microcytic red cells late in disease; indices normal early, occasional thrombocytosis
  - Serum iron low, total iron-binding capacity increased; absent marrow iron; serum ferritin < 15 ng/mL classically, but concomitant illness may elevate it
  - Newer tests include increased serum soluble transferrin receptor and transferrin receptor:log ferritin ratio
  - Occult blood loss invariably causative in adults; malabsorption or dietary insufficiency rarely causes deficiency

- Differential Diagnosis
  - Anemia of chronic disease
  - Myelodysplasia
  - Thalassemia
  - Sideroblastic anemias, including lead intoxication

- Treatment
  - Oral ferrous sulfate or ferrous gluconate three times daily for 6–12 months
  - Parenteral iron for selected patients with severe, clinically significant iron deficiency with continuing chronic blood loss
  - Evaluation for occult blood loss

- Pearl

Remember iron deficiency as a treatable cause of obesity; ice cream craving is one of many associated picas.

Reference

Hershko C, Skikne B. Pathogenesis and management of iron deficiency anemia: emerging role of celiac disease, Helicobacter pylori, and autoimmune gastritis. Semin Hematol 2009;46:339. [PMID: 19786202]

Multiple Myeloma

- **Essentials of Diagnosis**
  - Weakness, weight loss, recurrent infection, bone (especially back) pain, often resulting in pathologic fractures
  - Pallor, bony tenderness; spleen is not enlarged
  - Anemia; accelerated sedimentation rate; elevated serum calcium, renal insufficiency; normal alkaline phosphatase; elevated B_2 microglobulin; narrowed anion gap in most
  - Nephrotic syndrome (with associated amyloidosis causing albuminuria or by light chains in urine)
  - Elevated serum globulin with monoclonal spike on serum or urine protein electrophoresis
  - Infiltration of bone marrow with clonal proliferation of plasma cells
  - Lytic bone lesions with negative bone scan

- **Differential Diagnosis**
  - Benign monoclonal gammopathy of undetermined significance
  - Metastatic cancer
  - Lymphoproliferative disorder with associated monoclonal spike
  - Hyperparathyroidism
  - Primary amyloidosis

- **Treatment**
  - Pamidronate or zoledronic acid for patients with extensive bone disease or hypercalcemia
  - Novel therapies, including thalidomide, lenalidomide, and bortezomib, offer significant response rates with minimal side effects; newer front-line regimens combine novel agents with conventional chemotherapy
  - Autologous bone marrow transplant, though unlikely to be curative, results in improved disease control and survival rates
  - Avoid alkylating agents as first-line therapy for patients eligible for transplantation
  - Radiation therapy limited to areas of local bone pain or pathologic fractures

- **Pearl**

No fever, no increased alkaline phosphatase, and no splenomegaly; all true of myeloma, all usually characteristic of other liquid tumors.

Reference

Reece DE. Recent trends in the management of newly diagnosed multiple myeloma. Curr Opin Hematol 2009;16:306. [PMID: 19491669]

Myelodysplastic Syndromes

- ■ Essentials of Diagnosis
  - • Clonal hematopoietic disorder characterized by ineffective hematopoiesis leading to dyshematopoiesis with a variable presence of blasts and peripheral blood cytopenias
  - • Subtypes include: Refractory anemia (RA), refractory anemia with ringed sideroblasts (RARS), refractory anemia with excess blasts (RAEB), and chronic myelomonocytic leukemia (CMML)
  - • Evolution to acute leukemia may occur within months (RAEB) to many years (RA, RARS)
  - • Morphologic dysplasia frequently seen in cells of myeloid lineage (eg, Pelger-Huët anomaly, hypogranular-hypolobulated neutrophils, giant platelets, macrocytosis, and acanthocytosis)
  - • Previous chemotherapy predisposes (especially alkylating agents such as cyclophosphamide and topoisomerase II inhibitors such as etoposide)

- ■ Differential Diagnosis
  - • Acute myeloid leukemia
  - • Aplastic anemia
  - • Anemia of chronic disease
  - • Alcohol-induced sideroblastic anemia
  - • Other causes of specific cytopenias
  - • Other causes of macrocytic anemias

- ■ Treatment
  - • Supportive care with red cell or platelet transfusions
  - • Erythropoietin (epoetin alfa), filgrastim (G-CSF), and lenalidomide may benefit selected patients
  - • Low-dose DNA hypomethylating agents (azacitidine, decitabine) may improve blood counts and delay onset of AML
  - • Allogeneic bone marrow transplantation for appropriate patients

- ■ Pearl

In anemia extensively evaluated with no cause being found, this is the cause.

Reference

Garcia-Manero G. Progress in myelodysplastic syndromes. Clin Lymphoma Myeloma 2009;9(suppl 3):S286. [PMID: 19778854]

Myelofibrosis

- **Essentials of Diagnosis**
  - Fatigue, abdominal discomfort, bleeding, bone pain
  - Massive splenomegaly, variable hepatomegaly
  - Approximately 60% of cases have JAK2V617F mutation, resulting in constitutive activation of tyrosine kinase–dependent cellular signaling pathways and ultimately cytokine-independent growth of hematopoietic cells
  - Anemia, leukocytosis or leukopenia; leukoerythroblastic peripheral smear with marked poikilocytosis, tear-drop cells, nucleated red cells, giant platelets, left-shifted myeloid series
  - Dry tap on bone marrow aspiration
  - Bone marrow with megakaryocyte proliferation, reticulin, and/or collagen fibrosis

- **Differential Diagnosis**
  - Chronic myelocytic leukemia
  - Other myeloproliferative disorders; if JAK2 mutation–positive, use other constellation of signs and/or symptoms to distinguish polycythemia vera versus essential thrombocytosis versus primary myelofibrosis
  - Hemolytic anemias
  - Lymphoma
  - Metastatic cancer involving bone marrow
  - Hairy cell leukemia

- **Treatment**
  - Red blood cell transfusion support
  - Androgenic steroids, thalidomide ± prednisone, lenalidomide for del(5q) patients, and interferon alfa may decrease transfusion requirements and reduce spleen size
  - Erythropoietin may be of benefit in selected patients
  - Splenectomy for painful splenomegaly, severe thrombocytopenia, or extraordinary red blood cell requirements, but carries significant mortality risk
  - Allogeneic hematopoietic stem-cell transplantation in select patients; only treatment with curative potential
  - Hydroxyurea can be used for excessive leukocytosis, thrombocytosis, or progressive splenomegaly

- **Pearl**

Hilar adenopathy, transverse myelitis, and any mass lesion complicating this disorder are likely foci of extramedullary hematopoiesis.

Reference

Kröger N, Mesa RA. Choosing between stem cell therapy and drugs in myelofibrosis. Leukemia 2008;22:474. [PMID: 18185525]

Non-Hodgkin's Lymphoma

■ Essentials of Diagnosis

- Fever, night sweats, weight loss in many
- Common in HIV infection, where isolated central nervous system lymphoma and other extranodal involvement are typical
- Variable hepatosplenomegaly; enlarged lymph nodes
- Elevated LDH in many, bone marrow positive in one-third
- Lymph node or involved extranodal tissue biopsies diagnostic; along with flow cytometry; non-Hodgkin's lymphomas are separated into low, intermediate, and aggressive groups based on immunophenotype, cell morphology, nodal architecture, and cytogenetics

■ Differential Diagnosis

- Hodgkin's disease
- Metastatic cancer
- Infectious mononucleosis
- Cat-scratch disease
- Pseudolymphoma caused by phenytoin
- Sarcoidosis
- Primary HIV infection

■ Treatment

- Staging with CT scans of the chest, abdomen, and pelvis; PET-CT scan; bone marrow biopsy and lumbar puncture in selected cases
- With indolent disease, radiation therapy for localized disease; chemotherapy for more advanced disease at symptoms, cytopenias or end-organ effects
- Combination chemotherapy immediately for intermediate and aggressive lymphomas, with goal for cure
- Monoclonal antibody therapy (rituximab) added to combination chemotherapy has improved response rates and survival outcomes
- Autologous bone marrow transplantation effective in relapsed intermediate and highly aggressive lymphoma

■ Pearl

An increasingly commonly encountered lymphoma given the HIV/AIDS epidemic; don't forget extranodal disease, particularly gastrointestinal and intracranial.

Reference

Lugtenburg PJ, Sonneveld P. Treatment of diffuse large B-cell lymphoma in the elderly: strategies integrating oncogeriatric themes. Curr Oncol Rep 2008;10:412. [PMID: 18706269]

Paroxysmal Nocturnal Hemoglobinuria

■ Essentials of Diagnosis

- Episodic red-brown urine, especially on first morning specimen
- Variable anemia with or without leukopenia, thrombocytopenia; reticulocytosis; positive urine hemosiderin, elevated serum LDH
- Triad of hemolysis (Coombs negative, intravascular), venous thrombosis (unusual sites including mesenteric, hepatic, portal, and intracranial veins), and cytopenias
- Flow cytometry of red blood cells or white blood cells (if recently transfused) negative for CD55 or CD59 (glycosylphosphatidylinositol [GPI]-linked antigens), positive sucrose hemolysis test or Ham's test
- Iron deficiency often concurrent

■ Differential Diagnosis

- Hemolytic anemia
- DIC or hypercoagulable state
- Myelodysplasia
- Aplastic anemia

■ Treatment

- Prednisone for moderate to severe cases
- Oral iron replacement if iron-deficient and oral folic acid if hemolytic anemia evident
- Allogeneic bone marrow transplantation or immunosuppression with ATG and cyclosporine for severe cases
- Trial of eculizumab (monoclonal antibody to C5 component of complement) for patients with transfusion dependence, disabling symptoms, and/or thrombotic events
- Long-term anticoagulation for thrombotic events

■ Pearl

Hypercoagulability despite pancytopenia; the mechanism remains poorly understood.

Reference

Bessler M, Hiken J. The pathophysiology of disease in patients with paroxysmal nocturnal hemoglobinuria. Hematol Am Soc Hematol Educ Program 2008:104. [PMID: 19074066]

5

Polycythemia Vera

■ Essentials of Diagnosis

- Pruritus (especially following a hot shower), tinnitus, blurred vision in some
- Venous thromboses, often in uncommon sites (eg, splenic or portal vein thromboses); plethora, splenomegaly
- Erythrocytosis (elevated hemoglobin) and elevated total red blood cell mass are major criteria for diagnosis
- Normal PO_2; subnormal serum Epo level
- More than 95% of cases have JAK2V617F mutations, resulting in cytokine-independent growth of hematopoietic cells
- JAK2V617F mutation clearly establishes a diagnosis of a clonal myeloproliferative neoplasm and rules out a reactive erythrocytosis, thrombocytosis, or myelofibrosis
- Can transform to post-polycythemic myelofibrosis ("spent" phase) or acute leukemia late in course; higher incidence of peptic ulcer

■ Differential Diagnosis

- Hypoxemia (pulmonary or cardiac disease, high altitude)
- Carboxyhemoglobin (tobacco use)
- Certain hemoglobinopathies characterized by tight O_2 binding
- Congenital erythrocytosis (mutations of Epo receptor or VHL gene)
- Erythropoietin-secreting tumors
- Cystic renal disease
- Spurious erythrocytosis with decreased plasma volume and high normal red cell mass (Gaisböck's syndrome)
- Other myeloproliferative disorders

■ Treatment

- Phlebotomy to Hct < 45% in men and < 42% in women
- Hydroxyurea if elevated WBC and platelet count or if patient cannot tolerate phlebotomy
- Myelosuppressive therapy with radiophosphorus (^{32}P) or alkylating agents only for patients with high phlebotomy requirements, intractable pruritus, or marked thrombocytosis
- Avoidance of medicinal iron; low-iron diet
- Aspirin 81–100 mg a day safe and effective in reducing thrombotic risk in all patients without substantially increasing risk of bleeding
- Deep venous thrombosis prophylaxis for any surgical procedure or prolonged period of immobilization

■ Pearl

The only disease in medicine with iron deficiency despite polycythemia.

Reference

Basquiera AL, Soria NW, Ryser R, et al. Clinical significance of V617F mutation of the JAK2 gene in patients with chronic myeloproliferative disorders. Hematology 2009;14:323. [PMID: 19941738]

Pure Red Cell Aplasia

■ Essentials of Diagnosis

- Autoimmune disease in which IgG antibody attacks erythroid precursors
- Lassitude, malaise; nonspecific examination except for pallor
- Severe anemia with normal red blood cell morphology; myeloid and platelet lines unaffected; low or absent reticulocyte count
- Reduced or absent erythroid precursors in normocellular marrow
- Rare associations with thymoma, SLE, chronic lymphocytic leukemia, non-Hodgkin's lymphoma, myasthenia gravis, and large granular lymphocytic leukemia

5

■ Differential Diagnosis

- Aplastic anemia
- Myelodysplastic syndromes
- Drug-induced red cell aplasia (phenytoin, trimethoprim-sulfamethoxazole, zidovudine)
- Parvovirus B19 infection
- Anti-erythropoietin antibodies in patient receiving recombinant erythropoietin

■ Treatment

- Evaluate for underlying disease
- Red cell transfusions for symptomatic anemia
- Immunosuppressive therapy with prednisone, cyclophosphamide, and/or cyclosporine
- For refractory or relapsed cases, trial of antithymocyte globulin, tacrolimus, rituximab, alemtuzumab (monoclonal antibody to CD52), daclizumab (monoclonal antibody to IL-2 receptor), high-dose intravenous immune globulin, or hematopoietic stem-cell transplantation
- Thymectomy in patients with thymoma may be beneficial

■ Pearl

When associated with arthritis, ask about a child in the family with fever followed by a facial rash; parvovirus B19 infection is your diagnosis.

Reference

Malhotra P, Muralikrishna GK, Varma N, et al. Spectrum of pure red cell aplasia in adult population of north-west India. Hematology 2008;13:88. [PMID: 18616874]

Sickle Cell Anemia

- ### Essentials of Diagnosis
  - Caused by substitution of valine for glutamine in the sixth position on the beta chain
  - Recurrent episodes of fever with pain in arms, legs, or abdomen starting in early childhood
  - Splenomegaly in early childhood *only;* jaundice, pallor; adults are functionally asplenic
  - Anemia and elevated reticulocyte count with irreversibly sickled cells on peripheral smear; elevated indirect bilirubin, LDH; positive sickling test; hemoglobin S and F on electrophoresis
  - Complications include *Salmonella* osteomyelitis, remarkably high incidence of encapsulated infections, and ischemic complications
  - Five types of crises: Pain, aplastic, megaloblastic, sequestration, hemolytic

- ### Differential Diagnosis
  - Other hemoglobinopathies
  - Acute rheumatic fever
  - Osteomyelitis
  - Acute abdomen due to any cause
  - If hematuria present, renal stone or tumor

- ### Treatment
  - Chronic oral folic acid supplementation
  - Hydration and analgesics
  - Hydroxyurea for patients with frequent crises
  - Partial exchange transfusions for intractable vaso-occlusive crises, acute chest syndrome, stroke or transient ischemic attack, priapism
  - Transfusion for hemolytic or aplastic crises and during third trimester of pregnancy
  - Pneumonia vaccination
  - Genetic counseling
  - Hematopoietic stem-cell transplantation is the only curative therapy, but of limited use given toxicity and limited candidacy of patients with severe pulmonary and neurologic vasculopathy

- ### Pearl

  Pneumococcal meningitis is 200 times as common in SS; vaccinate, vaccinate, vaccinate.

Reference

Lanzkron S, Strouse JJ, Wilson R, et al. Systematic review: hydroxyurea for the treatment of adults with sickle cell disease. Ann Intern Med 2008;148:939. [PMID: 18458272]

Sideroblastic Anemia

■ Essentials of Diagnosis

- Dimorphic (ie, normal and hypochromic) red blood cell population on smear
- Hematocrit may reach 20%
- Most often result of clonal stem cell disorder, though rarely may be drugs, lead, or alcohol; may be a megaloblastic component
- Elevated serum iron with high percentage saturation; marrow is diagnostic with abnormal ringed sideroblasts (iron deposits encircling red blood cell precursor nuclei)
- Minority progress to acute leukemia

5

■ Differential Diagnosis

- Iron deficiency anemia
- Post-transfusion state
- Anemia of chronic disease
- Thalassemia

■ Treatment

- Remove offending toxin if present
- Chelation therapy for lead toxicity
- Pyridoxine 200 mg/d occasionally helpful

■ Pearl

Most nucleated red cells in the bone marrow contain iron, and if seen in a ring about the nucleus, alcohol may have impaired entry of the metal into hemoglobin production, otherwise think myelodysplasia.

Reference

Moyo V, Lefebvre P, Duh MS, Yektashenas B, Mundle S. Erythropoiesis-stimulating agents in the treatment of anemia in myelodysplastic syndromes: a meta-analysis. Ann Hematol 2008;87:527. [PMID: 18351340]

Thalassemia Major

- **Essentials of Diagnosis**
  - Severe anemia from infancy; positive family history
  - Massive splenomegaly
  - Hypochromic, microcytic red cells with severe poikilocytosis, target cells, acanthocytes, and basophilic stippling on smear
  - Mentzer's index (MCV/RBC) < 13
  - Greatly elevated hemoglobin F level

- **Differential Diagnosis**
  - Other hemoglobinopathies
  - Congenital nonspherocytic hemolytic anemia

- **Treatment**
  - Regular red blood cell transfusions
  - Oral folic acid supplementation
  - Splenectomy for secondary hemolysis due to hypersplenism
  - Deferoxamine to avoid iron overload
  - Allogeneic bone marrow transplantation in selected cases

- **Pearl**

If greater than 100 red cell transfusions have been given, an iron overload syndrome indistinguishable from hemochromatosis occurs; chelating is essential to avoid it.

Reference

Delea TE, Edelsberg J, Sofrygin O, Thomas SK, Baladi JF, Phatak PD, Coates TD. Consequences and costs of noncompliance with iron chelation therapy in patients with transfusion-dependent thalassemia: a literature review. Transfusion 2007;47:1919. [PMID: 17880620]

Thrombotic Thrombocytopenic Purpura (TTP)

■ Essentials of Diagnosis

- Petechial rash, mucosal bleeding, fever, altered mental status, renal failure; many cases in HIV infection
- Laboratory reports are notable for anemia, dramatically elevated LDH, normal prothrombin and partial thromboplastin times, fibrin degradation products, and thrombocytopenia
- Most cases probably related to acquired inhibitor of von Willebrand factor (vWF)–cleaving protease; may also be secondary to drugs, chemotherapy, or cancer
- Demonstrating decreased activity of vWF-cleaving protease inhibitor (ADAMTS13) may be diagnostic

■ Differential Diagnosis

- Disseminated intravascular coagulation
- Pre-eclampsia–eclampsia
- Other microangiopathic hemolytic anemias
- Catastrophic antiphospholipid antibody syndrome
- Hemolytic-uremic syndrome

■ Treatment

- Immediate plasmapheresis
- Fresh-frozen plasma infusions help if plasmapheresis not readily available
- Splenectomy and immunosuppressive or cytotoxic medications for refractory cases

■ Pearl

HIV/AIDS has doubled the incidence; few conditions cause LDH this high.

Reference

Elliott MA, Heit JA, Pruthi RK, Gastineau DA, Winters JL, Hook CC. Rituximab for refractory and or relapsing thrombotic thrombocytopenic purpura related to immune-mediated severe ADAMTS13-deficiency: a report of four cases and a systematic review of the literature. Eur J Haematol 2009;83:365. [PMID: 19508684]

Vitamin B$_{12}$ Deficiency

■ Essentials of Diagnosis

- Dyspnea on exertion, nonspecific gastrointestinal symptoms
- Constant symmetric numbness and tingling of the feet; later, poor balance and dementia manifest
- Pallor, mild jaundice, decreased vibratory and position sense
- Pancytopenia with oval macrocytes and hypersegmented neutrophils, increased MCV, megaloblastic bone marrow; low serum vitamin B$_{12}$
- Both homocysteine and methylmalonic acid levels are elevated in vitamin B$_{12}$ deficiency; send these tests when B$_{12}$ level equivocal
- Positive anti-intrinsic factor antibodies, diagnostic of pernicious anemia; positive antiparietal cell antibodies less sensitive and less specific
- Neurologic manifestations occur without anemia in rare cases, including dementia
- Hematologic response to pharmacologic doses of folic acid
- History of total gastrectomy, bowel resection, bacterial overgrowth, fish tapeworm, Crohn's disease, or autoimmune endocrinopathies (eg, diabetes mellitus, hypothyroidism)

■ Differential Diagnosis

- Folic acid deficiency
- Myelodysplastic syndromes
- Occasional hemolytic anemias with megaloblastic red cell precursors in marrow
- Infiltrative granulomatous or malignant processes causing pancytopenia
- Hypersplenism
- Paroxysmal nocturnal hemoglobinuria
- Acute leukemia

■ Treatment

- Vitamin B$_{12}$ 100 μg intramuscularly daily during first week, then weekly for 1 month
- Lifelong B$_{12}$ 100 μg intramuscularly every month thereafter (or 1–2 mg [high-dose] oral B$_{12}$)
- Hypokalemia may complicate early therapy
- Gastrointestinal work-up if GI symptoms or young age

■ Pearl

An arrest in reticulocytosis shortly after institution of therapy means concealed iron deficiency until proved otherwise.

Reference

Dali-Youcef N, Andrès E. An update on cobalamin deficiency in adults. QJM 2009;102:17. [PMID: 18990719]

von Willebrand's Disease

■ Essentials of Diagnosis

- History of lifelong excessive bruising and mucosal bleeding; excessive bleeding during previous surgery, dental extraction, or childbirth
- Usually prolonged bleeding time, especially after aspirin, but platelet count normal
- Variable abnormalities in factor VIII level, von Willebrand factor (vWF), or ristocetin cofactor activity
- Prolonged partial thromboplastin time when factor VIII levels decreased

■ Differential Diagnosis

- Qualitative platelet disorders
- Waldenström's macroglobulinemia
- Aspirin ingestion
- Hemophilias
- Dysfibrinogenemia

■ Treatment

- Avoid aspirin
- vWF and factor VIII concentrates for severe bleeding or for surgical procedures in most cases
- Desmopressin acetate in type I disease may be sufficient to raise vWF and factor VIII to acceptable levels
- Antifibrinolytic agents, such as aminocaproic acid, and topical agents (topical thrombin, fibrin sealant) are used for bleeding not responsive to other interventions

■ Pearl

Remember this with past histories of erratic bleeding after surgery; aspirin may have been given in some circumstances, other analgesics under different conditions.

Reference

James AH, Manco-Johnson MJ, Yawn BP, Dietrich JE, Nichols WL. Von Willebrand disease: key points from the 2008 National Heart, Lung, and Blood Institute guidelines. Obstet Gynecol 2009;114:674. [PMID: 19701049]

Waldenström's Macroglobulinemia

5

- **Essentials of Diagnosis**
  - Fatigue, symptoms of hyperviscosity (altered mental status, bleeding, or thrombosis)
  - Variable hepatosplenomegaly and lymphadenopathy; boxcar retinal vein engorgement
  - Anemia with rouleaux formation; monoclonal IgM paraprotein; increased serum viscosity; narrowed anion gap
  - Lymphoplasmacytoid infiltrate in marrow
  - Absence of bone lesions

- **Differential Diagnosis**
  - Benign monoclonal gammopathy
  - Chronic lymphocytic leukemia with M spike
  - Multiple myeloma
  - Lymphoma

- **Treatment**
  - Emergency plasmapheresis for severe hyperviscosity (stupor or coma)
  - Start treatment when symptomatic or progression of disease (lymphadenopathy, hepatomegaly, splenomegaly, cytopenias)
  - Chemotherapy including chlorambucil, cyclophosphamide, fludarabine, cladribine
  - Monoclonal antibody therapy (rituximab) may be effective

- **Pearl**

There's rouleaux and then there's rouleaux; some can be found on any blood smear, but they are in every field in Waldenström's and myeloma.

Reference

Treon SP, Ioakimidis L, Soumerai JD, et al. Primary therapy of Waldenström macroglobulinemia with bortezomib, dexamethasone, and rituximab: WMCTG clinical trial 05-180. J Clin Oncol 2009;27:3830. [PMID: 19506160]

6

Rheumatologic & Autoimmune Disorders

Adult Still's Disease

- **Essentials of Diagnosis**
  - Occurs in younger adults, with some patients older than 50 years
  - Fevers > 39°C, daily peak with return to normal temperature, may antedate seronegative arthritis by months; occasional cases entirely nonarticular; sore throat common
  - Proximal interphalangeal and metacarpophalangeal joints, wrists, knees, hips, and shoulders are most commonly involved
  - Evanescent, salmon-colored, nonpruritic maculopapular rash involving the trunk and extremities during fever spikes; may be elicited by mechanical irritation (Koebner's phenomenon)
  - Additional findings include hepatosplenomegaly, hepatitis, lymphadenopathy, pleuropericarditis, leukocytosis, thrombocytosis, anemia, and elevations of the erythrocyte sedimentation rate, C-reactive protein level, and ferritin

- **Differential Diagnosis**
  - Leukemia or lymphoma
  - Viral syndrome such as acute HIV, parvovirus B19, hepatitis B and C
  - Chronic bacterial infection (eg, Lyme disease, culture-negative endocarditis)
  - Granulomatous diseases (eg, sarcoidosis, Crohn's disease)
  - Acute, early rheumatoid arthritis
  - Systemic vasculitis; systemic lupus erythematosus (SLE)

- **Treatment**
  - Aspirin often dramatically lyses fever
  - NSAIDs (eg, ibuprofen 800 mg three times daily)
  - Corticosteroids, hydroxychloroquine, methotrexate, azathioprine, and other immunosuppressive agents are used as second-line agents

- **Pearl**

One of three diseases in all of medicine with biquotidian fever spikes; kala azar and gonococcal endocarditis are the others.

Reference

Fautrel B. Adult-onset Still disease. Best Pract Res Clin Rheumatol 2008;22:773. [PMID: 19028363]

Amyloidosis

■ Essentials of Diagnosis
- A group of disorders characterized by deposition in tissues of ordinarily soluble peptides; can be systemic or localized
- Four groups when systemic: AL, AA, AB_2M, and genetic
- AL derived from immunoglobulin light chain associated with plasma cell dyscrasias; peripheral neuropathy, nephrotic syndrome, cardiomyopathy, gut hypomotility, hepatosplenomegaly, malabsorption, carpal tunnel syndrome, macroglossia, arthropathy, postural hypotension, and cutaneous lesions
- AA derived from serum amyloid A; seen in chronic poorly controlled inflammatory disorders (eg, untreated osteomyelitis, leprosy, aggressive rheumatoid arthritis and seronegative spondyloarthropathies); nephrotic syndrome and hepatic involvement common
- AB_2M derived from B_2 microglobulin that is not filtered in chronic hemodialysis patients; carpal tunnel syndrome common
- Genetic amyloid derived from numerous mutant proteins rendered insoluble; many syndromes
- Beta amyloid protein found in Alzheimer's plaques (localized disease)
- Green birefringence under polarizing microscope after Congo red staining seen in all tissues infiltrated by amyloid; biopsy of same thus diagnostic

■ Differential Diagnosis
- Hemochromatosis
- Subacute bacterial endocarditis
- Chronic bacterial infection (eg, tuberculosis, leprosy)
- Sarcoidosis
- Waldenström's macroglobulinemia
- Metastatic neoplasm
- Other causes of nephrotic syndrome

■ Treatment
- Preventive colchicine in familial Mediterranean fever to prevent AA deposits
- Melphalan, prednisone, marrow transplantation (treat AL associated with multiple myeloma)
- Treat underlying disease if present

■ Pearl

When nephrotic syndrome and hepatosplenomegaly are noted in an adult, obtain a serum protein electrophoresis; amyloidosis associated with multiple myeloma may give you the answer.

Reference

Sideras K, Gertz MA. Amyloidosis. Adv Clin Chem 2009;47:1. [PMID: 19634775]

Ankylosing Spondylitis

- **Essentials of Diagnosis**
  - Gradual onset of backache in adults under age 40, absent history of trauma, with progressive limitation of back motion and chest expansion
  - Diminished anterior flexion of lumbar spine, loss of lumbar lordosis, inflammation at tendon insertions
  - Peripheral arthritis and anterior uveitis in many
  - Aortic insufficiency with cardiac conduction defects in some
  - Cauda equina syndrome, apical pulmonary fibrosis are late complications
  - HLA-B27 histocompatibility antigen present in > 90% of patients; rheumatoid factor absent
  - Radiographic evidence of bilateral sacroiliac joint sclerosis; demineralization and squaring of the vertebral bodies with calcification of the anterior and lateral spinal ligaments (bamboo spine)

- **Differential Diagnosis**
  - Rheumatoid arthritis
  - Osteoporosis
  - Reactive arthritis
  - Arthritis associated with inflammatory bowel disease
  - Psoriatic arthritis
  - Diffuse idiopathic skeletal hyperostosis
  - Synovitis-acne-pustulosis-hyperostosis-osteitis syndrome

- **Treatment**
  - Physical therapy to maintain posture and mobility
  - NSAIDs (eg, indomethacin 50 mg three times daily) often marginally effective
  - Sulfasalazine reported effective in some patients for peripheral arthritis
  - Intra-articular corticosteroids for synovitis; ophthalmic corticosteroids for uveitis
  - Institute methotrexate in those with persistent arthritis; if symptoms progress or are debilitating initiate anti–tumor necrosis factor (TNF) agents
  - Surgery for severely affected joints

- **Pearl**

Tuberculosis was once thought to be more common in this disorder; in fact, an idiopathic biapical pulmonary fibrosis is the answer.

Reference

Goh L, Samanta A. A systematic MEDLINE analysis of therapeutic approaches in ankylosing spondylitis. Rheumatol Int 2009;29:1123. [PMID: 19562344]

Arthritis Associated with Inflammatory Bowel Disease

- **Essentials of Diagnosis**
  - Peripheral arthritis: Asymmetric oligoarthritis that typically involves the knees, ankles, and occasionally the upper extremities; in some patients with ulcerative colitis, severity of findings can parallel bowel disease activity
  - Spondylitis: Clinically identical to ankylosing spondylitis; also with bilateral sacroiliitis; HLA-B27 antigen present in most patients in a male:female ratio of 4:1
  - Articular features may precede intestinal symptoms, especially in Crohn's disease
  - Extra-articular manifestations may also occur in Crohn's disease (erythema nodosum) and in ulcerative colitis (pyoderma gangrenosum)

- **Differential Diagnosis**
  - Reactive arthritis
  - Ankylosing spondylitis
  - Psoriatic arthritis
  - Rheumatoid arthritis

- **Treatment**
  - Treat underlying intestinal inflammation
  - Aspirin, other NSAIDs (eg, indomethacin 50 mg three times daily)
  - Physical therapy for spondylitis

- **Pearl**

The younger the patient, the fewer the GI complaints; thus arthritis in adolescence should prompt a search for IBD despite absence of symptoms.

Reference

De Vos M. Joint involvement in inflammatory bowel disease: managing inflammation outside the digestive system. Expert Rev Gastroenterol Hepatol 2010;4:81. [PMID: 20136591]

Behçet's Syndrome

- **Essentials of Diagnosis**
  - Usually occurs in young adults from Mediterranean countries or Japan; incidence decreases if patient's descendants emigrate elsewhere
  - Most common: Recurrent painful oral aphthous ulcerations (99%) and genital ulcers (80%), ocular lesions in half (uveitis, hypopyon, iritis, keratitis, optic neuritis), and skin lesions (erythema nodosum, superficial thrombophlebitis, cutaneous hypersensitivity, folliculitis)
  - Less common: Gastrointestinal erosions, epididymitis, glomerulonephritis, pulmonary artery aneurysms, cranial nerve palsies, aseptic meningitis, and focal neurologic lesions
  - Pathergy test—a papule or a pustule forms 24–48 hours after simple trauma such as a needle prick
  - Diagnosis is clinical
  - HLA-B5 histocompatibility antigen often present

- **Differential Diagnosis**
  - HLA-B27 spondyloarthropathies
  - Inflammatory bowel disease
  - Small vessel vasculitis (eg, anti-neutrophil cytoplasmic antibody [ANCA]–associated)
  - Oral aphthous ulcers
  - Herpes simplex infection
  - Erythema multiforme
  - SLE
  - HIV infection
  - Infective endocarditis

- **Treatment**
  - Local mydriatics in all patients with eye findings to prevent synechiae from forming; close follow-up by experienced ophthalmologist critical
  - Corticosteroids
  - Colchicine (for erythema nodosum and arthralgia)
  - Chlorambucil, azathioprine commonly used; cyclosporine occasionally successful in those with eye disease

- **Pearl**

Stroke in a young native Japanese woman is Behçet's unless proven otherwise.

Reference

Mendes D, Correia M, Barbedo M, Vaio T, Mota M, Gonçalves O, Valente J. Behçet's disease—a contemporary review. J Autoimmun 2009;32:178. [PMID: 19324519]

Carpal Tunnel Syndrome

- ■ Essentials of Diagnosis
  - The most common entrapment neuropathy, caused by compression of the median nerve (which innervates the flexor muscles of the wrist and fingers)
  - Middle-aged women and those with a history of repetitive use of the hands commonly affected
  - Pain classically worse at night (sleep with hands curled into the body) and exacerbated by hand movement
  - Initial symptoms of pain or paresthesias in thumb, index, middle, and lateral part of ring finger; progression to thenar eminence wasting
  - Pain radiation to forearm, shoulder, neck, chest, or other fingers of the hand not uncommon
  - Positive Tinel's sign
  - Usually idiopathic; in bilateral onset consider secondary causes including rheumatoid arthritis, amyloidosis, sarcoidosis, hypothyroidism, diabetes, pregnancy, acromegaly, gout
  - Diagnosis is primarily clinical; detection of deficits by electrodiagnostic testing (assessing nerve conduction velocity) very helpful to guide referral for surgical release

- ■ Differential Diagnosis
  - C6 or C7 cervical radiculopathy
  - Thoracic outlet syndrome leading to brachial plexus neuropathy
  - Mononeuritis multiplex
  - Syringomyelia
  - Multiple sclerosis
  - Angina pectoris, especially when left-sided

- ■ Treatment
  - Conservative measures initially, including hand rest, nocturnal splinting of wrists, anti-inflammatory medications
  - Steroid injection into the carpal tunnel occasionally
  - Surgical decompression in a few who have nerve conduction abnormalities; best done before development of thenar atrophy

- ■ Pearl

Carpal tunnel affects the radial three and one-half fingers, myocardial ischemia the ulnar one and one-half; remember this in evaluating arm pain—and hope it's the right arm.

Reference

Dahlin LB, Salö M, Thomsen N, Stütz N. Carpal tunnel syndrome and treatment of recurrent symptoms. Scand J Plast Reconstr Surg Hand Surg 2010;44:4. [PMID: 20136467]

Chondrocalcinosis and Pseudogout (Calcium Pyrophosphate Dihydrate Deposition Disease)

- **Essentials of Diagnosis**
  - Subacute, recurrent, and under-appreciated cause of chronic arthritis, usually involving large joints (especially knees, shoulders, and wrists) and almost always accompanied by chondrocalcinosis of the affected joints
  - May be hereditary, idiopathic, or associated with metabolic disorders, including hemochromatosis, hypoparathyroidism, osteoarthritis, ochronosis, diabetes mellitus, hypothyroidism, Wilson's disease, and gout
  - Identification of calcium pyrophosphate rhomboidal crystals (strong positive birefringence) in the joint fluid is diagnostic; however, much more challenging to see on slide than urate crystals
  - Radiographs may reveal chondrocalcinosis or signs of degenerative joint disease at the following sites: Knee (medial meniscus), fibrocartilaginous portion of the symphysis pubica, glenohumeral joint and articular disk of the wrist with calcium in the triangular ligament

- **Differential Diagnosis**
  - Gout
  - Calcium phosphate disease (hydroxyapatite arthropathy)
  - Calcium oxalate deposition disease
  - Degenerative joint disease
  - Rheumatoid arthritis

- **Treatment**
  - Treat underlying disease if present
  - Aspirin, other NSAIDs (eg, indomethacin 50 mg three times daily)
  - Intra-articular injection of corticosteroids (eg, triamcinolone 10–40 mg)
  - Colchicine, 0.6 mg twice daily, occasionally useful for prophylaxis

- **Pearl**

Pseudogout is the clinical syndrome, chondrocalcinosis the radiologic finding; the latter does not diagnose the former.

Reference

Announ N, Guerne PA. Treating difficult crystal pyrophosphate dihydrate deposition disease. Curr Rheumatol Rep 2008;10:228. [PMID: 18638432]

Churg-Strauss Vasculitis (Allergic Granulomatosis and Angiitis)

- **Essentials of Diagnosis**
  - Granulomatous vasculitis of small- and medium-sized blood vessels
  - Four of the following have a sensitivity of 85% and specificity of 100% for diagnosis: new-onset asthma; allergic rhinitis; transient pulmonary infiltrates; palpable purpura or extravascular eosinophils; mononeuritis multiplex; and peripheral blood eosinophilia

- **Differential Diagnosis**
  - Wegener's granulomatosis
  - Eosinophilic pneumonia
  - Polyarteritis nodosa (often overlaps)
  - Hypersensitivity vasculitis

- **Treatment**
  - Rheumatology consult to advise on managing toxic medications
  - Corticosteroids
  - Cyclophosphamide

- **Pearl**

New onset of reactive airways disease in an adult with peripheral eosinophilia and mononeuritis multiplex...think Churg-Strauss.

Reference

Zwerina J, Axmann R, Jatzwauk M, Sahinbegovic E, Polzer K, Schett G. Pathogenesis of Churg-Strauss syndrome: recent insights. Autoimmunity 2009;42:376. [PMID: 19811306]

Cryoglobulinemia

■ Essentials of Diagnosis

- Refers to any globulin precipitable at lower than body temperature
- Any elevation of globulin may be associated
- Monoclonal gammopathies, reactive hypergammaglobulinemia, cryoprecipitable immune complexes are associated with acral cold symptoms because of higher titers of cryoproteins
- Essential mixed cryoglobulinemia occurs in patients serologically positive for hepatitis C
- Symptoms and signs depend on type; most common are palpable purpura, arthralgias, neuropathies, and nephritis
- Low erythrocyte sedimentation rate

■ Differential Diagnosis

- Multiple myeloma, Waldenström's macroglobulinemia
- Any small vessel vasculitis
- Chronic inflammatory diseases such as endocarditis, sarcoidosis, rheumatoid arthritis, Sjögren's syndrome

■ Treatment

- Entirely dependent on cause

■ Pearl

In a patient whose blood "clots" in the CBC test tube, it may be caused by a cryoprecipitable M-spike; do a serum protein electrophoresis at 37 degrees in such patients.

Reference

Chan AO, Lau JS, Chan CH, Shek CC. Cryoglobulinaemia: clinical and laboratory perspectives. Hong Kong Med J 2008;14:55. [PMID: 18239245]

Degenerative Joint Disease (Osteoarthritis)

- ■ Essentials of Diagnosis
  - Progressive degeneration of articular cartilage and hypertrophy of bone at the articular margin
  - Affects almost all joints, especially weight-bearing and frequently used joints; hips, knees, and first carpometacarpal joint (thumb on dominant hand) most common
  - Primary degenerative joint disease most commonly affects the terminal interphalangeal joints (Heberden's nodes), hips, and first carpometacarpal joints
  - Morning stiffness brief; pain worse with use
  - Radiographs reveal narrowing of the joint spaces, osteophytes, subchondral sclerosis, and cyst formation

- ■ Differential Diagnosis
  - Rheumatoid arthritis
  - Seronegative spondyloarthropathies
  - Crystal-induced arthritides
  - Hyperparathyroidism
  - Multiple myeloma
  - Hemochromatosis

- ■ Treatment
  - Weight reduction; exercise to strengthen periarticular muscle
  - NSAIDs or acetaminophen
  - Glucosamine and chondroitin sulfate possibly effective for some individuals
  - Topical capsaicin cream on large affected joints may help some
  - Intra-articular corticosteroid injection (eg, triamcinolone 10–40 mg) in selected patients (up to three times yearly)
  - Surgery for severely affected joints, especially hip and knee; timing dictated by debilitating pain

- ■ Pearl

Morning stiffness lasts more than an hour in rheumatoid arthritis, 15 minutes or less in degenerative joint disease.

Reference

Crosby J. Osteoarthritis: managing without surgery. J Fam Pract 2009;58:354. [PMID: 19607772]

Eosinophilic Fasciitis

- ■ Essentials of Diagnosis
  - Occurs predominantly in men
  - Pain, swelling, stiffness, and tenderness of the hands, forearms, feet, or legs, evolving to woody induration and retraction of subcutaneous tissue within days to weeks
  - Associated with peripheral eosinophilia, polyarthralgias, arthritis, carpal tunnel syndrome; no Raynaud's phenomenon
  - Biopsy of deep fascia is diagnostic
  - Association with aplastic anemia, thrombocytopenia

- ■ Differential Diagnosis
  - Systemic sclerosis
  - Eosinophilia myalgia syndrome
  - Hypothyroidism
  - Trichinosis
  - Mixed connective tissue disease

- ■ Treatment
  - NSAIDs
  - Short course of corticosteroids
  - Antimalarials

- ■ Pearl

The only noninfectious disease in medicine confined to the fascia.

Reference

Boin F, Hummers LK. Scleroderma-like fibrosing disorders. Rheum Dis Clin North Am 2008;34:199; ix. [PMID: 18329541]

Fibrositis (Fibromyalgia)

■ Essentials of Diagnosis

- Most frequent in women ages 20–50
- Chronic aching pain and stiffness of trunk and extremities, especially around the neck, shoulder, low back, and hips
- Elicit pain with mild palpation (enough pressure to blanch your fingernail) at 11 of 18 bilateral tender points: Occiput, low cervical, trapezius, supraspinatus, second rib at costochondral junction, lateral epicondyle, gluteal region, greater trochanter, and medial fat pad of the knee
- Associated with fatigue, headaches, subjective numbness, irritable bowel symptoms; often occurs after a physically or emotionally traumatic event
- Nearly universal description of nonrestful sleep
- Absence of objective signs of inflammation; normal laboratory studies, including erythrocyte sedimentation rate
- A diagnosis of exclusion after you work through the following differential diagnosis

■ Differential Diagnosis

- Metabolic-Hypothyroidism, hypocalcemia, vitamin D deficiency
- Neoplasm-Lymphoma or paraneoplastic syndrome
- Rheumatic-Rheumatoid arthritis, SLE, Polymyalgia rheumatica
- Depression, physical abuse
- HIV disease
- Chronic fatigue syndrome

■ Treatment

- Reassure patient that you have ruled out cancer or chronic infection; despite the pain, this is a nonlethal disease
- Patients who improve are those who identify some physical activity they enjoy and can do without exertion
- Aspirin, other NSAIDs
- Tricyclics offer transient relief related to anti-insomniac effect; cyclobenzaprine, chlorpromazine
- Injection of trigger points with corticosteroids works for some

■ Pearl

Consider the diagnosis in patients who exhibit the "wince reflex": they wince each time you touch them during the exam; however, be sure the erythrocyte sedimentation rate is normal before making this diagnosis.

Reference

Clauw DJ. Fibromyalgia: an overview. Am J Med 2009;122(suppl):S3. [PMID: 19962494]

Gonococcal Arthritis

■ Essentials of Diagnosis

- Two clinical scenarios: (1) Septic joint with mono- or oligoarticular involvement and no skin changes; or (2) a systemic process with oligoarticular arthritis, tenosynovitis, and characteristic purpuric or pustular skin lesions on the distal extremities (commonly called disseminated gonococcal infection [DGI])
- Septic joint variant: White cell count in synovial fluid 20,000–50,000/μL; synovial fluid Gram's stain and culture more likely to be positive
- Systemic presentation variant: Lower synovial cell counts, negative Gram stain and culture of joint fluid because signs secondary to inflammation due to bacterial debris, not direct infection
- Urethral, cervical, throat, skin lesion, and rectal cultures on chocolate or Thayer-Martin agar for *Neisseria gonorrhoeae* have higher yield, may be positive in the absence of symptoms
- Recurrent disseminated gonococcal infection seen with congenital complement component deficiencies

■ Differential Diagnosis

- Nongonococcal bacterial arthritis
- Reactive arthritis; Lyme disease; viral hepatitis
- Sarcoidosis; infective endocarditis
- Meningococcemia with arthritis
- Seronegative spondyloarthropathy

■ Treatment

- Obtain Venereal Disease Research Laboratory (VDRL) test and HIV testing
- Intravenous ceftriaxone or ceftizoxime for 7 days followed by oral cefixime or ciprofloxacin
- Perform washout of joints exhibiting mono-articular septic picture.
- Avoid NSAIDs early in treatment of DGI. If the arthritis improves within 72 hours after initiating antibiotics, the diagnosis is DGI; if you treat with both NSAIDs and antibiotics you will not know if the improving patient had reactive arthritis or DGI

■ Pearl

An infectious arthritis causing very little cartilage damage may in fact be an autoimmune phenomenon.

Reference

García-De La Torre I, Nava-Zavala A. Gonococcal and nongonococcal arthritis. Rheum Dis Clin North Am 2009;35:63. [PMID: 19480997]

Gout

■ Essentials of Diagnosis

- Especially common among native Pacific Islanders
- Broad spectrum of disease, including recurrent arthritic attacks, tophi, interstitial nephropathy, and uric acid nephrolithiasis
- First attack typically nocturnal and usually monarticular 90% of time involving the foot, ankle, or knee, with pain "worsened by the weight of the bedsheet"; may become polyarticular with repeated attacks
- Affects in descending order of frequency: The first metatarsophalangeal joint (podagra), mid foot, ankle, knee, wrist, elbow; hips and shoulders typically spared
- Hyperuricemia may be primary (caused by overproduction [10%] or underexcretion [90%] of uric acid) or secondary to diuretic use, cyclosporine, myeloproliferative disorders, multiple myeloma, chronic renal disease
- After long periods of untreated gout, tophi (monosodium urate deposits with an associated foreign body reaction) develop in subcutaneous tissues, cartilage, ears, and other tissues
- Identification of weakly negatively birefringent, needlelike sodium urate crystals in joint fluid or tophi is diagnostic

■ Differential Diagnosis

- Cellulitis; septic arthritis
- Pseudogout
- Rheumatoid arthritis
- Chronic lead intoxication (saturnine gout)

■ Treatment

- Treat the acute arthritis first and the hyperuricemia later
- For acute attacks: Dramatic therapeutic response to NSAIDs (eg, indomethacin 50 mg three times daily), intra-articular or systemic corticosteroids; never use colchicine in acute gout
- For chronic prophylaxis in patients with frequent acute attacks, tophaceous deposits, or renal damage: Allopurinol and probenecid (uricosuric agent) with concomitant oral colchicine
- Avoid thiazides and loop diuretics

■ Pearl

When operating on the back for an epidural "abscess," if the lesion appears chalky, be sure to stain for uric acid crystals; tophi may occur in the spine.

Reference

Conway N, Schwartz S. Diagnosis and management of acute gout. Med Health R I 2009;92:356. [PMID: 19999893]

Hypersensitivity Vasculitis

- **Essentials of Diagnosis**
  - Necrotizing vasculitis of small blood vessels
  - Palpable purpura of lower extremities the predominant feature; glomerulonephritis; peripheral polyneuropathy
  - Most commonly occurs in response to a new antigen: Numerous medications, neoplasms, serum sickness, viral or bacterial infection, or congenital complement deficiency
  - On occasion associated with fever, arthralgias, abdominal pain with or without gastrointestinal bleeding, pulmonary infiltrates, kidney involvement with hematuria
  - Skin biopsy reveals leukocytoclastic vasculitis

- **Differential Diagnosis**
  - Polyarteritis nodosa
  - Henoch-Schönlein purpura
  - Essential mixed cryoglobulinemia
  - ANCA-associated vasculitides (eg, Wegener's, microscopic polyangiitis)
  - Meningococcemia
  - Gonococcemia

- **Treatment**
  - Treat underlying disease if present
  - Discontinue offending drug
  - Corticosteroids in severe cases

- **Pearl**

The palpable purpura of this lesion is dependent; thus it is more prominent on the legs of the ambulatory patient, but seen on the lower back in those who are bed bound.

Reference

Chen KR, Carlson JA. Clinical approach to cutaneous vasculitis. Am J Clin Dermatol 2008;9:71. [PMID: 18284262]

Infectious Osteomyelitis

- ■ Essentials of Diagnosis
  - Infection usually occurs via hematogenous seeding of the bone; metaphyses of long bones and vertebrae most frequently involved
  - Subacute vague pain and tenderness of affected bone or back with little or no fever in adults; more acute presentation in children
  - Organisms include *Staphylococcus aureus,* coagulase-negative staphylococci, group A streptococci, gram-negative rods, anaerobic and polymicrobial infections, tuberculosis, brucellosis, histoplasmosis, coccidioidomycosis, blastomycosis
  - Blood cultures may be negative; biopsy of bone is diagnostic
  - Radiographs early in the course are often negative, but periostitis may be detected 2–3 weeks into the course, followed by periarticular demineralization and erosion of bone
  - Radionuclide bone scan is 90% sensitive and may be positive within 2 days after onset of symptoms, though offers no information regarding pathogen

- ■ Differential Diagnosis
  - Acute bacterial arthritis
  - Rheumatic fever
  - Cellulitis
  - Multiple myeloma
  - Ewing's sarcoma
  - Metastatic neoplasia

- ■ Treatment
  - Intravenous antibiotics after appropriate cultures have been obtained
  - Oral ciprofloxacin, 750 mg twice daily for 6–8 weeks, may be effective in limited osteomyelitis
  - In older patients, treat with broad-spectrum antibiotics as for a gram-negative bacteremia as a consequence of urinary, biliary, intestinal, and lower respiratory infections
  - Débridement if response to antibiotics is poor

- ■ Pearl

In chronic osteomyelitis: once an osteo, always an osteo.

Reference

Sia IG, Berbari EF. Infection and musculoskeletal conditions: osteomyelitis. Best Pract Res Clin Rheumatol 2006;20:1065. [PMID: 17127197]

Microscopic Polyangiitis (MPAN)

- **■ Essentials of Diagnosis**
  - Necrotizing vasculitis affecting arterioles, capillaries, and venules
  - Presents with rapidly progressive glomerulonephritis (RPGN), often with palpable purpura; diffuse alveolar hemorrhage in some
  - 80% of cases are ANCA-associated, most often in the perinuclear (P-ANCA) pattern with antimyeloperoxidase antibodies; like all ANCA-associated vasculitides, affects men and women equally, with predilection for whites more than blacks
  - Diagnosis most often made on renal biopsy showing pauci-immune RPGN

- **■ Differential Diagnosis**
  - Polyarteritis nodosa
  - Wegener's granulomatosis
  - Churg-Strauss vasculitis
  - Goodpasture's syndrome
  - Cryoglobulinemic vasculitis

- **■ Treatment**
  - Institute intravenous steroids acutely with cytotoxic agents such as cyclophosphamide
  - Maintenance therapy can include steroids, with cyclophosphamide or azathioprine

- **■ Pearl**

The ANCA is highly valuable, but to make the diagnosis, tissue is the issue.

Reference

Jayne D. Challenges in the management of microscopic polyangiitis: past, present and future. Curr Opin Rheumatol 2008;20:3. [PMID: 18281850]

Polyarteritis Nodosa

- **Essentials of Diagnosis**
  - Systemic illness causing inflammation and necrosis of medium-sized arteries
  - Distribution of affected arteries dictates clinical manifestations, which include fever, hypertension, abdominal pain, arthralgias, myalgias, cotton-wool spots and microaneurysms in fundus, pericarditis, myocarditis, palpable purpura, mononeuritis multiplex, livedo reticularis, ischemic bowel, and nonglomerulonephritic renal failure
  - Acceleration of sedimentation rate in most; serologic evidence of new-onset hepatitis B in 30–50%
  - P-ANCA positive in < 10% of cases
  - Diagnosis confirmed by deep-muscle biopsy or selected visceral angiography

- **Differential Diagnosis**
  - Wegener's granulomatosis
  - Churg-Strauss vasculitis
  - Hypersensitivity vasculitis
  - Subacute endocarditis
  - Essential mixed cryoglobulinemia
  - Microscopic polyangiitis (MPAN)
  - Cholesterol atheroembolic disease
  - Paraneoplastic syndrome

- **Treatment**
  - Corticosteroids with cyclophosphamide for systemic vasculitis; azathioprine is used as a maintenance immunosuppressant

- **Pearl**

In clinical cholecystitis in a patient with systemic illness, consider this diagnosis; the cystic artery is very commonly involved and causes acalculous cholecystitis.

Reference

Pettigrew HD, Teuber SS, Gershwin ME. Polyarteritis nodosa. Compr Ther 2007;33:144. [PMID: 18004029]

Polymyalgia Rheumatica and Giant Cell Arteritis

- **Essentials of Diagnosis**

  - Patients usually over age 50
  - Polymyalgia rheumatica characterized by pain and stiffness (often morning stiffness), not weakness, of the shoulder and pelvic girdle lasting 1 month or more without evidence of infection or malignancy
  - Associated with fever, little if any joint swelling, sedimentation rate > 40 mm/h, and dramatic response to prednisone 15 mg/d
  - Giant cell (temporal) arteritis frequently coexists with polymyalgia rheumatica; headache, jaw claudication, temporal artery tenderness
  - Monocular vision changes represent medical emergencies; blindness is permanent
  - Diagnosis confirmation by 5-cm temporal artery biopsy remains reliable for 1–2 weeks after starting steroids

- **Differential Diagnosis**

  - Multiple myeloma
  - Chronic infection (eg, endocarditis, visceral abscess)
  - Neoplasm
  - Rheumatoid arthritis
  - Depression
  - Myxedema
  - Carotid plaque with embolic amaurosis fugax
  - Carotid Takayasu's arteritis

- **Treatment**

  - Prednisone 10–20 mg/d for polymyalgia rheumatica
  - Prednisone 60 mg/d immediately on suspicion of temporal arteritis; treat for at least 4 months depending on response of symptoms—not sedimentation rate
  - Methotrexate or azathioprine spares steroids in some patients with side effects on high doses

- **Pearl**

Most patients with giant cell arteritis first have polymyalgia rheumatica; when the latter is diagnosed, the patient should be instructed to keep 60 mg of prednisone with them and take it immediately in the event of any visual symptom.

Reference

Salvarani C, Cantini F, Hunder GG. Polymyalgia rheumatica and giant-cell arteritis. Lancet 2008;372:234. [PMID: 18640460]

Polymyositis-Dermatomyositis

■ Essentials of Diagnosis
- Bilateral proximal muscle weakness for both entities
- Dermatomyositis characterized by true weakness and skin changes: periorbital edema and a purplish (heliotrope) rash over the upper eyelids in many; violaceous, scaly papules overlying the interphalangeal joints of the hands (Gottron's papules)
- Serum CK and aldolase elevated (500-5000 range)
- Muscle biopsy and characteristic electromyographic (EMG) pattern are diagnostic; MRI of affected muscles replaces EMG study
- When associated with rheumatoid arthritis, SLE, scleroderma, it is called an overlap syndrome
- Dermatomyositis associated with increased incidence of malignancy; may precede or follow detection of cancer

■ Differential Diagnosis
- Endocrine myopathies (eg, hyperthyroidism, Cushing's)
- Polymyalgia rheumatica; parasitic myositis
- Myasthenia gravis; Eaton-Lambert syndrome
- Muscular dystrophy; rhabdomyolysis
- Drug-induced myopathies (eg, corticosteroids, alcohol, colchicine, statins, zidovudine, hydroxychloroquine)
- Adult glycogen storage disease; mitochondrial myopathy

■ Treatment
- Corticosteroids are cornerstone initially
- Methotrexate or azathioprine spares steroids; start early in therapy
- Intravenous immune globulin for some cases of dermatomyositis; consider when weakness compromises the airway
- Search for malignancy should encompass age-appropriate cancer screening and follow-up on abnormalities detected on physical exam or basic laboratory evaluation

■ Pearl
The heliotropic skin rash is named for its similarity to the color of orchid of the same name.

Reference

Wiendl H. Idiopathic inflammatory myopathies: current and future therapeutic options. Neurotherapeutics 2008;5:548. [PMID: 19019306]

Psoriatic Arthritis

- ■ Essentials of Diagnosis
  - Classically a destructive arthritis of distal interphalangeal joints; many patients also have peripheral arthritis involving shoulders, elbows, wrists, knees, and ankles, often asymmetrically
  - Sacroiliitis (unilateral) in B27-positive patients
  - Occurs in 15–20% of patients with psoriasis; small number experience inflammatory arthritis absent characteristic skin changes
  - Psoriatic arthritis associated with nail pitting, onycholysis, sausage digits, arthritis mutilans (severe deforming arthritis)
  - Rheumatoid factor negative; serum uric acid may be elevated
  - Radiographs may reveal irregular destruction of joint spaces and bone, pencil-in-cup deformity of the phalanges, sacroiliitis, or severely disfiguring process of wrists and fingers

- ■ Differential Diagnosis
  - Rheumatoid arthritis
  - Ankylosing spondylitis
  - Arthritis associated with inflammatory bowel disease
  - Reactive arthritis
  - Juvenile spondyloarthropathy

- ■ Treatment
  - NSAIDs (eg, ibuprofen 800 mg three times daily)
  - Sulfasalazine reportedly effective in patients with symmetric polyarthritis
  - Intra-articular corticosteroid injection; sterilize skin carefully as psoriatic lesions are colonized with staphylococci and streptococci
  - Avoid systemic corticosteroids, which when tapered can trigger a flare of pustular psoriasis
  - Methotrexate useful; institute early
  - Anti-TNF agents very effective
  - Treatment of psoriasis helpful in many but not in sacroiliitis

- ■ Pearl

In a seronegative inflammatory arthritis, look for signs of psoriasis in the intergluteal folds, the umbilicus, and along the hairline; the arthritis may dominate the clinical picture.

Reference

Anandarajah AP, Ritchlin CT; Medscape. The diagnosis and treatment of early psoriatic arthritis. Nat Rev Rheumatol 2009;5:634. [PMID: 19806150]

Reactive Arthritis

- **Essentials of Diagnosis**
  - Predominantly diagnosed in young men but also occurs in women (painless vaginal mucosal lesions often not appreciated)
  - Triad of urethritis, conjunctivitis (or uveitis), and arthritis occur synchronously in 10% of cases (Reiter's syndrome); conjunctivitis may be subtle and evanescent
  - Follows invasive dysenteric infection (with *Shigella, Salmonella, Yersinia, Campylobacter*) or sexually transmitted infection (with *Chlamydia*)
  - Asymmetric, oligoarticular arthritis typically involving the knees and ankles; look for tendinitis and plantar fasciitis
  - Associated with fever, mucocutaneous lesions, stomatitis, optic neuritis, circinate balanitis, prostatitis, keratoderma blennorrhagicum (nearly indistinguishable from psoriatic lesions), pericarditis, and aortic regurgitation
  - HLA-B27 histocompatibility antigen in most

- **Differential Diagnosis**
  - Gonococcal arthritis
  - Rheumatoid arthritis
  - Ankylosing spondylitis
  - Psoriatic arthritis
  - Arthritis associated with inflammatory bowel disease
  - Juvenile spondyloarthropathy

- **Treatment**
  - NSAIDs (eg, indomethacin 50 mg three times daily); often ineffective
  - Tetracycline for associated *Chlamydia trachomatis* infection; obtain VDRL, perform HIV testing
  - Methotrexate when NSAIDs insufficient to control inflammation
  - Sulfasalazine may help in some patients
  - Intra-articular corticosteroids for arthritis; ophthalmic corticosteroids for uveitis

- **Pearl**

In "gonococcal arthritis" that does not respond promptly to antibiotics, this is your likely diagnosis.

Reference

Carter JD, Hudson AP. Reactive arthritis: clinical aspects and medical management. Rheum Dis Clin North Am 2009;35:21. [PMID: 19480995]

Reflex Sympathetic Dystrophy (Complex Regional Pain Syndrome)

■ Essentials of Diagnosis

- Severe pain and tenderness, most commonly of the hand or foot, associated with vasomotor instability, skin atrophy, edema, and hyperhidrosis; atrophic, nonfunctional hand or foot seen late in disease
- Usually follows direct trauma to the hand, foot, or knee; stroke; peripheral nerve injury; or arthroscopic knee surgery
- Shoulder-hand variant with restricted ipsilateral shoulder movement common after neck or shoulder injuries or after myocardial infarction
- Characteristic disparity between degree of injury (usually modest) and degree of pain (debilitating)
- Triple-phase bone scan reveals increased uptake in the early phases of the disease; radiographs show severe osteopenia (Sudeck's atrophy) late in the course

■ Differential Diagnosis

- Rheumatoid arthritis
- Polymyositis
- Scleroderma
- Gout, pseudogout
- Acromegaly
- Multiple myeloma
- Osteoporosis due to other causes

■ Treatment

- Supportive care
- Physical therapy is critical to salvage extremity function; active and passive exercises combined with benzodiazepines
- Stellate ganglion or lumbar sympathetic block
- Short course of corticosteroids given early in course

■ Pearl

Once called the shoulder-hand syndrome, extreme osteopenia in a young person with it suggests the diagnosis.

Reference

Hsu ES. Practical management of complex regional pain syndrome. Am J Ther 2009;16:147. [PMID: 19300041]

Rheumatoid Arthritis

■ Essentials of Diagnosis

- Disproportionately affects women of child-bearing age
- Symmetric, inflammatory, destructive polyarthritis of peripheral joints, often involving wrists and hands; ulnar deviation common
- Symptoms of stiffness worse with disuse (eg, morning stiffness)
- Rheumatoid factor present in up to 85%; 20% of seropositive patients have subcutaneous nodules; presence of antibodies to cyclic-citrullinated peptide (anti-CCP) 80% specific for RA
- Extra-articular manifestations, most common among strongly seropositive patients with nodules, include systemic vasculitis, pleural exudative effusion (low in glucose), scleritis, sicca symptoms
- Radiographic findings include juxta-articular and sometimes generalized osteopenia, narrowing of the joint spaces, and bony erosions, particularly of the MCPs and ulnar styloid

■ Differential Diagnosis

- SLE; polymyalgia rheumatica
- Degenerative joint disease
- Polyarticular gout or pseudogout
- Serum sickness; inflammatory osteoarthritis
- Parvovirus B19 infection; acute hepatitis B

■ Treatment

- Pharmacologic doses of aspirin, other NSAIDs
- Disease-modifying anti-rheumatic drugs, including methotrexate, sulfasalazine, hydroxychloroquine, azathioprine, and leflunomide (alone or in combination) in patients with moderate disease activity
- Anti-TNF therapy (infliximab or etanercept, after assessing risk of tuberculosis and other infections) indicated early in disease if erosive arthritis or severe inflammation present
- Surgery for severely affected joints

■ Pearl

A flare of a single joint in a patient with established RA is a septic joint until proved otherwise.

Reference

Goronzy JJ, Weyand CM. Developments in the scientific understanding of rheumatoid arthritis. Arthritis Res Ther 2009;11:249. [PMID: 19835638]

Septic Arthritis (Nongonococcal Acute Bacterial Arthritis)

- ■ Essentials of Diagnosis
  - Acute pain, swelling, erythema, warmth, and limited movement of joints
  - Typically monarticular; knee, hip, wrist, shoulder, or ankle most often involved
  - Infection usually occurs via hematogenous seeding of the synovium
  - Previous joint damage (eg, degenerative joint disease, erosive arthritis) and intravenous drug abuse predispose
  - Most common organisms: *Staphylococcus aureus,* group A streptococci, *Escherichia coli,* and *Pseudomonas aeruginosa; Haemophilus influenzae* in children under 5 years of age; *Staphylococcus epidermidis* after arthroscopy or joint surgery
  - White cell count in synovial fluid > 25,000/μL; synovial fluid culture positive in 50–75%, blood culture in 50%; cell count and culture results affected by use of antibiotics by patients before presentation

- ■ Differential Diagnosis
  - Gonococcal arthritis
  - Microcrystalline synovitis
  - Rheumatoid arthritis
  - Still's disease
  - Infective endocarditis (may be associated)

- ■ Treatment
  - Intravenous antibiotics should be administered empirically; tailor antibiotic selection with culture results to complete 4–6 weeks of therapy
  - When orthopedic surgery is available, each septic joint requires irrigation and drainage in the operating room; if orthopedic surgery support unavailable, joint will require serial draining procedures by needle aspiration
  - Rest, immobilization, and elevation
  - Removal of prosthetic joint or other foreign implants to prevent development of osteomyelitis

- ■ Pearl

An ongoing cause of disagreement between orthopedists and rheumatologists regarding serial arthrocenteses versus surgical drains; the latter is agreed upon by all, however, in a septic hip.

Reference

García-Lechuz J, Bouza E. Treatment recommendations and strategies for the management of bone and joint infections. Expert Opin Pharmacother 2009;10:35. [PMID: 19236181]

Sjögren's Syndrome

- ■ Essentials of Diagnosis
    - Destruction of exocrine glands, leading to mucosal and conjunctival dryness secondary to inflammatory infiltrate
    - Dry mouth (xerostomia) and dry eyes (keratoconjunctivitis sicca), decreased tear production, parotid enlargement, severe dental caries, loss of taste and smell
    - Occasionally associated with glomerulonephritis, renal tubular acidosis type IV, biliary cirrhosis, pancreatitis, neuropsychiatric dysfunction, transverse myelitis, polyneuropathy, interstitial pneumonitis, thyroiditis, cardiac conduction defects
    - More than 50% have cytoplasmic antibodies, anti-Ro (SS-A), and anti-La (SS-B)
    - Decreased lacrimation measured by Schirmer's filter paper test; biopsy of minor salivary glands of lower lip confirms diagnosis
    - Secondary form may also be observed in patients with rheumatoid arthritis, SLE, systemic sclerosis, polymyositis, or polyarteritis

- ■ Differential Diagnosis
    - Sarcoidosis
    - Sialolithiasis
    - Tuberculosis
    - Lymphoma
    - Waldenström's macroglobulinemia
    - Anticholinergic medications
    - Chronic irritation from smoking

- ■ Treatment
    - Symptomatic relief of dryness with artificial tears, chewing gum, sialagogues
    - Cholinergic drugs such as pilocarpine
    - Meticulous care of teeth and avoidance of sugar-containing candies
    - Corticosteroids or azathioprine; cyclophosphamide for peripheral neuropathy, interstitial pneumonitis, glomerulonephritis, and vasculitis

- ■ Pearl

    Dry mouth is a remarkably common primary care syndrome, and most cases are not Sjögren's syndrome; if you give pilocarpine for this, be sure that the ensuing enlarged salivary glands are not mistaken for lymphadenopathy.

Reference

Nikolov NP, Illei GG. Pathogenesis of Sjögren's syndrome. Curr Opin Rheumatol 2009;21:465. [PMID: 19568172]

Systemic Lupus Erythematosus (SLE)

- ■ Essentials of Diagnosis
  - • Multisystem inflammatory autoimmune disorder with periods of exacerbation and remission, principally in young women
  - • Four or more of the following 11 criteria must be present: malar and discoid rashes; photosensitivity; oral ulcers; arthritis; serositis; renal and neurologic disease; immune hematologic disorders (eg, Coombs-positive hemolytic anemia and thrombocytopenia); positive antinuclear antibody or other immunopathies (eg, antibody to native double-stranded DNA or Sm antigen, false-positive rapid plasma reagin)
  - • Also associated with fever, myositis, alopecia, myocarditis, vasculitis, lymphadenopathy, conjunctivitis, antiphospholipid antibodies with hypercoagulability, and miscarriages
  - • Renal involvement includes crescentic, mesangial, and less commonly, membranous glomerulonephritis
  - • Syndrome may be drug-induced (eg, procainamide, hydralazine), primarily serosal and cutaneous, not renal or neurologic

- ■ Differential Diagnosis
  - • Rheumatoid arthritis
  - • Vasculitis
  - • Sjögren's syndrome
  - • Systemic sclerosis
  - • Endocarditis
  - • Lymphoma
  - • Glomerulonephritis due to other cause

- ■ Treatment
  - • Mild disease (ie, arthralgias with dermatologic findings) often responds to hydroxychloroquine and NSAIDs
  - • Moderate disease activity (ie, refractory to antimalarials): Corticosteroids and azathioprine, methotrexate, or mycophenolate mofetil
  - • Corticosteroids and cyclophosphamide for lupus cerebritis and lupus nephritis
  - • Avoid sun exposure

- ■ Pearl

A lupus "anticoagulant" is in fact associated with hypercoagulability; it is an antibody to phospholipid, which produces in vitro prolongation of the PTT in many cases.

Reference

Francis L, Perl A. Pharmacotherapy of systemic lupus erythematosus. Expert Opin Pharmacother 2009;10:1481. [PMID: 19505215]

Systemic Sclerosis (Scleroderma)

- **Essentials of Diagnosis**
  - Diffuse systemic sclerosis (20%): Proximal skin thickening; interstitial lung disease; greater risk of hypertensive renal crisis
  - Limited disease (80%) or CREST syndrome (calcinosis cutis, Raynaud's phenomenon, esophageal hypomotility, sclerodactyly, and telangiectasia): Skin tightening in distal extremities and feet; lower risk of renal disease; more commonly develop pulmonary hypertension and biliary cirrhosis
  - For both forms, Raynaud's phenomenon present at time of diagnosis 85% of the time; if severe can lead to acral ulceration
  - ANA abnormal 60% of cases; anticentromere antibody positive in 1% of patients with diffuse scleroderma and 50% of those with limited form; antitopoisomerase I (Scl-70) in one-third of patients with diffuse systemic sclerosis and 20% of those with limited form and a poor prognostic factor

- **Differential Diagnosis**
  - Eosinophilic fasciitis
  - Graft-versus-host disease
  - Amyloidosis; Raynaud's disease

- **Treatment**
  - Focus on symptomatic relief as no effective disease modifiers exist
  - Angiotensin-converting enzyme blockers to treat hypertensive crisis when seen in patients with diffuse systemic sclerosis
  - Corticosteroids not helpful and may even precipitate renal crisis; penicillamine also not helpful
  - Cyclophosphamide may provide benefit in those with interstitial lung disease
  - Warm clothing, smoking cessation, and extended-release calcium channel blockers for Raynaud's phenomenon; intravenous iloprost may be helpful for digital ulcers
  - H_2-receptor antagonists or omeprazole for esophageal reflux, which can be highly morbid

- **Pearl**

  Malabsorption in systemic sclerosis is due to bacterial overgrowth, not intestinal fibrosis; hypomotility causes it.

Reference
Hachulla E, Launay D. Diagnosis and classification of systemic sclerosis. Clin Rev Allergy Immunol 2010 Feb 10 [epub ahead of print]. [PMID: 20143182]

Takayasu's Arteritis ("Pulseless Disease")

- **Essentials of Diagnosis**
  - Large vessel vasculitis involving the aortic arch and its major branches
  - Seen most commonly in the third to fifth decade of life with predominance in women
  - Associated most commonly with absent peripheral pulses; may see myalgias, arthralgias, headaches, angina, claudication, erythema nodosum–like lesions, hypertension, bruits, cerebrovascular insufficiency, aortic insufficiency
  - Angiography reveals narrowing, stenosis, and aneurysms of the aortic arch and its major branches
  - Bruits may be heard over the subclavian arteries or aorta in up to 40% of patients; additionally, there may be a > 10 mm Hg difference in systolic blood pressure in the two arms
  - Rich collateral flow visible in the shoulder, chest, and neck areas

- **Differential Diagnosis**
  - Giant cell arteritis
  - Syphilitic aortitis
  - Severe atherosclerosis

- **Treatment**
  - Corticosteroids
  - Cyclophosphamide or methotrexate added for severe disease
  - Surgical bypass or reconstruction of affected vessels

- **Pearl**

A three-phase illness: nonspecific systemic symptoms, early signs of arterial insufficiency, and intense fibrosis of evolved arteries.

Reference

Ogino H, Matsuda H, Minatoya K, et al. Overview of late outcome of medical and surgical treatment for Takayasu arteritis. Circulation 2008;118:2738. [PMID: 19106398]

Thromboangiitis Obliterans (Buerger's Disease)

- ■ Essentials of Diagnosis
  - • Inflammatory disease involving small- and medium-sized arteries and veins of the distal upper and lower extremities
  - • Described first in young men who were heavy cigarette smokers, but since observed in men and women alike of any age
  - • Associated with migratory superficial segmental thrombophlebitis of superficial veins, absent peripheral pulses, claudication, numbness, paresthesias, Raynaud's phenomenon, ulceration and gangrene of fingertips and toes
  - • Angiography reveals multiple occluded segments in the small- and medium-sized arteries of the arms and legs

- ■ Differential Diagnosis
  - • Atherosclerosis
  - • Raynaud's disease
  - • Livedo reticularis due to other cause
  - • Antiphospholipid antibody syndrome
  - • Cholesterol atheroembolic disease
  - • Limited systemic sclerosis

- ■ Treatment
  - • Smoking cessation is essential
  - • Warm clothing, nifedipine for Raynaud's phenomenon
  - • Surgical sympathectomy of some value
  - • Amputation required in some, though surgery often begets more surgery as wounds heal poorly with diminished perfusion

- ■ Pearl

A notable decline of this condition has been observed in recent years, likely a result of efforts at smoking cessation.

Reference

Paraskevas KI, Liapis CD, Briana DD, Mikhailidis DP. Thromboangiitis obliterans (Buerger's disease): searching for a therapeutic strategy. Angiology 2007;58:75. [PMID: 17351161]

Wegener's Granulomatosis

- ■ Essentials of Diagnosis
  - Vasculitis associated with glomerulonephritis and necrotizing granulomas of upper and lower respiratory tracts
  - Slight male predominance with peak incidence in fourth and fifth decades
  - Ninety percent present with upper or lower respiratory tract symptoms, including perforation of nasal septum, chronic sinusitis, otitis media, mastoiditis, cough, dyspnea, hemoptysis
  - Proptosis, scleritis, arthritis, purpura, or neuropathy (mononeuritis multiplex) may also be present
  - Cytoplasmic ANCA (C-ANCA) in 90% correlates with anti–proteinase 3 antibodies
  - Biopsy in the correct clinical setting yields the diagnosis: Sinus, nonspecific; lung, granulomatous necrotizing vasculitis; renal, focal glomerulonephritis
  - Eosinophilia not a feature
  - Chest film may reveal large nodular densities; urinalysis may show hematuria, red cell casts; CT scans of sinuses may reveal bony erosion

- ■ Differential Diagnosis
  - Polyarteritis nodosa
  - Churg-Strauss vasculitis
  - Goodpasture's syndrome
  - Takayasu's arteritis
  - Microscopic polyarteritis
  - Lymphomatoid granulomatosis
  - Lymphoproliferative disorders (especially angiocentric T-cell lymphoma)
  - Heavy intranasal cocaine use

- ■ Treatment
  - Corticosteroids
  - Primarily oral cyclophosphamide or methotrexate; chronic cyclophosphamide therapy predisposes to bladder cancer, and therefore significant fluid intake during therapy to irrigate the bladder is important
  - Trimethoprim-sulfamethoxazole effective in mild disease; given to all patients not allergic to sulfonamides

- ■ Pearl

In only 10% of renal biopsies does one see a granulomatous vasculitis; in the rest, the glomerulonephritis noted is not specific for Wegener's.

Reference

Seo P. Wegener's granulomatosis: managing more than inflammation. Curr Opin Rheumatol 2008;20:10. [PMID: 18281851]

7

Endocrine Disorders

Acromegaly

- **Essentials of Diagnosis**
  - Excessive growth of hands (increased glove size), feet (increased shoe size), jaw (protrusion), face, and tongue; coarse facial features; deep voice
  - Headache, visual field defects, amenorrhea, diminished libido, excessive sweating
  - Hyperglycemia, hypogonadotropic hypogonadism
  - Elevated serum insulin-like growth factor-1
  - Growth hormone levels do not suppress with an oral glucose load
  - Enlarged sella, thickened skull; MRI demonstrates a pituitary tumor in most cases

- **Differential Diagnosis**
  - Physiologic growth spurt
  - Familial coarse features
  - Myxedema

- **Treatment**
  - Transsphenoidal resection of adenoma is successful in many patients, medical therapy is necessary for those with residual disease
  - The majority of patients respond to treatment with somatostatin analogues (eg, octreotide or lanreotide) or growth hormone receptor antagonist (eg, pegvisomant)
  - Pituitary irradiation may be necessary if patients are not cured by surgical and medical therapy
  - Hormone replacement for residual panhypopituitarism

- **Pearl**

The only noninvasive biopsy in medicine may make the diagnosis; the "wallet biopsy" will likely reveal an older photograph of the patient on his driver's license.

Reference

Giustina A, Barkan A, Chanson P, et al; Pituitary Society; European Neuroendocrine Association. Guidelines for the treatment of growth hormone excess and growth hormone deficiency in adults. J Endocrinol Invest 2008;31:820. [PMID: 18997495]

Adult Hypothyroidism and Myxedema

■ Essentials of Diagnosis

- Fatigue, cold intolerance, constipation, muscle cramps, weight gain, depression, altered mentation, menstrual irregularity
- Hypothermia, bradycardia, dry skin with yellow tone (carotenemia); nonpitting edema, macroglossia, delayed relaxation of deep tendon reflexes
- Low serum free thyroxine (FT_4); thyroid-stimulating hormone (TSH) elevated in primary hypothyroidism; anemia, hypercholesterolemia
- Myxedema coma may be associated with obtundation, profound hypothermia, hypoventilation, hypotension, striking bradycardia; pleural and pericardial effusions
- Associated with other autoimmune endocrinopathies

■ Differential Diagnosis

- Chronic fatigue syndrome
- Congestive heart failure
- Primary amyloidosis
- Depression
- Exposure hypothermia
- Parkinson's disease

■ Treatment

- Levothyroxine replacement starting with low doses and increasing gradually until euthyroid
- Treat myxedema coma with intravenous levothyroxine; if adrenal insufficiency is suspected, add intravenous hydrocortisone

■ Pearl

Myxedema masks the commonly associated Addison's disease; add steroids to thyroid hormone until adrenal cortical insufficiency is excluded.

Reference

Vaidya B, Pearce SH. Management of hypothyroidism in adults. BMJ 2008;337:a801. [PMID: 18662921]

Diabetes Insipidus

■ Essentials of Diagnosis

- Polyuria with volumes of 2–20 L/d, nocturia; polydipsia, intense thirst
- Serum osmolality > urine osmolality
- Low urine-specific gravity with inappropriate urinary fluid loss
- Inability to concentrate urine with fluid restriction, resulting in hypernatremia
- Central diabetes insipidus (vasopressin-deficient) caused by hypothalamic or pituitary disease
- Nephrogenic diabetes insipidus (vasopressin-resistant) may be familial or caused by lithium, chronic renal disease, hypokalemia, hypercalcemia, demeclocycline
- Vasopressin challenge establishes central cause

■ Differential Diagnosis

- Psychogenic polydipsia
- Osmotic diuresis
- Diabetes mellitus
- Beer potomania

■ Treatment

- Ensure adequate free water intake
- Intranasal or oral desmopressin acetate for central diabetes insipidus
- Hydrochlorothiazide or indomethacin for nephrogenic diabetes insipidus

■ Pearl

Tetracycline can cause mild nephrogenic diabetes insipidus which is permanent; inquire about remote use for teenage acne.

Reference

Behan LA, Phillips J, Thompson CJ, Agha A. Neuroendocrine disorders after traumatic brain injury. J Neurol Neurosurg Psychiatry 2008;79:753. [PMID: 18559460]

Diabetic Ketoacidosis

■ Essentials of Diagnosis

- Polyuria and polydipsia, marked fatigue, nausea and vomiting, abdominal pain
- Fruity breath, Kussmaul's respirations; dehydration, hypotension, if severe volume depletion occurs; coma
- Hyperglycemia > 250 mg/dL, ketonemia, anion gap metabolic acidosis with blood pH < 7.3 and serum bicarbonate typically < 15 mEq/L; glycosuria and ketonuria; total body potassium depleted despite elevation in serum potassium
- Due to insulin deficiency or increased insulin requirements in a patient with type 1 diabetes (eg, in association with myocardial ischemia, surgery, infection, gastroenteritis, intra-abdominal disease, or medical noncompliance)

■ Differential Diagnosis

- Alcoholic ketoacidosis
- Uremia
- Lactic acidosis
- Sepsis

■ Treatment

- Intravenous regular insulin replacement with careful laboratory monitoring
- Aggressive volume resuscitation with saline; dextrose should be added to intravenous fluids once glucose reaches 250–300 mg/dL
- Potassium, magnesium, and phosphate replacement
- Identify and treat precipitating cause

■ Pearl

Take the low pH and hyperkalemia seriously, but remember that hyperosmolality is a worse prognostic sign.

Reference

Solá E, Garzón S, García-Torres S, Cubells P, Morillas C, Hernández-Mijares A. Management of diabetic ketoacidosis in a teaching hospital. Acta Diabetol 2006;43:127. [PMID: 17211563]

Gynecomastia

- ### Essentials of Diagnosis
  - Glandular enlargement of the male breast
  - Often asymmetric or unilateral and may be tender
  - Common in puberty and among elderly men
  - In questionable cases, gynecomastia can be confirmed by mammography or ultrasound
  - Multiple causes include obesity, chronic liver disease, hypogonadism, Klinefelter's syndrome, androgen resistance, adrenal tumors, testicular tumors and those producing human chorionic gonadotropin (hCG), hyperthyroidism, and drugs (eg, estrogens, phytoestrogens, spironolactone, flutamide, ketoconazole, cimetidine, diazepam, digoxin, tricyclic antidepressants, isoniazid, alcohol, marijuana, heroin)

- ### Differential Diagnosis
  - Associations noted above
  - Benign or malignant tumors of the breast
  - Pseudogynecomastia due to increased adiposity

- ### Treatment
  - Careful testicular examination; measurement of liver and thyroid function as well as hCG, luteinizing hormone (LH), testosterone, and estradiol to determine underlying disorder
  - Remove offending drug or treat underlying condition; reassurance if idiopathic
  - Consider needle biopsy of suspicious areas of breast enlargement
  - Consider surgical correction for severe cases

- ### Pearl

One percent of breast cancer occurs in men; although its biologic traits are similar to this disorder in women, there is commonly a delay in diagnosis and a poorer prognosis because of it.

Reference

Johnson RE, Murad MH. Gynecomastia: pathophysiology, evaluation, and management. Mayo Clin Proc 2009;84:1010. [PMID: 19880691]

Hirsutism and Virilizing Diseases of Women

- ■ Essentials of Diagnosis
  - Oligo/amenorrhea, hirsutism, acne
  - Virilization may occur; increased muscularity, temporal balding, deepening of voice, clitoral enlargement, male escutcheon
  - Occasionally a pelvic mass is palpable if due to ovarian tumor
  - Serum testosterone and androstenedione often elevated; serum dehydroepiandrosterone sulfate elevated in adrenal disorders
  - May be due to polycystic ovary syndrome, congenital adrenal hyperplasia, ovarian or adrenal tumors, adrenocorticotropic hormone (ACTH)–dependent Cushing's syndrome

- ■ Differential Diagnosis
  - Familial, idiopathic, or drug-related hirsutism
  - Cushing's syndrome
  - Exogenous androgen ingestion

- ■ Treatment
  - Surgical removal of ovarian or adrenal tumor if present
  - Oral contraceptives to suppress ovarian androgen excess and normalize menses
  - Glucocorticoids for congenital adrenal hyperplasia
  - Spironolactone or cyproterone acetate to ameliorate hirsutism; finasteride and flutamide may help in refractory cases
  - Consider metformin for women with polycystic ovary syndrome

- ■ Pearl

Be sure to check the prescription drug history before expensive endocrinological testing; it may be the cause, and the condition may be reversible.

Reference

Costello MF, Shrestha B, Eden J, Johnson NP, Sjoblom P. Metformin versus oral contraceptive pill in polycystic ovary syndrome: a Cochrane review. Hum Reprod 2007;22:1200. [PMID: 17261574]

Hypercortisolism (Cushing's Syndrome)

■ Essentials of Diagnosis

- Weakness, muscle wasting, weight gain, central obesity, psychosis, hirsutism, acne, menstrual irregularity, hypogonadism
- Moon facies, buffalo hump, thin skin, easy bruisability, purple striae, poor wound healing, hypertension, osteoporosis
- Hyperglycemia, glycosuria, leukocytosis; may have hypokalemia with ectopic ACTH secretion
- Elevated plasma cortisol and urinary free cortisol; failure to suppress plasma cortisol with exogenous dexamethasone (overnight low-dose dexamethasone test)
- A normal or high ACTH level indicates ACTH-dependent Cushing's disease (pituitary adenoma or ectopic ACTH syndrome); a low ACTH level indicates adrenal tumor; imaging studies should be targeted accordingly
- Adrenal CT will reveal adrenal tumor if present
- Obtain pituitary MRI for ACTH-dependent Cushing's, followed by petrosal sinus sampling for ACTH if MRI is negative or equivocal

■ Differential Diagnosis

- Chronic alcoholism
- Depression
- Diabetes mellitus
- Exogenous glucocorticoid administration
- Severe obesity

■ Treatment

- Transsphenoidal resection of pituitary adenoma if present; radiation therapy for residual disease
- Resection of adrenal tumor if present
- Resection of ectopic ACTH-producing tumor if able to localize (eg, carcinoid, small-cell carcinoma of the lung)
- Ketoconazole or metyrapone to suppress cortisol in unresectable cases
- Bilateral adrenalectomy for adrenal hyperplasia in refractory cases of ACTH-dependent Cushing's syndrome

■ Pearl

A disease of women in its classical iteration; elevated cortisol in men constitutes 10% of classic Cushing's, a rare disease to begin with.

Reference

Boscaro M, Arnaldi G. Approach to the patient with possible Cushing's syndrome. J Clin Endocrinol Metab 2009;94:3121. [PMID: 19734443]

Hyperosmotic Nonketotic Diabetic Coma

- **Essentials of Diagnosis**
  - Gradual onset of polyuria, polydipsia, dehydration, and weakness; in severe cases, may progress to obtundation and coma
  - Occurs in patients with type 2 diabetes, typically in elderly patients with reduced fluid intake or precipitating factors
  - Profound hyperglycemia (> 600 mg/dL), hyperosmolality (> 310 mOsm/kg); pH > 7.3, serum bicarbonate > 15 mEq/L; ketosis and acidosis are usually absent

- **Differential Diagnosis**
  - Cerebrovascular accident or head trauma
  - Diabetes insipidus
  - Hypoglycemia
  - Hyperglycemia

- **Treatment**
  - Aggressive volume resuscitation with normal saline until patient is euvolemic, then with hypotonic saline
  - Initial intravenous regular insulin followed by subcutaneous insulin
  - Careful monitoring of serum sodium, osmolality, and glucose
  - Dextrose-containing fluids when glucose is 250–300 mg/dL
  - Potassium and phosphate replacement as needed

- **Pearl**

As in diabetic ketoacidosis, osmolality is the best predictor of outcome; the prognosis is worse than that of ketoacidosis, as patients seek medical care early because of the hyperventilation of acidemia.

Reference

Scott A. Hyperosmolar hyperglycaemic syndrome. Diabet Med 2006;23(suppl):22. [PMID: 16805880]

Hyperprolactinemia

■ Essentials of Diagnosis

- Women: Menstrual disturbance (oligomenorrhea, amenorrhea), galactorrhea, infertility
- Men: Hypogonadism; decreased libido and erectile dysfunction; galactorrhea; infertility
- May be caused by primary hypothyroidism or dopamine antagonist drugs
- Serum prolactin > 100 ng/mL usually suggests a prolactin-secreting pituitary adenoma
- Pituitary adenoma often demonstrated by MRI

7

■ Differential Diagnosis

- Primary hypothyroidism
- Use of prolactin-stimulating drugs (eg, certain antipsychotic drugs)
- Pregnancy or lactation
- Hypothalamic disease
- Cirrhosis; renal failure
- Chronic nipple stimulation; chest wall injury

■ Treatment

- Dopamine agonists (eg, bromocriptine or cabergoline) usually shrink pituitary adenoma and restore fertility
- Transsphenoidal resection for large pituitary tumors refractory to dopamine agonists

■ Pearl

In patients with suspected prolactinoma, ask about visits to a mental health provider; most psychotropic agents cause hyperprolactinemia.

Reference

Prabhakar VK, Davis JR. Hyperprolactinaemia. Best Pract Res Clin Obstet Gynaecol 2008;22:341. [PMID: 17889620]

Hyperthyroidism

■ Essentials of Diagnosis

- Sweating, weight loss, heat intolerance, irritability, weakness, increased number of bowel movements, menstrual irregularity
- Sinus tachycardia or atrial fibrillation, tremor, warm moist skin, eye findings (stare, lid lag); diffuse goiter, thyroid bruit and exophthalmos in Graves' disease
- Serum FT_4 and FT_3 increased; TSH low or undetectable
- Radioiodine uptake scan will differentiate Graves' disease, toxic nodule, and thyroiditis; may also be useful in identifying rare ectopic thyroid tissue (ovarian teratoma)
- Thyroid-stimulating immunoglobulin and thyroid autoantibodies are often positive in Graves' disease

■ Differential Diagnosis

- Anxiety, neurosis, or mania
- Pheochromocytoma
- Exogenous thyroid administration
- Catabolic illness
- Chronic alcoholism

■ Treatment

- Supportive care for patients with thyroiditis
- Propranolol for symptomatic relief of catecholamine-mediated symptoms
- Antithyroid drugs (methimazole or propylthiouracil) for patients with Graves' disease; chance of remission greater for milder cases/smaller goiters, whereas more severe cases may eventually require radioactive iodine treatment
- Radioactive iodine ablation provides definitive therapy and is indicated for refractory Graves' disease and in patients with toxic nodular disease; in older patients or those with severe hyperthyroidism, treat first with antithyroid drugs
- Subtotal thyroidectomy for failure of medical therapy if radioactive iodine is contraindicated (eg, pregnancy) or for very large nodular goiters; euthyroid state should be achieved medically before surgery

■ Pearl

In patients older than 60, when you think hyperthyroidism, it's usually hypothyroidism, and when you think hypothyroidism, it's usually hyperthyroidism; the diseases become increasingly atypical with age.

Reference

Brent GA. Clinical practice. Graves' disease. N Engl J Med 2008;358:2594. [PMID: 18550875]

Hypoglycemia in the Adult

- **Essentials of Diagnosis**
  - Blurred vision, diplopia, headache, slurred speech, weakness, sweating, palpitations, tremulousness, altered mentation; focal neurologic signs common
  - Plasma glucose < 40 mg/dL
  - Causes include alcoholism, postprandial hypoglycemia (eg, post-gastrectomy), insulinoma, medications (insulin, sulfonylureas, pentamidine), adrenal insufficiency

- **Differential Diagnosis**
  - Central nervous system disease
  - Hypoxia
  - Psychoneurosis
  - Pheochromocytoma

- **Treatment**
  - Intravenous glucose (oral glucose for patients who are conscious and able to swallow)
  - Intramuscular glucagon if no intravenous access available
  - Diagnosis and treatment of underlying disease (eg, insulinoma) or removal of offending agent (eg, alcohol, sulfonylureas)
  - For patients with postprandial (reactive) hypoglycemia, eating small frequent meals with reduced proportion of carbohydrates may help

- **Pearl**

In alcoholic hypoglycemia, blood glucose determinations as low as 6 have been reported; symptoms are atypical, because rate of glucose fall is slower than that produced by insulin.

Reference

Murad MH, Coto-Yglesias F, Wang AT, et al. Clinical review: drug-induced hypoglycemia: a systematic review. J Clin Endocrinol Metab 2009;94:741. [PMID: 19088166]

Hypoparathyroidism

- **Essentials of Diagnosis**
  - Tetany, carpopedal spasms, tingling of lips and hands; altered mentation
  - Positive Chvostek's sign (facial muscle contraction on tapping the facial nerve) and Trousseau's phenomenon (carpal spasm after application of arm cuff); dry skin and brittle nails; cataracts
  - Serum calcium low; serum phosphate high; serum parathyroid hormone low to absent
  - Long ST segment resulting in long QT interval on ECG
  - History of previous thyroidectomy or neck surgery in patients with surgical hypoparathyroidism

- **Differential Diagnosis**
  - Pseudohypoparathyroidism
  - Vitamin D deficiency syndromes
  - Acute pancreatitis
  - Hypomagnesemia
  - Chronic renal failure
  - Hypoalbuminemia

- **Treatment**
  - For acute tetany, intravenous calcium gluconate, followed by oral calcium and vitamin D derivatives
  - Correct concurrent hypomagnesemia
  - Chronic therapy includes high-calcium diet in addition to calcium and vitamin D supplements
  - Avoid phenothiazines (prolonged QT interval) and furosemide (increases calciuria)

- **Pearl**

Radiotherapy causes hypothyroidism, but almost never hypoparathyroidism; parathyroids are among the most resistant tissues in the body to radiation injury.

Reference

Shoback D. Clinical practice. Hypoparathyroidism. N Engl J Med 2008;359:391. [PMID: 18650515]

Male Hypogonadism

■ Essentials of Diagnosis
- Diminished libido and impotence
- Sparse growth of male body hair
- Testes may be small or normal in size; serum testosterone is usually decreased
- Serum gonadotropins (LH and follicle-stimulating hormone [FSH]) are decreased in hypogonadotropic hypogonadism; they are increased in primary testicular failure (hypergonadotropic hypogonadism)
- Causes of hypogonadotropic hypogonadism include chronic illness, malnutrition, drugs, pituitary tumor, Cushing's syndrome, hyperprolactinemia, congenital syndromes (eg, Kallmann's syndrome)
- Causes of hypergonadotropic hypogonadism include Klinefelter's syndrome, anorchia or cryptorchidism, testicular trauma, orchitis, hemochromatosis, gonadal dysgenesis, and defects in testosterone biosynthesis

■ Differential Diagnosis
- Conditions noted above
- Androgen insensitivity
- Neurogenic or vascular erectile dysfunction
- Hypothyroidism

■ Treatment
- Evaluate and treat underlying disorder
- Testosterone replacement (intramuscular or transdermal)

■ Pearl

A reason to check the first cranial nerve; anosmia is a feature of Kallman's syndrome.

Reference

Theodoraki A, Bouloux PM. Testosterone therapy in men. Menopause Int 2009;15:87. [PMID: 19465676]

Osteoporosis

- **Essentials of Diagnosis**
  - Asymptomatic or associated with back pain from vertebral fractures; loss of height; kyphosis
  - Demineralization of spine, hip, and pelvis by radiograph; vertebral compression fractures often discovered incidentally
  - Bone mineral density at or more than 2.5 SD below the average value for a young adult

- **Differential Diagnosis**
  - Osteomalacia
  - Multiple myeloma
  - Metastatic carcinoma
  - Hypophosphatemic disorders
  - Osteogenesis imperfecta
  - Secondary osteoporosis due to glucocorticoids, hyperthyroidism, hypogonadism, alcoholism, renal or liver disease

- **Treatment**
  - Diet adequate in calcium and vitamin D with supplements to achieve 1200–1500 mg elemental calcium and at least 800–1000 IU vitamin D daily
  - Regular exercise
  - Fall prevention strategies
  - Effective antiresorptive therapies include bisphosphonates (eg, alendronate, risedronate, ibandronate, zoledronic acid), selective estrogen receptor modulators (SERMs; eg, raloxifene), and calcitonin
  - Effective anabolic therapy includes recombinant parathyroid hormone (eg, teriparatide)
  - Men with hypogonadism are treated with testosterone

- **Pearl**

Easily the most debilitating nonmalignant disease of bone.

Reference

Rahmani P, Morin S. Prevention of osteoporosis-related fractures among postmenopausal women and older men. CMAJ 2009;181:815. [PMID: 19841053]

Paget's Disease (Osteitis Deformans)

- **Essentials of Diagnosis**
  - Often asymptomatic or associated with bone pain, fractures, and bone deformity (bowing, kyphosis)
  - Serum calcium and phosphate normal; alkaline phosphatase elevated; urinary hydroxyproline elevated
  - Dense, expanded bones on x-ray resulting from accelerated bone turnover and disruption of normal architecture; osteolytic lesions in the skull and extremities; vertebral fractures; fissure fractures in the long bones
  - May have neurologic sequelae due to nerve compression as pagetic bones enlarge (eg, deafness)

- **Differential Diagnosis**
  - Osteogenic sarcoma
  - Multiple myeloma
  - Fibrous dysplasia
  - Metastatic carcinoma
  - Osteitis fibrosa cystica (hyperparathyroidism)

- **Treatment**
  - No treatment for asymptomatic patients
  - Treat symptomatic disease with inhibitors of osteoclastic resorption (bisphosphonates or calcitonin)
  - The role of prophylactic treatment to prevent bone deformities or neurologic sequelae is not well established

- **Pearl**

  Was Paget's disease the cause of Beethoven's deafness? Only his pictures suggest it, as no alkaline phosphatase determinations were available between 1770 and 1828.

Reference

Ralston SH, Langston AL, Reid IR. Pathogenesis and management of Paget's disease of bone. Lancet 2008;372:155. [PMID: 18620951]

Panhypopituitarism

■ Essentials of Diagnosis

- Sexual dysfunction, weakness, easy fatigability; poor resistance to stress, cold, or fasting; axillary and pubic hair loss
- Hypotension, often orthostatic; visual field defects if pituitary tumor present
- Deficient cortisol response to ACTH; low serum T_4 with low or low-normal TSH; serum prolactin level may be elevated
- Low serum testosterone in men; amenorrhea; FSH and LH are low or low-normal
- MRI may reveal a pituitary or hypothalamic lesion

■ Differential Diagnosis

- Anorexia nervosa or severe malnutrition
- Hypothyroidism
- Addison's disease
- Cachexia due to other causes (eg, carcinoma or tuberculosis)
- Empty sella syndrome

■ Treatment

- Surgical removal of pituitary tumor if present and indicated; pituitary irradiation may be necessary for residual invasive tumor but increases likelihood of permanent hypopituitarism
- Lifelong endocrine replacement therapy with corticosteroids, thyroid hormone, sex hormones, and in some instances, growth hormone

■ Pearl

When you suspect this in a woman, ask about a complicated delivery in the past; hypopituitarism results from the hypotension of postpartum bleeding, causing pituitary apoplexy.

Reference

Filipsson H, Johannsson G. GH replacement in adults: interactions with other pituitary hormone deficiencies and replacement therapies. Eur J Endocrinol 2009;161(suppl):S85. [PMID: 19684055]

Pheochromocytoma

■ Essentials of Diagnosis

- Paroxysmal or sustained hypertension; postural hypotension
- Episodes of palpitations, perspiration, and headache; anxiety, nausea, chest or abdominal pain, pallor
- Hypermetabolism with normal thyroid tests; mild hyperglycemia may be present
- Elevated urinary catecholamines, metanephrines, and vanillyl-mandelic acid are diagnostic; elevated plasma free metanephrines helpful in high-risk subgroups
- CT or MRI can confirm and localize pheochromocytoma; metaiodobenzylguanidine (MIBG) scan may help to localize tumors

■ Differential Diagnosis

- Essential hypertension
- Thyrotoxicosis
- Panic attacks
- Acute intermittent porphyria

■ Treatment

- Surgical removal of tumor or tumors
- Alpha blockade with phenoxybenzamine before surgery
- Beta-adrenergic receptor blockade can be added after effective alpha blockade to help control tachycardia
- Adequate volume replenishment mandatory before surgery
- Long-term alpha blockade for symptomatic treatment in patients with inoperable tumors; metastatic pheochromocytoma may be treated with chemotherapy or ^{131}I-MIBG

■ Pearl

Rule of tens: 10% bilateral, 10% malignant, 10% extra-adrenal, 10% familial, and 10% normotensive.

Reference

Karagiannis A, Mikhailidis DP, Athyros VG, Harsoulis F. Pheochromocytoma: an update on genetics and management. Endocr Relat Cancer 2007;14:935. [PMID: 18045948]

Primary Adrenal Insufficiency (Addison's Disease)

■ Essentials of Diagnosis

- Weakness, anorexia, weight loss, abdominal pain, nausea and vomiting; increased skin pigmentation
- Hypotension, dehydration; postural symptoms
- Hyponatremia, hyperkalemia, hypoglycemia, lymphocytosis, and eosinophilia; increased serum urea nitrogen and calcium may be present
- Serum cortisol levels low to absent and ACTH elevated; cortisol level fails to rise after cosyntropin (ACTH) stimulation
- Often associated with other autoimmune endocrinopathies; may also be due to trauma, infection (especially tuberculosis, histoplasmosis), adrenal hemorrhage, or adrenoleukodystrophy

■ Differential Diagnosis

- Secondary adrenal insufficiency
- Anorexia nervosa
- Malignancy
- Infection
- Salt-wasting nephropathy
- Hemochromatosis

■ Treatment

- In acute adrenal crisis, treat immediately with intravenous hydrocortisone (100 mg intravenously every 8 hours) once the diagnosis is suspected; provide appropriate volume resuscitation and blood pressure support; consider empiric antibiotics
- In chronic adrenal insufficiency, maintenance therapy includes glucocorticoids (hydrocortisone) and mineralocorticoids (fludrocortisone)
- Increase glucocorticoid dose for trauma, surgery, infection, or stress

■ Pearl

If the systolic blood pressure is over 100, classic Addison's disease is unlikely.

Reference

Vaidya B, Chakera AJ, Dick C. Addison's disease. BMJ 2009;339:b2385. [PMID: 19574315]

Primary Aldosteronism

- **Essentials of Diagnosis**
  - Hypertension, polyuria, fatigue, and weakness
  - Hypokalemia, metabolic alkalosis
  - Elevated plasma and urine aldosterone levels with suppressed plasma renin activity level
  - May be associated with adrenocortical adenoma or bilateral adrenocortical hyperplasia
  - Rarely due to glucocorticoid-remediable aldosteronism
  - Adrenal mass often demonstrated by CT

- **Differential Diagnosis**
  - Essential hypertension
  - Periodic paralysis
  - Congenital adrenal hyperplasia (11- or 17-hydroxylase deficiency)
  - Pseudohyperaldosteronism: Licorice ingestion, Liddle's syndrome
  - Chronic diuretic use or laxative abuse
  - Unilateral renovascular disease
  - Cushing's syndrome

- **Treatment**
  - Surgical resection of unilateral adenoma secreting aldosterone (Conn's syndrome)
  - Medical management with mineralocorticoid antagonist therapy (spironolactone or eplerenone) for hyperaldosteronism due to bilateral adrenal hyperplasia
  - Dexamethasone for glucocorticoid-remediable aldosteronism
  - Antihypertensive therapy as necessary

- **Pearl**

If the sodium is less than 140 mEq/dL and a spot urine potassium is less than 40 mEq/dL, this condition is far less likely.

Reference

Patel SM, Lingam RK, Beaconsfield TI, Tran TL, Brown B. Role of radiology in the management of primary aldosteronism. Radiographics 2007;27:1145. [PMID: 17620472]

Primary Hyperparathyroidism

- ■ Essentials of Diagnosis
  - Renal stones, bone pain, mental status changes, constipation ("stones, bones, moans, and abdominal groans"), polyuria; many patients are asymptomatic
  - Serum and urine calcium elevated; low-normal to low serum phosphate; high-normal or elevated serum parathyroid hormone level; alkaline phosphatase often elevated
  - Bone radiographs show cystic bone lesions (brown tumors) and subperiosteal resorption of cortical bone, especially the phalanges (osteitis fibrosa cystica); may have osteoporosis and pathologic fractures
  - History of renal stones, nephrocalcinosis, recurrent peptic ulcer disease, or recurrent pancreatitis may be present

- ■ Differential Diagnosis
  - Familial hypocalciuric hypercalcemia
  - Hypercalcemia of malignancy
  - Renal failure
  - Vitamin D intoxication or milk-alkali syndrome
  - Sarcoidosis, granulomatous disorders
  - Multiple myeloma

- ■ Treatment
  - Parathyroidectomy for patients with elevated calcium level (> 1.0 mg/dL above normal range), creatinine clearance < 60 mL/min, osteoporosis by bone mineral density or fragility fracture or age < 50 years
  - For patients with mild asymptomatic disease: Maintain adequate fluid intake and avoid immobilization and thiazide diuretics; follow for disease progression

- ■ Pearl

The difficulty in obtaining long-term follow-up of patients with this disorder suggests it is generally—but not always—benign.

Reference

Suliburk JW, Perrier ND. Primary hyperparathyroidism. Oncologist 2007;12:644. [PMID: 17602056]

Simple and Nodular Goiter

- ■ Essentials of Diagnosis
  - Single or multiple thyroid nodules found on thyroid palpation
  - Large multinodular goiters may be associated with compressive symptoms (dysphagia, cough, stridor)
  - Measurement of free thyroxine (FT_4) and TSH; radioiodine uptake scan helpful in selected cases for distinguishing cold from hot nodules

- ■ Differential Diagnosis
  - Graves' disease (diffuse toxic goiter)
  - Autoimmune thyroiditis
  - Carcinoma of the thyroid

- ■ Treatment
  - Fine-needle biopsy for solitary or dominant nodules meeting size or imaging criteria; carcinomas or suspicious cold lesions require surgery
  - Levothyroxine treatment may suppress growth and cause regression in benign nodules or multinodular goiter; contraindicated if TSH is low
  - Surgery for severe compressive symptoms

- ■ Pearl

Pharmacologic amounts of iodine may cause hyperthyroidism in patients with a goiter; inquire about recent diagnostic studies done for other reasons in a newly hyperthyroid patient.

Reference

Albino CC, Graf H, Sampaio AP, Vigário A, Paz-Filho GJ. Thiamazole as an adjuvant to radioiodine for volume reduction of multinodular goiter. Expert Opin Investig Drugs 2008;17:1781. [PMID: 19012495]

Thyroiditis

■ Essentials of Diagnosis

- Painful enlarged thyroid gland in acute and subacute forms; painless enlargement in chronic form
- Generally classified as chronic lymphocytic (Hashimoto's) thyroiditis and subacute (granulomatous) thyroiditis; suppurative thyroiditis and Riedel's thyroiditis are uncommon
- Thyroid function tests variable, with serum T_4 and T_3 levels often transiently high in acute forms and low in chronic disease
- Elevated erythrocyte sedimentation rate and reduced radioiodine uptake in subacute thyroiditis
- Thyroid autoantibodies positive in Hashimoto's thyroiditis

■ Differential Diagnosis

- Endemic goiter
- Graves' disease (diffuse toxic goiter)
- Carcinoma of the thyroid
- Pyogenic infections of the neck

■ Treatment

- Antibiotics for suppurative thyroiditis
- Nonsteroidal anti-inflammatory drugs for subacute thyroiditis; prednisone in severe cases; symptomatic treatment with propranolol
- Levothyroxine replacement for Hashimoto's thyroiditis
- Partial thyroidectomy for local severe pressure or adhesions in Riedel's thyroiditis

■ Pearl

The patient can be hyper-, hypo-, or euthyroid depending on when in the clinical course this is tested.

Reference

Lazúrová I, Benhatchi K, Rovenský J, et al. Autoimmune thyroid disease and autoimmune rheumatic disorders: a two-sided analysis. Ann N Y Acad Sci 2009;1173:211. [PMID: 19758153]

Type 1 Diabetes Mellitus

■ Essentials of Diagnosis

- Crisp onset, no family history
- Polyuria, polydipsia, weight loss
- Fasting plasma glucose $\geq$ 126 mg/dL; random plasma glucose $\geq$ 200 mg/dL with symptoms; glycosuria
- Associated with ketosis in untreated state; may present as medical emergency (diabetic ketoacidosis)
- Long-term risks include retinopathy, nephropathy, neuropathy, and cardiovascular disease

■ Differential Diagnosis

- Nondiabetic glycosuria (eg, Fanconi's syndrome)
- Diabetes insipidus
- Acromegaly
- Cushing's disease or syndrome
- Pheochromocytoma
- Medications (eg, glucocorticoids, niacin)

■ Treatment

- Insulin treatment is required
- Patient education is crucial, emphasizing dietary management, intensive insulin therapy, self-monitoring of blood glucose, hypoglycemia awareness, foot and eye care

■ Pearl

The autoimmune nature of this condition was signaled by a European study years ago showing improvement with immunosuppressives when type 1 diabetes appeared abruptly.

Reference

Isermann B, Ritzel R, Zorn M, Schilling T, Nawroth PP. Autoantibodies in diabetes mellitus: current utility and perspectives. Exp Clin Endocrinol Diabetes 2007;115:483. [PMID: 17853330]

Type 2 Diabetes Mellitus

- **Essentials of Diagnosis**
  - Most patients are older and tend to be obese
  - Gradual onset of polyuria, polydipsia; often asymptomatic
  - Candidal vaginitis in women, chronic skin infection, blurred vision
  - Fasting plasma glucose $\geq$ 126 mg/dL; random plasma glucose $\geq$ 200 mg/dL with symptoms; glycosuria; elevated glycosylated hemoglobin (A_{1c}); ketosis rare
  - Family history often present; frequently associated with hypertension, hyperlipidemia, and atherosclerosis
  - May present as a medical emergency (especially in the elderly) as nonketotic hyperosmolar coma
  - Long-term risks include retinopathy, nephropathy, neuropathy, and cardiovascular disease

- **Differential Diagnosis**
  - Nondiabetic glycosuria (eg, Fanconi's syndrome)
  - Diabetes insipidus
  - Acromegaly
  - Cushing's disease or syndrome
  - Pheochromocytoma
  - Medications (eg, glucocorticoids, niacin)
  - Severe insulin resistance syndromes
  - Altered mental status due to other cause

- **Treatment**
  - Patient education is important, emphasizing dietary management, exercise, weight loss, self-monitoring of blood glucose, hypoglycemia awareness, foot and eye care
  - Mild cases may be controlled initially with diet, exercise, and weight loss
  - Metformin or alternative oral agents if diet is ineffective; insulin may be required if combination oral agents fail

- **Pearl**

When untreated, the weight loss in this condition may seem desirable for some patients, but runs the risk of resulting in hyperosmolar nonketotic coma.

Reference

Rodbard HW, Jellinger PS, Davidson JA, et al. Statement by an American Association of Clinical Endocrinologists/American College of Endocrinology consensus panel on type 2 diabetes mellitus: an algorithm for glycemic control. Endocr Pract 2009;15:540. [PMID: 19858063]

8

Infectious Diseases

BACTERIAL INFECTIONS

Actinomycosis

- **Essentials of Diagnosis**
  - Due to anaerobic gram-positive rod (*Actinomyces* species) part of the normal mouth flora; becomes pathogenic when introduced into traumatized tissue
  - Chronic suppurative lesion of the skin (cervicofacial in 60%) with sinus tract formation; thoracic or abdominal abscesses seen; pelvic disease associated with intrauterine devices
  - Accelerated sedimentation rate; anemia, thrombocytosis
  - Isolation of *Actinomyces* species or sulfur granule from pus by anaerobic culture
  - Sulfur granules show branching, gram-positive filaments on smear

- **Differential Diagnosis**
  - Lung cancer
  - Other causes of cervical adenitis
  - Scrofula
  - Nocardiosis
  - Crohn's disease
  - Pelvic inflammatory disease of other cause

- **Treatment**
  - Long-term penicillin
  - Surgical drainage necessary in selected cases

- **Pearl**

Poor dental hygiene in the face of the above clinical scenario suggests the diagnosis.

Reference

Hall V. Actinomyces—gathering evidence of human colonization and infection. Anaerobe 2008;14:1. [PMID: 18222714]

Anthrax (*Bacillus anthracis*)

■ Essentials of Diagnosis

- History of industrial or agricultural exposure (farmer, veterinarian, tannery or wool worker); a potential agent in biologic warfare and bioterrorism
- Persistent necrotic ulcer on exposed surface
- Regional adenopathy, fever, malaise, headache, nausea and vomiting
- Inhalation of spores causes hemorrhagic mediastinitis as spores are taken up by alveolar macrophages and transported to mediastinal lymph nodes
- Hematologic spread with profound toxicity and cardiovascular collapse may complicate either cutaneous or pulmonary form
- Confirmation of diagnosis by culture or specific fluorescent antibody test, but clinical picture highly suggestive

■ Differential Diagnosis

- Skin lesions: Staphylococcal or streptococcal infection
- Pulmonary disease: Tuberculosis, sarcoidosis, lymphoma with mediastinal adenopathy, plague, tularemia

■ Treatment

- Therapy for postexposure prophylaxis is oral doxycycline or oral ciprofloxacin
- Optimal therapy for confirmed disease due to a susceptible strain is oral or intravenous ciprofloxacin or oral doxycycline
- Mortality rate is high despite proper therapy, especially in pulmonary disease

■ Pearl

Considerable recent interest in anthrax has emerged because of its potential use in germ warfare.

Reference

Frankel AE, Kuo SR, Dostal D, et al. Pathophysiology of anthrax. Front Biosci 2009;14:4516. [PMID: 19273366]

Bacillary Dysentery (Shigellosis)

■ Essentials of Diagnosis

- Fever, malaise, toxicity, diarrhea (typically bloody), cramping, abdominal pain
- Positive fecal leukocytes; organism isolated in stool; in immunosuppressed patients, blood culture often positive

■ Differential Diagnosis

- *Campylobacter* and *Salmonella* infection
- Amebiasis
- Ulcerative colitis
- Viral gastroenteritis
- Food poisoning

■ Treatment

- Supportive care
- Antibiotics determined based on sensitivities of local *Shigella* species; trimethoprim-sulfamethoxazole and ciprofloxacin are the usual drugs of choice, although resistance to these agents is increasing

■ Pearl

The first organism associated with reactive arthritis.

Reference

Ashida H, Ogawa M, Mimuro H, Sasakawa C. Shigella infection of intestinal epithelium and circumvention of the host innate defense system. Curr Top Microbiol Immunol 2009;337:231. [PMID: 19812985]

Botulism (*Clostridium botulinum*)

- **Essentials of Diagnosis**
  - History of recent ingestion of home-canned, smoked, or vacuum-packed foods; intravenous drug users also at risk (see below)
  - Sudden onset of cranial nerve paralysis, diplopia, dry mouth, dysphagia, dysphonia, and progressive muscle weakness
  - Fixed and dilated pupils in 50%
  - In infants: Irritability, weakness, and hypotonicity
  - Demonstration of toxin in serum or food

- **Differential Diagnosis**
  - Bulbar poliomyelitis
  - Myasthenia gravis
  - Posterior cerebral circulation ischemia
  - Tick paralysis
  - Guillain-Barré syndrome or variant
  - Inorganic phosphorus poisoning

8

- **Treatment**
  - Removal of unabsorbed toxin from gut
  - Specific antitoxin
  - Vigilant support, including attention to respiratory function
  - Penicillin for wound botulism

- **Pearl**

Regional outbreaks among intravenous drug users suggest "black tar" heroin is being sold in the area.

Reference

Smith LA. Botulism and vaccines for its prevention. Vaccine 2009;27(suppl):D33. [PMID: 19837283]

Brucellosis (*Brucella* Species)

- **Essentials of Diagnosis**
    - Invariable history of animal exposure (veterinarian, slaughter-house) or ingestion of unpasteurized milk or cheese
    - Vectors are cattle, hogs, and goats
    - Insidious onset of fever, diaphoresis, anorexia, fatigue, headache, back pain
    - Cervical and axillary lymphadenopathy, hepatosplenomegaly
    - Lymphocytosis with normal total white blood cell count; positive blood, cerebrospinal fluid, or bone marrow culture after days to weeks; serologic tests positive in second week of illness; molecular testing also available
    - Osteomyelitis, epididymitis, meningitis, and endocarditis may complicate

- **Differential Diagnosis**
    - Lymphoma
    - Infective endocarditis
    - Tuberculosis
    - Q fever
    - Typhoid fever
    - Tularemia
    - Malaria
    - Other causes of osteomyelitis

- **Treatment**
    - Rifampin and doxycycline required for at least 21 days
    - Prolonged treatment for osteoarticular disease, neurologic involvement, and endocarditis

- **Pearl**

A favorite on the FUO list of clinicians, but the epidemiology must be there to consider it seriously.

Reference

Al-Tawfiq JA. Therapeutic options for human brucellosis. Expert Rev Anti Infect Ther 2008;6:109. [PMID: 18251668]

Campylobacter Enteritis (*Campylobacter jejuni*)

■ Essentials of Diagnosis

- Outbreaks associated with consumption of raw milk
- Fever, abdominal pain, bloody diarrhea
- Fecal leukocytes present; presumptive diagnosis by darkfield or phase contrast microscopy of stool wet mount
- Definitive diagnosis by stool culture

■ Differential Diagnosis

- Shigellosis
- Salmonellosis
- Viral gastroenteritis
- Amebic dysentery
- Food poisoning
- Ulcerative colitis

■ Treatment

- Erythromycin or ciprofloxacin will shorten the duration of illness by approximately 1 day, although quinolone resistance is increasing
- Disease is self-limited but can be severe; antimicrobial therapy recommended only for immunocompromised or severely ill patients

■ Pearl

Although it is uncommon to isolate a bacterium in dysentery, this one is found most often; still, it accounts for less than 5% of all dysentery.

Reference

Young KT, Davis LM, Dirita VJ. *Campylobacter jejuni*: molecular biology and pathogenesis. Nat Rev Microbiol 2007;5:665. [PMID: 17703225]

Cat-Scratch Disease (*Bartonella henselae*)

- ### Essentials of Diagnosis
  - History of cat scratch or contact with cats; may be forgotten by patient
  - Primary lesion (papule, pustule, conjunctivitis) at site of inoculation in one-third of cases
  - One to three weeks after scratch: fever, malaise, and headache accompanied by regional lymphadenopathy
  - Sterile pus from node aspirate
  - Biopsy consistent with cat-scratch disease showing necrotizing lymphadenitis; positive serology for bacteria; molecular testing also available
  - Bacillary angiomatosis and peliosis hepatis in immunosuppressed patients

- ### Differential Diagnosis
  - Lymphadenitis due to other bacterial infections
  - Lymphoma
  - Tuberculosis
  - Toxoplasmosis
  - Kikuchi's disease

- ### Treatment
  - Nonspecific; exclusion of similar diseases most important
  - Erythromycin in immunocompromised patients

- ### Pearl

The involved vector is usually an asymptomatic kitten adopted from an animal shelter; such animals, when blood cultured, have enormous organism burdens.

Reference

Florin TA, Zaoutis TE, Zaoutis LB. Beyond cat scratch disease: widening spectrum of *Bartonella henselae* infection. Pediatrics 2008;121:e1413. [PMID: 18443019]

Chancroid (*Haemophilus ducreyi*)

- ### Essentials of Diagnosis

  - A sexually transmitted disease with an incubation period of 3–5 days
  - Painful, tender genital ulcer
  - Inguinal adenitis with erythema or fluctuance and multiple genital ulcers often develop
  - Balanitis, phimosis frequent complications
  - Some women have no external signs of infection

- ### Differential Diagnosis

  - Behçet's syndrome
  - Syphilis
  - Pyogenic infection of lower extremity with regional lymphadenitis
  - Genital ulcers of other cause

- ### Treatment

  - Appropriate antibiotic (azithromycin, ceftriaxone, or ciprofloxacin)
  - Rapid plasma reagin (RPR) for all, HIV when appropriate

- ### Pearl

Tender (inguinal) lymphadenopathy in overweight patients may not be lymph nodes at all; an incarcerated femoral hernia may be the problem.

Reference

Rosen T, Vandergriff T, Harting M. Antibiotic use in sexually transmissible diseases. Dermatol Clin 2009;27:49. [PMID: 18984368]

Cholera (*Vibrio cholerae*)

- ■ Essentials of Diagnosis
  - Acute diarrheal illness leading to profound hypovolemia and death if not addressed promptly
  - History of travel to endemic area or contact with infected person
  - Occurs in epidemics under conditions of crowding and famine; acquired via ingestion of contaminated food or water
  - Sudden onset of frequent, high-volume diarrhea
  - Liquid ("rice water") stool is gray, turbid
  - Rapid development of hypotension, marked dehydration, acidosis, and hypokalemia
  - Positive stool culture confirmatory; serologic testing useful after first week

- ■ Differential Diagnosis
  - Other small intestinal diarrheal illness (eg, salmonellosis, enterotoxigenic *E. coli*)
  - Viral gastroenteritis
  - Vasoactive intestinal peptide (VIP)–producing pancreatic tumor (pancreatic cholera)

- ■ Treatment
  - Vaccine less than 50% effective and is no longer recommended for travelers
  - Rapid replacement of fluid and electrolytes, especially potassium; can be done either orally or intravenously
  - Cola beverages inhibit cyclic adenosine monophosphate (cAMP) and reduce diarrhea, adjunctive to standard volume repletion
  - Tetracycline and many other antibiotics may shorten duration of *Vibrio* excretion

- ■ Pearl

Deaths in epidemics do not come from toxicity, but rather from the effects of severe dehydration, including hyperviscosity and venous thrombosis.

Reference

Nelson EJ, Harris JB, Morris JG Jr, Calderwood SB, Camilli A. Cholera transmission: the host, pathogen and bacteriophage dynamic. Nat Rev Microbiol 2009;7:693. [PMID: 19756008]

Clostridial Myonecrosis (Gas Gangrene)

- **Essentials of Diagnosis**

  - Sudden onset of pain, swelling in an area of wound contamination
  - Severe systemic toxicity and rapid progression of involved tissue
  - Brown or blood-tinged watery exudate with surrounding skin discoloration
  - Gas in tissue by palpation, auscultated crepitus, or x-ray
  - *Clostridium perfringens* in anaerobic culture or smear of exudate is the classic—but not the only—cause

- **Differential Diagnosis**

  - Other gas-forming infections (mixed aerobic and anaerobic enteric organisms)
  - Cellulitis due to staphylococcal or streptococcal infection

- **Treatment**

  - Immediate surgical débridement and exposure of infected areas
  - Hyperbaric oxygen of uncertain benefit
  - Intravenous penicillin with clindamycin
  - Tetanus prophylaxis

- **Pearl**

A condition in which a relatively low-grade fever belies the extraordinary systemic toxicity the clinician witnesses.

Reference

Hickey MJ, Kwan RY, Awad MM, et al. Molecular and cellular basis of microvascular perfusion deficits induced by *Clostridium perfringens* and *Clostridium septicum*. PLoS Pathog 2008;4:e1000045. [PMID: 18404211]

Diphtheria (*Corynebacterium diphtheriae*)

■ Essentials of Diagnosis

- An acute infection spread by respiratory secretions
- Sore throat, rhinorrhea, hoarseness, malaise, relatively unimpressive fever (usually < 37.8°C)
- Some cases confined to the skin
- Tenacious gray membrane at portal of entry
- Toxin-induced myocarditis and neuropathy may complicate, due to an exotoxin; more common in pharyngeal than cutaneous diphtheria
- Smear and culture confirm diagnosis; testing for toxin production should also be performed

■ Differential Diagnosis

- Other causes of pharyngitis (streptococcal, infectious mononucleosis, adenovirus)
- Necrotizing gingivostomatitis
- Candidiasis
- Myocarditis from other causes
- Myasthenia gravis
- Botulism

■ Treatment

- Active immunization (usually as diphtheria-tetanus-pertussis [DTP]) is preventive
- Diphtheria antitoxin
- Penicillin or erythromycin
- Exposures of susceptible individuals call for throat cultures, active immunization, antibiotics, and daily throat inspections

■ Pearl

Don't forget cutaneous diphtheria in the differential of leg ulcers in homeless patients, especially if these ulcers are hyperesthetic.

Reference

Mokrousov I. *Corynebacterium diphtheriae*: genome diversity, population structure and genotyping perspectives. Infect Genet Evol 2009;9:1. [PMID: 19007916]

Enteric Fever (Typhoid Fever)

- **Essentials of Diagnosis**
  - Caused by several *Salmonella* species; in "typhoid fever," serotype *Salmonella typhi* is causative and accompanied by bacteremia
  - Transmitted by contaminated food or drink; incubation period is 5–21 days
  - Gradual onset of malaise, headache, and abdominal pain, followed by diarrhea, or with *S. typhi*, constipation; stepladder rise of fever to a maximum of 40°C over 7–10 days, then slow return to normal with little diurnal variation
  - Rose spots, relative bradycardia, splenomegaly, abdominal distention and tenderness
  - Leukopenia; blood, stool, and urine cultures positive for *S. typhi* (group D) or other salmonellae

- **Differential Diagnosis**
  - Brucellosis
  - Tuberculosis
  - Infectious endocarditis
  - Q fever
  - Yersiniosis
  - Hepatitis
  - Lymphoma
  - Adult Still's disease

- **Treatment**
  - Active immunization helpful for travelers to endemic areas or for household contacts of persons with the disease
  - Ciprofloxacin or third-generation cephalosporin pending susceptibility results
  - Cholecystectomy may be necessary for relapsed cases
  - Complications in one-third of untreated patients include intestinal hemorrhage or perforation, cholecystitis, nephritis, and meningitis

- **Pearl**

Relative leukopenia and bradycardia are the rule; if tachycardia and leukocytosis develop several days into the infection, strongly consider ileal perforation.

Reference

Thaver D, Zaidi AK, Critchley J, Azmatullah A, Madni SA, Bhutta ZA. A comparison of fluoroquinolones versus other antibiotics for treating enteric fever: meta-analysis. BMJ 2009;338:b1865. [PMID: 19493939]

Gonorrhea (*Neisseria gonorrhoeae*)

■ Essentials of Diagnosis

- A common communicable venereal disease; incubation period is 2–8 days
- Purulent profuse urethral discharge (men); vaginal discharge rare (women); may be asymptomatic in both sexes
- Disseminated disease causes intermittent fever, skin lesions (few in number and peripherally located), tenosynovitis in numerous joints, and usually monarticular arthritis involving the knee, ankle, or wrist
- Conjunctivitis, pharyngitis, proctitis, endocarditis, meningitis also occur
- Gram-negative intracellular diplococci on smear or culture from urethra, cervix, rectum, or pharynx; DNA probe of urethral or cervical swab; molecular testing of first 10 mL of urine superior to urethral cultures
- Synovial fluid cultures seldom positive early, may become positive later in disease course

■ Differential Diagnosis

- Cervicitis, vaginitis, or urethritis due to other causes
- Other causes of pelvic inflammatory disease
- Reactive arthritis
- Meningococcemia

■ Treatment

- Rapid plasma reagin (RPR) obtained in all, HIV in selected cases
- Ceftriaxone intramuscularly for suspected cases; treat all sexual partners
- Oral antibiotics for concurrent chlamydial infection also recommended
- Intravenous antibiotics required for salpingitis, prostatitis, arthritis, or endocarditis

■ Pearl

Treat empirically for this in a young patient with an inflammatory arthritis despite a negative Gram stain and culture; the sexual history may be difficult to verify.

Reference

Hosenfeld CB, Workowski KA, Berman S, et al. Repeat infection with Chlamydia and gonorrhea among females: a systematic review of the literature. Sex Transm Dis 2009;36:478. [PMID: 19617871]

Granuloma Inguinale (Donovanosis) (*Klebsiella* [formerly *Calymmatobacterium*] *granulomatis*)

■ Essentials of Diagnosis

- A chronic relapsing granulomatous anogenital infection; incubation period is 1–12 weeks
- Ulcerative lesions on the skin or mucous membranes of the genitalia or perianal area
- Donovan bodies revealed by Wright's or Giemsa's stain of ulcer scrapings

■ Differential Diagnosis

- Genital ulcers of other cause
- Syphilis
- Herpes simplex
- Reactive arthritis
- Behçet's disease

■ Treatment

- Appropriate antibiotic (azithromycin or tetracycline) for at least 21 days
- Surveillance and counseling for other sexually transmitted infections (STIs) (eg, syphilis, gonorrhea, HIV)

■ Pearl

The most indolent of the major sexually transmitted diseases—unless one includes tertiary syphilis.

Reference

Velho PE, Souza EM, Belda Junior W. Donovanosis. Braz J Infect Dis 2008;12:521. [PMID: 19287842]

Legionnaires' Disease

- **Essentials of Diagnosis**
  - Caused by *Legionella pneumophila* and a common cause of community-acquired pneumonia in some areas
  - Seen in patients who are immunocompromised or have chronic lung disease
  - Malaise, fever, headache, pleuritic chest pain, toxic appearance, cough
  - Chest x-ray with patchy infiltrates often unimpressive early; subsequent development of effusion or multiple lobar involvement common
  - Purulent sputum without organisms seen by Gram's stain; diagnosis confirmed by culture or special silver stains or direct fluorescent antibodies, urinary antigen

- **Differential Diagnosis**
  - Other infectious pneumonias
  - Pulmonary embolism
  - Pleurodynia
  - Myocardial infarction

- **Treatment**
  - Azithromycin at high doses; quinolones are an effective alternative

- **Pearl**

Hyponatremia and intestinal symptomatology are not diagnostic; many atypical pneumonias share these clinical manifestations.

Reference

Cunha BA. Atypical pneumonias: current clinical concepts focusing on Legionnaires' disease. Curr Opin Pulm Med 2008;14:183. [PMID: 18427241]

Leprosy (*Mycobacterium leprae*)

■ Essentials of Diagnosis

- A chronic infection due to *M. leprae*
- Pale, anesthetic macular (tuberculoid or paucibacillary) or infiltrative erythematous (lepromatous or multibacillary) skin lesions
- Superficial nerve thickening with associated sensory changes; progression slow and symmetric (lepromatous) or sudden and asymmetric (tuberculoid)
- History of residence in endemic area during childhood; mode of transmission probably is respiratory
- Acid-fast bacilli in skin lesions or nasal scrapings; characteristic histologic nerve biopsy
- Lepromatous type occurs in patients with defective cellular immunity, organisms numerous in tissue specimens; bacilli sparse in tuberculoid disease

■ Differential Diagnosis

- Lupus erythematosus
- Sarcoidosis
- Syphilis
- Erythema nodosum
- Erythema multiforme
- Vitiligo
- Neuropathy due to other causes, particularly amyloidosis
- Cutaneous tuberculosis or atypical mycobacterial infection
- Scleroderma
- Syringomyelia

■ Treatment

- Combination therapy for months or years, including dapsone, rifampin, and clofazimine

■ Pearl

How this was learned remains a puzzle to most, but M. leprae *can be grown experimentally only in the footpad of the armadillo.*

Reference

Wilder-Smith EP, Van Brakel WH. Nerve damage in leprosy and its management. Nat Clin Pract Neurol 2008;4:656. [PMID: 19002133]

Leptospirosis (*Leptospira* Species)

- ### Essentials of Diagnosis
  - An acute and often severe infection transmitted to humans by exposure to water or soil contaminated by the urine of reservoir animals (rats, dogs, cattle, swine)
  - Abrupt onset of high fever, headache, myalgias, and conjunctival injection after incubation period of 2–26 days
  - Jaundice, conjunctival hemorrhages, meningeal signs, abdominal tenderness
  - Renal insufficiency, acalculous cholecystitis may occur
  - Variable renal function abnormalities, elevated creatinine phosphokinase level, abnormal cerebrospinal fluid in more than 50% after 7 days of illness due to host immune response
  - Culture of organism from blood, cerebrospinal fluid, or urine, or direct darkfield microscopy of urine or cerebrospinal fluid is diagnostic
  - Serologic tests positive after first week; rapid enzyme-linked immunosorbent assay (ELISA) for immunoglobulin M (IgM) now available

- ### Differential Diagnosis
  - Aseptic meningitis due to other causes
  - Hepatitis
  - Lymphoma
  - Cholecystitis due to other causes
  - Hepatorenal syndrome
  - Halogenated hydrocarbon ingestion

- ### Treatment
  - Early treatment with penicillin or doxycycline may shorten course
  - Herxheimer reaction may appear after therapy
  - Doxycycline effective as prophylaxis for exposures

- ### Pearl

The social history may be diagnostic here; jaundice and conjunctivitis in a homeless patient who lives near brackish water is leptospirosis until proven otherwise.

Reference

Vijayachari P, Sugunan AP, Shriram AN. Leptospirosis: an emerging global public health problem. J Biosci 2008;33:557. [PMID: 19208981]

Lyme Disease (*Borrelia burgdorferi*)

■ Essentials of Diagnosis

- History of exposure to *Ixodes* species of tick in endemic area; most US cases occur in the Northeast and upper Midwest
- Stage I (early localized disease): Early flulike syndrome, erythema migrans (flat macular rash and erythema with central clearing); usually occurs about 1 week after tick bite
- Stage II (early disseminated disease): Neurologic (Bell's palsy, meningoencephalitis, aseptic meningitis, peripheral neuropathy, transverse myelitis)
- Stage III (late disease): Musculoskeletal, usually arthritis, monarticular or oligoarticular
- Overlap between clinical stages often observed
- Mild carditis may occur
- Serologic diagnosis is possible after 2–4 weeks of illness; rarely, organism can be cultured from blood, cerebrospinal fluid, or rash aspirate

■ Differential Diagnosis

- Stage I: Other causes of viral exanthems; rheumatic fever
- Stage II: Other causes of peripheral neuropathy, transverse myelitis, encephalitis, aseptic meningitis, Bell's palsy
- Stage III: Autoimmune disease, particularly seronegative spondyloarthropathies, Still's disease
- Other causes of myocarditis, arrhythmias, and heart block
- Chronic fatigue syndrome

■ Treatment

- Antibiotic chosen depends on stage of disease
- Prophylaxis of tick bites not recommended

■ Pearl

A disease many patients believe they have, but only a small minority do.

Reference

Bratton RL, Whiteside JW, Hovan MJ, Engle RL, Edwards FD. Diagnosis and treatment of Lyme disease. Mayo Clin Proc 2008;83:566. [PMID: 18452688]

Lymphogranuloma Venereum
(*Chlamydia trachomatis* Types L1–L3)

■ Essentials of Diagnosis

- A sexually transmitted disease with an incubation period of 3–12 days
- Evanescent primary genital lesion
- Inguinal lymphadenopathy and suppuration with draining sinuses
- Proctitis; rectal stricture; systemic joint, eye, or central nervous system involvement may occur
- Serologic tests positive in second to third week of illness

■ Differential Diagnosis

- Syphilis
- Genital herpes
- Chancroid
- Bacterial lymphadenitis of other cause (eg, tuberculosis, tularemia)
- Cancer of rectosigmoid
- Rectal stricture due to other causes

■ Treatment

- Obtain rapid plasma reagin (RPR) test, consider HIV testing
- Tetracyclines; erythromycin in pregnancy
- Dilation or surgical repair of rectal stricture

■ Pearl

Early anorectal symptoms in women and in men having sex with men may simulate inflammatory bowel disease.

Reference

White JA. Manifestations and management of lymphogranuloma venereum. Curr Opin Infect Dis 2009;22:57. [PMID: 19532081]

Meningococcal Meningitis (*Neisseria meningitidis*)

- ## Essentials of Diagnosis
  - Fever, headache, vomiting, confusion, delirium, or seizures; typically epidemic in young adults; onset may be astonishingly abrupt
  - Petechial or ecchymotic rash of skin and mucous membranes
  - May have positive Kernig's and Brudzinski's signs
  - Purulent spinal fluid with gram-negative intracellular and extracellular diplococci
  - Culture of cerebrospinal fluid, blood, or petechial aspirate confirms diagnosis
  - Disseminated intravascular coagulation and shock may complicate

- ## Differential Diagnosis
  - Meningitis due to other causes
  - Petechial rash due to rickettsial, viral, or other bacterial infection
  - Idiopathic thrombocytopenic purpura

- ## Treatment
  - Active immunization available for selected susceptible groups (military recruits, college dormitory residents)
  - Penicillin or ceftriaxone
  - Mannitol and corticosteroids for elevated intracranial pressure
  - Ciprofloxacin (single dose) or rifampin (2 days) therapy for intimate exposures; resistance to ciprofloxacin has been reported

- ## Pearl

Despite the impression many younger clinicians have of this condition, it was the bacterial meningitis from which survival was most likely in the pre-antibiotic era.

Reference

Stephens DS. Biology and pathogenesis of the evolutionarily successful, obligate human bacterium *Neisseria meningitidis*. Vaccine 2009;27(suppl):B71. [PMID: 19477055]

Nocardiosis

■ Essentials of Diagnosis

- *Nocardia asteroides* and *Nocardia brasiliensis* are aerobic soil bacteria causing pulmonary and systemic disease
- Malaise, weight loss, fever, night sweats, cough
- Pulmonary consolidation or thin-walled abscess; invasion through chest wall possible
- Lobar infiltrates, air-fluid level, effusion by chest x-ray
- Delicate branching, gram-positive filaments by Gram's stain, weakly positive acid-fast staining; culture identifies specific organism
- Disseminated form may occur with abscess in any organ; brain, subcutaneous nodules most frequent
- Solid organ or bone marrow transplant, corticosteroid use, and malignancy predispose to infection
- The above are all due to *N. asteroides; N. brasiliensis* causes lymphangitis after skin inoculation and is common among gardeners

■ Differential Diagnosis

- Actinomycosis
- Tuberculosis or atypical mycobacterial infections
- Other causes of pyogenic lung abscess
- Lymphoma
- Coccidioidomycosis
- Histoplasmosis
- Sporotrichosis (*N. brasiliensis*)
- Herpetic whitlow (*N. brasiliensis*)
- Bacterial lymphangitis (*N. brasiliensis*)

■ Treatment

- Parenteral and then oral trimethoprim-sulfamethoxazole for many months; shorter, oral course acceptable for *N. brasiliensis*
- Surgical drainage and resection may be needed

■ Pearl

May mimic both tuberculosis and lung cancer; N. asteroides *has a peculiar affinity for the lung in pulmonary alveolar proteinosis.*

Reference

Agterof MJ, van der Bruggen T, Tersmette M, ter Borg EJ, van den Bosch JM, Biesma DH. Nocardiosis: a case series and a mini review of clinical and microbiological features. Neth J Med 2007;65:199. [PMID: 17587645]

Pertussis (*Bordetella pertussis*)

- ■ Essentials of Diagnosis
  - An acute infection of the respiratory tract spread by respiratory droplets
  - History of declined diphtheria-pertussis-tetanus (DPT) vaccination
  - Two-week prodromal catarrhal stage of malaise, cough, coryza, and anorexia; seen predominantly in infants under age 2
  - Paroxysmal cough ending in high-pitched inspiratory "whoop" (whooping cough) in children; prolonged cough in adults
  - Absolute lymphocytosis with extremely high white blood cell counts possible
  - Culture or molecular testing confirms diagnosis

- ■ Differential Diagnosis
  - Viral pneumonia
  - Foreign body aspiration
  - Acute bronchitis
  - Acute leukemia (when leukocytosis is marked)

- ■ Treatment
  - Active immunization preventive (as part of DTP)
  - Erythromycin in selected patients
  - Antibiotic prophylaxis for close contacts

- ■ Pearl

Along with Clostridium difficile *colitis, the cause of the highest white counts in clinical medicine caused by benign disease.*

Reference

Wood N, McIntyre P. Pertussis: review of epidemiology, diagnosis, management and prevention. Paediatr Respir Rev 2008;9:201. [PMID: 18694712]

Plague (*Yersinia pestis*)

- **Essentials of Diagnosis**
  - History of exposure to rodents in endemic area of southwestern United States; transmitted by bites of fleas or contact with infected rodents; human-to-human transmission with pneumonic plague only
  - Sudden onset of high fever, severe malaise, myalgias; stunning systemic toxicity
  - Regional lymphangitis and lymphadenitis with suppuration of nodes
  - Bacteremia, pneumonitis, or meningitis complicate
  - Positive smear and culture from aspirate or blood; striking leukopenia with marked left shift

- **Differential Diagnosis**
  - Tularemia
  - Lymphadenitis with bacterial disease of extremity
  - Lymphogranuloma venereum
  - Other bacterial pneumonia or meningitis
  - Typhoid fever
  - Various rickettsial diseases

- **Treatment**
  - Streptomycin or tetracyclines
  - Tetracycline prophylaxis for persons exposed to patients with pneumonic plague
  - Strict isolation of those with pneumonic disease

- **Pearl**

Empiric treatment should be administered in any suspected meningitis in such locales such as the desert Southwest United States, where it is rare but endemic.

Reference

Butler T. Plague into the 21st century. Clin Infect Dis 2009;49:736. [PMID: 19606935]

Pneumococcal Infections

- ■ Essentials of Diagnosis
    - Pneumonia characterized by initial chill, severe pleuritis, fever without diurnal variation; signs of consolidation and lobar infiltrate on x-ray ensue rapidly
    - Leukocytosis, hyperbilirubinemia
    - Gram-positive diplococci in sputum; lancet-shaped only on stained culture colonies
    - Meningitis: Rapid onset of fever, altered mental status, and headache; cerebrospinal fluid polymorphonuclear leukocytosis with elevated protein and decreased glucose; gram-stained smear of fluid obtained before receipt of antimicrobial therapy positive in 90% of cases
    - Endocarditis, empyema, pericarditis, and arthritis may also complicate, with empyema most common
    - Predisposition to bacteremia in children under 24 months of age or in asplenic or immunocompromised adults (eg, AIDS, elderly)

- ■ Differential Diagnosis
    - Pneumonia, meningitis of other cause
    - Pulmonary embolism
    - Myocardial infarction
    - Acute exacerbation of chronic bronchitis
    - Acute bronchitis
    - Gram-negative septicemia

- ■ Treatment
    - Blood culture before antibiotics
    - Third-generation cephalosporin for severe disease; add empiric vancomycin for meningitis pending culture results
    - Adults older than 50 years with any serious medical illness, patients with sickle cell disease, and asplenic patients should receive pneumococcal vaccine
    - Penicillin unreliable pending results of susceptibility testing

- ■ Pearl

Pneumonia was once treated with 10,000 units of penicillin daily for 3 days; no such luck anymore with increasing numbers of resistant strains being isolated.

Reference

van der Poll T, Opal SM. Pathogenesis, treatment, and prevention of pneumococcal pneumonia. Lancet 2009;374:1543. [PMID: 19880020]

Psittacosis (*Chlamydophila* [formerly *Chlamydia*] *psittaci*)

- **Essentials of Diagnosis**
  - Contact with infected bird 7–15 days before onset of symptoms
  - Rapid onset of fever, chills, malaise, headache, dry cough, epistaxis
  - Temperature-pulse dissociation, meningismus, erythematous macular rash (Horder's spots), dry crackles, splenomegaly
  - Slightly delayed appearance of signs of pneumonitis; culture-negative endocarditis may occur
  - Serologic diagnosis by second week of illness; organism rarely isolated by culture of respiratory secretions

- **Differential Diagnosis**
  - Other atypical pneumonias (eg, viral, mycoplasmal)
  - Typhoid fever
  - Lymphoma
  - Tuberculosis
  - Other culture-negative endocarditis

- **Treatment**
  - Tetracycline

- **Pearl**

The history of bird contact may be difficult to obtain; many cases are transmitted by illegally imported parrots valued by patients as loyal pets.

Reference

Beeckman DS, Vanrompay DC. Zoonotic *Chlamydophila psittaci* infections from a clinical perspective. Clin Microbiol Infect 2009;15:11. [PMID: 19220335]

Rat-Bite Fever (*Streptobacillus moniliformis* [United States] or *Spirillum minus* [Asia and Africa])

- **Essentials of Diagnosis**
  - History of rodent bite; 1 to several weeks after bite, the site becomes swollen, indurated, and painful (*S. minus*)
  - Fever, chills, nausea, vomiting, rash, headache, myalgia, and arthralgia; symptoms relapse at 24- to 48-hour intervals
  - Regional lymphangitis or adenopathy, splenomegaly
  - False-positive rapid plasma reagin (RPR) test
  - Diagnosis confirmed by culture (*S. moniliformis*) or Giemsa-stained darkfield examination of blood or exudates (*S. minus*)

- **Differential Diagnosis**
  - Malaria
  - Tularemia
  - Leptospirosis
  - Borreliosis
  - Rickettsial infection
  - Brucellosis
  - Lymphangitis caused by *Nocardia brasiliensis*

- **Treatment**
  - Penicillin or tetracycline

- **Pearl**

One of medicine's few relapsing fevers.

Reference

Elliott SP. Rat bite fever and *Streptobacillus moniliformis*. Clin Microbiol Rev 2007;20:13. [PMID: 17223620]

Relapsing Fever (*Borrelia recurrentis*)

■ Essentials of Diagnosis
- History of exposure to ticks or lice in endemic area
- Abrupt fever and chills, nausea, headache, arthralgia lasting 3–10 days with relapse at intervals of 1–2 weeks
- Tachycardia, hepatosplenomegaly, rash
- Spirochetes seen on blood smear during fever; serologic diagnosis is difficult and not widely available

■ Differential Diagnosis
- Malaria
- Leptospirosis
- Meningococcemia
- Yellow fever
- Typhus
- Rat-bite fever
- Hodgkin's disease with Pel-Ebstein fever

■ Treatment
- Single dose of tetracycline, erythromycin, or penicillin for louse-borne relapsing fever; 10 days of treatment for tick-borne relapsing fever
- Jarisch-Herxheimer reaction may occur after treatment with bactericidal agents

■ Pearl
One of the rare infectious diseases in which the pathogen may be seen on Wright's blood smear during fever.

Reference
Cutler SJ, Abdissa A, Trape JF. New concepts for the old challenge of African relapsing fever borreliosis. Clin Microbiol Infect 2009;15:400. [PMID: 19489922]

Salmonella Gastroenteritis
(Various *Salmonella* Species)

■ Essentials of Diagnosis

- The most common form of salmonellosis
- Nausea, headache, fever, high-volume diarrhea, usually without blood, and abdominal pain 8–72 hours after ingestion of contaminated food or liquid
- Positive fecal leukocytes
- Culture of organism from stool; bacteremia less common

■ Differential Diagnosis

- Viral gastroenteritis, especially enterovirus
- Dysenteric illness (*Shigella, Campylobacter,* amebic)
- Enterotoxigenic *E. coli* infection
- Inflammatory bowel disease

■ Treatment

- Rehydration and potassium repletion
- Antibiotics (ciprofloxacin or ceftriaxone) essential in those with sickle cell anemia, immunosuppression, or severe vascular disease
- In others, antimicrobials reduce symptoms by 1–2 days

■ Pearl

Continuous bacteremia with Salmonella *should raise the possibility of mycotic aortic aneurysm, especially in the HIV-infected patient.*

Reference

Crum-Cianflone NF. Salmonellosis and the gastrointestinal tract: more than just peanut butter. Curr Gastroenterol Rep 2008;10:424. [PMID: 18627657]

Staphylococcal Soft Tissue or Skin Infections

- ■ Essentials of Diagnosis
  - More often encountered in diabetics
  - Folliculitis, furunculosis, carbuncle, abscess, and cellulitis all seen
  - Culture of abscess is diagnostic; gram-stained smear positive for large gram-positive cocci (*Staphylococcus aureus*) in clusters

- ■ Differential Diagnosis
  - Streptococcal skin infections

- ■ Treatment
  - Penicillinase-resistant penicillin or first-generation cephalosporin; for suspected methicillin-resistant *S. aureus*, vancomycin, trimethoprim-sulfamethoxazole, or doxycycline
  - Drainage of abscess
  - Persistence of blood culture positivity suggests endocarditis or osteomyelitis

- ■ Pearl

Microbiologic etiology is seldom in doubt; given clinical appearance, treatment often requires incision and drainage in addition to antibiotics.

Reference

Stevens DL. Treatments for skin and soft-tissue and surgical site infections due to MDR Gram-positive bacteria. J Infect 2009;59(suppl):S32. [PMID: 19766887]

Staphylococcus aureus–Associated Toxic Shock Syndrome

- **Essentials of Diagnosis**
  - Association with tampon use, often postsurgical
  - Abrupt onset of fever, vomiting, diarrhea, sore throat, headache, myalgia
  - Toxic appearance, with tachycardia and hypotension
  - Diffuse maculopapular erythematous rash with desquamation on the palms and soles; nonpurulent conjunctivitis
  - Culture of nasopharynx, vagina, rectum, and wounds may yield staphylococci, but blood cultures usually negative
  - Usually caused by toxic shock syndrome toxin-1 (TSST-1)

- **Differential Diagnosis**
  - Streptococcal infection, particularly scarlet fever
  - Gram-negative sepsis
  - Rickettsial disease, especially Rocky Mountain spotted fever

- **Treatment**
  - Aggressive supportive care (eg, fluids, vasopressor medication, monitoring)
  - Antistaphylococcal antibiotics to eliminate source

- **Pearl**

Most patients with staphylococcal toxic shock syndrome do not have a clinically apparent tissue staph infection; this is purely a toxigenic phenomenon.

Reference

Lappin E, Ferguson AJ. Gram-positive toxic shock syndromes. Lancet Infect Dis 2009;9:281. [PMID: 19393958]

Streptococcal Pharyngitis

- ### Essentials of Diagnosis
  - Abrupt onset of sore throat, fever, malaise, nausea, headache
  - Pharynx erythematous and edematous with exudate; cervical adenopathy
  - Strawberry tongue
  - Throat culture or rapid antigen detection confirmatory
  - If erythrotoxin (scarlet fever) is produced, scarlatiniform rash that is red and papular with petechiae and fine desquamation will be present; prominent in axilla, groin, behind knees
  - Glomerulonephritis, rheumatic fever may complicate

- ### Differential Diagnosis
  - Viral pharyngitis
  - Mononucleosis
  - Diphtheria
  - With rash: Meningococcemia, toxic shock syndrome, drug reaction, viral exanthem

- ### Treatment
  - For two or more clinical criteria (cervical adenopathy, fever, exudate, and absence of rhinorrhea): Empiric penicillin
  - If equivocal, await culture or antigen confirmation
  - If history of rheumatic fever, continuous antibiotic prophylaxis for 5 years

- ### Pearl
Despite the clinical severity of pharyngeal diphtheria, fever is higher in strep throat.

Reference
Brook I, Dohar JE. Management of group A beta-hemolytic streptococcal pharyngotonsillitis in children. J Fam Pract 2006;55:S1. [PMID: 17137534]

Streptococcal Skin Infection

- **Essentials of Diagnosis**
    - Erysipelas: Rapidly spreading cutaneous erythema and edema with sharp borders
    - Impetigo: Rapidly spreading erythema with vesicular or denuded areas and golden-colored crust
    - Culture of wound or blood grows group A beta-hemolytic streptococci
    - Complication: Glomerulonephritis

- **Differential Diagnosis**
    - Other causes of infectious cellulitis (eg, staphylococcal)
    - Toxic shock syndrome
    - Beriberi (in setting of thiamin deficiency)

- **Treatment**
    - Penicillin for culture-proved streptococcal infection
    - Staphylococcal coverage (nafcillin, dicloxacillin) for empiric therapy or uncertain diagnosis

- **Pearl**

Group A cutaneous infections can result in subsequent glomerulonephritis, but are not associated with rheumatic fever.

Reference

Dryden MS. Skin and soft tissue infection: microbiology and epidemiology. Int J Antimicrob Agents 2009;34(suppl):S2. [PMID: 19560670]

Syphilis, Primary (*Treponema pallidum*)

■ Essentials of Diagnosis

- History of sexual contact, often of uncertain reliability or identity
- Painless ulcer (chancre) on genitalia, perianal region, oropharynx, or elsewhere 2–6 weeks after exposure
- Nontender regional adenopathy
- Fluid expressed from lesion positive, and infectious, by immuno-fluorescence or darkfield microscopy
- Rapid plasma reagin (RPR) positive in 60%

■ Differential Diagnosis

- Chancroid
- Lymphogranuloma venereum
- Genital herpes
- Lymphadenitis of other causes
- Lymphoma
- Drug eruption
- Reactive arthritis
- Behçet's syndrome

■ Treatment

- Benzathine penicillin, 2.4 million units intramuscularly
- With penicillin allergy, azithromycin or doxycycline acceptable

■ Pearl

Any painless genital or oral ulcer should be considered syphilitic until proved otherwise, and treated empirically.

Reference

Eccleston K, Collins L, Higgins SP. Primary syphilis. Int J STD AIDS 2008;19:145. [PMID: 18397550]

Syphilis, Secondary

■ Essentials of Diagnosis

- Develops coincident with, or more typically, 2 weeks to 6 months after appearance—and usually spontaneous disappearance—of chancre
- Fever, generalized maculopapular skin rash (including palms, soles, and mucous membranes, the latter highly contagious)
- Weeping papules (condyloma lata) in moist skin areas
- Generalized minimally tender lymphadenopathy
- Meningitis, hepatitis, osteitis, arthritis, or uveitis may occur
- Many treponemes in scrapings of mucous membranes or skin lesions by immunofluorescence or darkfield microscopy
- Rapid plasma reagin (RPR) test is uniformly positive in high titer; should be repeated 1–2 weeks later because of prozone effect with false negative

■ Differential Diagnosis

- Viral exanthems
- Pityriasis rosea
- Drug rash, especially erythema multiforme
- Multiple organ involvement may mimic meningitis, hepatitis, arthritis, uveitis, nephrotic syndrome of other etiology

■ Treatment

- Same as for primary syphilis; skin lesions may be temporarily exaggerated
- If central nervous system disease present, treat as neurosyphilis, with longer course of therapy
- Jarisch-Herxheimer reaction most common after bactericidal treatment of secondary syphilis

■ Pearl

Any dermatologic eruption involving the palms and soles should be considered secondary syphilis, irrespective of history or appearance, until proven otherwise.

Reference

Kent ME, Romanelli F. Reexamining syphilis: an update on epidemiology, clinical manifestations, and management. Ann Pharmacother 2008;42:226. [PMID: 18212261]

Syphilis, Tertiary (or Late)

- ■ Essentials of Diagnosis
  - • Many asymptomatic (latent)
  - • May occur at any time after secondary syphilis (occurs in one-third of untreated patients)
  - • Infiltrative tumors of skin, bone, liver (gummas); vascular disease with aortitis, ascending aortic aneurysms with aortic insufficiency
  - • Neurosyphilis, early: Meningovascular, with presenting symptoms of basilar meningitis or stroke
  - • Neurosyphilis, late: Tabes dorsalis; wide-based gait, fleeting abdominal or leg pain, bladder symptoms all due to dorsal column disease; general paresis; slowly progressive dementia; Argyll-Robertson pupils (miotic, nonreactive but accommodating)
  - • Tabes may result in severe knee arthropathy (Charcot's joint)

8

- ■ Differential Diagnosis
  - • Primary or secondary malignancy in any organ in which a gumma is involved
  - • Aortic insufficiency due to other causes
  - • Pernicious anemia (tabes)
  - • Surgical causes of acute abdomen (tabes)
  - • Viral or fungal meningitis (meningovascular)
  - • Other causes of neurogenic bladder (tabes)

- ■ Treatment
  - • Lumbar puncture for patients with syphilis longer than 1 year or with peripheral titers > 1:32 (unless asymptomatic), HIV-positive, or with neurologic signs
  - • For asymptomatic patients, treat with three doses 1 week apart of intramuscular benzathine penicillin
  - • For neurosyphilis with symptomatic or central nervous system abnormality: 10–14 days of parenteral penicillin
  - • Repeat lumbar puncture to follow cerebrospinal fluid abnormality to resolution
  - • Treatment in HIV neurosyphilis controversial

- ■ Pearl

Up to one-third of patients with tertiary lues are RPR-negative; if the disorder is being seriously considered, antitreponemal studies should be obtained.

Reference

Kent ME, Romanelli F. Reexamining syphilis: an update on epidemiology, clinical manifestations, and management. Ann Pharmacother 2008;42:226. [PMID: 18212261]

Tetanus (*Clostridium tetani*)

- **Essentials of Diagnosis**
  - History of nondebrided wound or contamination may or may not be obtained
  - Jaw stiffness followed by spasms (trismus)
  - Stiffness of neck or other muscles, dysphagia, irritability, hyper-reflexia; late, painful convulsions precipitated by minimal stimuli; fever is low-grade

- **Differential Diagnosis**
  - Infectious meningitis
  - Rabies
  - Strychnine poisoning
  - Malignant neuroleptic syndrome
  - Hypocalcemia

- **Treatment**
  - Active immunization preventive
  - Passive immunization with tetanus immune globulin and concurrent active immunization for all suspected cases
  - Chlorpromazine or diazepam for spasms or convulsions, with additional sedation by barbiturates as necessary
  - Vigorous supportive care with particular attention to airway and laryngospasm
  - Penicillin or metronidazole

- **Pearl**

Tetanus tops the list in "skin-popping" drug users with muscle spasm or even increased tone.

Reference

Gibson K, Bonaventure Uwineza J, Kiviri W, Parlow J. Tetanus in developing countries: a case series and review. Can J Anaesth 2009;56:307. [PMID: 19296192]

Tuberculosis (*Mycobacterium tuberculosis*)

- **Essentials of Diagnosis**
  - Most infections subclinical, with positive skin test only
  - Symptoms progressive and include cough, dyspnea, fever, night sweats, weight loss, and hemoptysis
  - In primary infection, mid-lung field infiltrates with regional lymphadenopathy; pleural effusion common
  - Apical fibronodular pulmonary infiltrate on chest film, with or without cavitation, is most typical in reactivated disease
  - Posttussive rales noted on auscultation
  - Most common extrapulmonary manifestations include meningitis, genitourinary infection, miliary disease, arthritis, with localized symptoms and signs

- **Differential Diagnosis**
  - Pneumonia of other cause; bacterial and fungal (histoplasmosis, coccidioidomycosis) most similar
  - Other mycobacterial infection
  - HIV infection (may be associated)
  - Prolonged fever of other cause
  - Urinary tract infection, oligoarticular arthritis of other cause
  - Carcinoma of the lung
  - Lung abscess

- **Treatment**
  - Four-drug regimens to include isoniazid and rifampin
  - Attention must be paid to sensitivity patterns due to increasing prevalence of drug-resistant strains

- **Pearl**

In HIV-infected patients, concerning tuberculosis and the clinical appearance in the lung: if it looks like TB, it's not, and if it doesn't, it is.

Reference

Hauck FR, Neese BH, Panchal AS, El-Amin W. Identification and management of latent tuberculosis infection. Am Fam Physician 2009;79:879. [PMID: 19496388]

Tuberculous Meningitis (*Mycobacterium tuberculosis*)

■ Essentials of Diagnosis

- Insidious onset of listlessness, irritability, headaches
- Meningeal signs, cranial nerve palsies
- Tuberculous focus evident elsewhere in half of patients
- Cerebrospinal fluid with lymphocytic pleocytosis, low glucose, and high protein; culture positive for acid-fast bacilli in many but not all; polymerase chain reaction (PCR) often helpful
- Chest x-ray may reveal abnormalities compatible with pulmonary tuberculosis

■ Differential Diagnosis

- Chronic lymphocytic meningitis due to fungi, brucellosis, leptospirosis, HIV infection, neurocysticercosis, sarcoidosis
- Carcinomatous meningitis
- Unsuspected head trauma with subdural hematoma
- Drug overdose
- Psychiatric disorder

■ Treatment

- Empiric antituberculous therapy essential in proper clinical setting
- Concomitant corticosteroids reduce long-term complications

■ Pearl

A highly elusive diagnosis, but most unlikely in patients with chronic meningitis and normal cerebrospinal fluid glucose.

Reference

Be NA, Kim KS, Bishai WR, Jain SK. Pathogenesis of central nervous system tuberculosis. Curr Mol Med 2009;9:94. [PMID: 19275620]

Tularemia (*Francisella tularensis*)

■ Essentials of Diagnosis

- History of contact with rabbits, other rodents, and biting arthropods (eg, ticks) in endemic areas; incubation period 2–10 days
- Fever, headache, nausea begin suddenly
- Papule progressing to ulcer at site of inoculation; the conjunctiva may be the site in occasional patients
- Prominent, tender regional lymphadenopathy, splenomegaly
- Diagnosis confirmed by serology; culture of ulcerated lesion, lymph node aspirate, or blood frequently negative
- Though primarily cutaneous, ocular, glandular, or typhoidal, only the very rare pneumonic form is transmissible between humans

■ Differential Diagnosis

- Cat-scratch disease
- Infectious mononucleosis
- Plague
- Typhoid fever
- Lymphoma
- Various rickettsial infections
- Meningococcemia

■ Treatment

- Streptomycin is the drug of choice; tetracycline is an alternative treatment option

■ Pearl

Rarely encountered in Tulare County, California, from whence its name comes, the most prominent epidemic was on Martha's Vineyard, documented in detail in The New Yorker.

Reference

Nigrovic LE, Wingerter SL. Tularemia. Infect Dis Clin North Am 2008;22:489. [PMID: 18755386]

FUNGAL INFECTIONS

Candidiasis (*Candida* Species)

- **Essentials of Diagnosis**
  - Plaquelike or ulcerative lesions of oral mucosa (thrush)
  - Vulvovaginitis, skin fold infections, or paronychia
  - Esophageal, central nervous system, or disseminated disease in immunosuppressed patients
  - Endocarditis in patients with prosthetic valves
  - A compatible clinical picture, susceptible host, and finding *Candida* in specimens establish diagnosis

- **Differential Diagnosis**
  - Severe atopic dermatitis
  - Herpetic or cytomegalovirus esophagitis in immunosuppressed patients
  - Other fungal or basilar meningitides
  - Prosthetic valve endocarditis of other cause

- **Treatment**
  - Nystatin, clotrimazole, miconazole for local lesions
  - Fluconazole for systemic infections
  - Amphotericin B or caspofungin for severe infection
  - Valve replacement obligatory in prosthetic valve endocarditis

- **Pearl**

An organism with a vast clinical spectrum from nail fungus to endocarditis.

Reference

Lewis RE. Overview of the changing epidemiology of candidemia. Curr Med Res Opin 2009;25:1732. [PMID: 19519284]

Coccidioidomycosis (*Coccidioides immitis*)

- ### Essentials of Diagnosis
    - Arthrospores in deserts of central and southern California and Arizona; highly infectious
    - Pulmonary form: Fever, pleuritis, dry cough, anorexia, weight loss, erythema nodosum, and erythema multiforme with arthralgias; "desert rheumatism or valley fever"
    - Incubation period 7–21 days; not contagious between humans
    - Disseminated lesions involve skin, bones, and meninges
    - Eosinophilia and leukocytosis
    - Sporangia in pus, sputum, or cerebrospinal fluid may be seen
    - Radiographic studies show nodular pulmonary infiltrates with thin-walled cavities and hilar adenopathy
    - Skin test of limited value, but serologic testing helpful both diagnostically and prognostically; persistence of IgG in higher titer indicates disseminated disease

- ### Differential Diagnosis
    - Tuberculosis
    - Histoplasmosis
    - Blastomycosis
    - Osteomyelitis from other causes
    - Aseptic meningitis from other causes
    - Sarcoidosis

- ### Treatment
    - Fluconazole in mild disease
    - Amphotericin B for disseminated disease

- ### Pearl
    When cultured from pathologic material, this fungus undergoes morphologic change to highly infectious arthrospores, endangering laboratory personnel; immunologic diagnosis is safer and more accurate.

Reference
Ampel NM. Coccidioidomycosis: a review of recent advances. Clin Chest Med 2009;30:241. [PMID: 19375631]

Cryptococcosis (*Cryptococcus neoformans*)

- ■ Essentials of Diagnosis
  - Opportunistic disease seen most commonly in AIDS patients or other immunocompromised patients
  - Findings subtle with fever, headache, photophobia, and neuropathies
  - Meningeal signs with positive Kernig's and Brudzinski's signs unusual
  - Subacute respiratory infection with low-grade fever, pleuritic pain, and cough seen as well
  - Spinal fluid findings include increased pressure, variable pleocytosis, increased protein, and decreased glucose
  - Large encapsulated yeasts by India ink mount of spinal fluid or cryptococcal antigen assay positive on both serum and spinal fluid

- ■ Differential Diagnosis
  - Other causes of meningitis
  - Lymphoma
  - Tuberculosis

- ■ Treatment
  - Amphotericin B and flucytosine for severe disease
  - Fluconazole can be used in many patients to complete therapy
  - All patients with serum antigen-positive and HIV disease should undergo lumbar puncture

- ■ Pearl

Ninety-five percent of patients with cryptococcal meningitis have positive serum cryptococcal antigen.

Reference

Ritter M, Goldman DL. Pharmacotherapy of cryptococcosis. Expert Opin Pharmacother 2009;10:2433. [PMID: 19708853]

Histoplasmosis (*Histoplasma capsulatum*)

- **Essentials of Diagnosis**
  - History of bird or bat exposure or of living near a river valley; house painters at risk
  - Often asymptomatic; variable cough, fever, malaise, chest pain in self-limited infections
  - Ulceration of naso- and oropharynx, hepatosplenomegaly, generalized lymphadenopathy in disseminated disease (1 in 250,000 cases) if not immunocompromised; this is the typical presentation in HIV disease
  - Acute pericarditis an uncommon presentation; adrenalitis also observed in systemic disease
  - Fibrosing mediastinitis a long-term complication; may cause superior vena cava syndrome
  - Skin test of limited value
  - Urinary *Histoplasma* antigen is diagnostic; small budding fungus cells found in reticuloendothelial cells; biopsy and culture of organism confirms diagnosis

- **Differential Diagnosis**
  - Tuberculosis
  - Blastomycosis
  - Coccidioidomycosis
  - Lymphoma
  - Sarcoidosis

- **Treatment**
  - Oral itraconazole for most infections
  - Amphotericin B in severe disease or in those who have failed itraconazole treatment

- **Pearl**

  Pulmonary calcifications on chest x-ray in patients whose Social Security number begins with 2, 3, or 4 is likely histoplasmosis.

Reference

Kauffman CA. Histoplasmosis. Clin Chest Med 2009;30:217. [PMID: 19375629]

Pneumocystosis
(*Pneumocystis jiroveci* [formerly *carinii*] Pneumonia [PCP])

- ■ Essentials of Diagnosis
  - Seen primarily in immunocompromised patients (AIDS, post–tissue transplantation, lymphoreticular malignancy); CD4 level < 200 is the rule
  - Fever, dyspnea, dry cough, often insidious onset
  - Dry crackles upon auscultation
  - Diffuse alveolar disease by chest x-ray; occasionally, small cavities
  - Large alveolar-arterial gradient; decreased single-breath diffusing capacity; elevated serum lactate dehydrogenase; abnormal gallium scan
  - Organism identified by silver stain, antibody staining, or PCR of secretions or biopsy
  - Extrapulmonary disease may be seen if patient is undergoing routine prophylactic therapy with pentamidine

- ■ Differential Diagnosis
  - Atypical pneumonia due to other causes
  - Congestive heart failure
  - Tuberculosis
  - Disseminated fungal disease

- ■ Treatment
  - Many drug regimens effective; trimethoprim-sulfamethoxazole is first-line therapy
  - Corticosteroids are adjunctive if moderate or severe hypoxemia present
  - Chemoprophylaxis recommended for immunocompromised patients at risk

- ■ Pearl

Although most cases occur in HIV/AIDS patients with CD4 counts of < 200, this doesn't hold true if antiretroviral treatment has raised the number to higher figures; the same is true of other opportunistic infections in that condition.

Reference

Krajicek BJ, Thomas CF Jr, Limper AH. Pneumocystis pneumonia: current concepts in pathogenesis, diagnosis, and treatment. Clin Chest Med 2009;30:265. [PMID: 19375633]

Sporotrichosis (*Sporothrix schenckii*)

■ Essentials of Diagnosis

- Ulcer after trauma to extremity
- Occupationally associated with exposure to plants or soil; thorn inoculation typical
- Nodules found along lymphatic drainage, which may ulcerate with a black eschar
- Culture is needed to establish diagnosis
- Serology helpful in disseminated disease (rare)

■ Differential Diagnosis

- Tularemia
- Anthrax
- Other mycotic infections
- Cutaneous tuberculosis

■ Treatment

- Itraconazole for several months is the treatment of choice for localized disease
- Amphotericin B used in severe systemic infection
- Potassium iodide solution orally in some cases

■ Pearl

Lymphadenopathy in a rose fancier—or at least someone who picks them—is sporotrichosis until proven otherwise.

Reference

Ramos-e-Silva M, Vasconcelos C, Carneiro S, Cestari T. Sporotrichosis. Clin Dermatol 2007;25:181. [PMID: 17350497]

HELMINTHIC INFECTIONS

Ascariasis (*Ascaris lumbricoides*)

■ Essentials of Diagnosis

- Pulmonary phase: Fever, cough, hemoptysis, wheezing, urticaria, and eosinophilia; fleeting pulmonary infiltrates may be seen (Löffler's pneumonia)
- Intestinal phase: Vague abdominal discomfort and colic, vomiting
- Inflammatory reactions in any organs and tissues invaded by wandering adult worms
- Pancreatitis, appendicitis, intestinal obstruction may all complicate infection
- Characteristic ascariatic ova in stool with larvae in sputum

■ Differential Diagnosis

- Pneumonitis due to other parasitic infiltrations (especially hookworm and *Strongyloides*)
- Bacterial or viral pneumonia
- Allergic disorders such as Löffler's syndrome, asthma, urticaria, allergic bronchopulmonary aspergillosis, Churg-Strauss syndrome
- Eosinophilic pneumonia
- Pancreatitis, peptic ulcer disease, appendicitis, and diverticulitis due to other causes

■ Treatment

- Mebendazole or albendazole

■ Pearl

Consider ascariasis in appendicitis or pancreatitis with eosinophilia.

Reference

Holland CV. Predisposition to ascariasis: patterns, mechanisms and implications. Parasitology 2009;136:1537. [PMID: 19450374]

Cysticercosis (*Taenia solium*)

■ Essentials of Diagnosis
- History of exposure in endemic area
- Infection by the larval (cysticercus) stage of *T. solium*; locations of cysts in order of frequency are central nervous system, subcutaneous tissue, striated muscle, globe of eye, and rarely, other tissues
- Seizure, headache, vomiting, blurred vision
- Focal neurologic abnormalities, papilledema, small subcutaneous or muscular nodules
- Lymphocytic and eosinophilic pleocytosis, elevated protein, and decreased glucose in cerebrospinal fluid
- Parasite seen upon histologic examination of skin or subcutaneous nodule
- Plain radiograph of soft tissue reveals oval or linear calcifications in nodules
- CT or MRI of the head reveals calcification of cysts and signs of elevated intracerebral pressure
- Serologic testing is helpful to differentiate cysticercosis from echinococcosis

■ Differential Diagnosis
- Echinococcosis
- Lymphoma
- Toxoplasmosis
- Brain abscess
- Brain tumor
- Coccidioidomycosis

■ Treatment
- Controversial in CNS disease
- Albendazole (or praziquantel)
- Concomitant treatment with steroids indicated to reduce inflammation
- Surgery in selected cases (orbital, retinal, spinal cord, or cisternal disease)

■ Pearl

The most common cause of seizures in young adults in Mexico.

Reference

Garcia HH, Moro PL, Schantz PM. Zoonotic helminth infections of humans: echinococcosis, cysticercosis and fascioliasis. Curr Opin Infect Dis 2007;20:489. [PMID: 17762782]

Echinococcosis (Hydatid Disease)

- ■ Essentials of Diagnosis
  - • A zoonosis in which humans are an intermediate host of the larval stage of the parasite
  - • History of close association with dogs in endemic area
  - • Often asymptomatic; signs of local obstruction or cyst rupture and leakage (pain, fever, or anaphylaxis)
  - • Avascular cystic tumor of liver, lung, bone, brain, or other organs
  - • Eosinophilia; serologic tests positive after 2–4 weeks

- ■ Differential Diagnosis
  - • Bacterial or amebic liver abscess
  - • Tuberculosis
  - • Other lung, bone, or brain tumors
  - • Obstructive jaundice due to other causes
  - • Cirrhosis from other causes
  - • Anaphylaxis or eosinophilia from other causes

- ■ Treatment
  - • Percutaneous aspiration or surgical removal of cysts if location permits
  - • Albendazole (or mebendazole) may be effective if surgery not possible
  - • Treat pet dogs prophylactically (with praziquantel) in endemic areas

- ■ Pearl

Be wary of aspirating liver cysts; when this organism causes peritonitis, it may be a devastating and fatal illness.

Reference

Garcia HH, Moro PL, Schantz PM. Zoonotic helminth infections of humans: echinococcosis, cysticercosis and fascioliasis. Curr Opin Infect Dis 2007;20:489. [PMID: 17762782]

Enterobiasis (Pinworm; *Enterobius vermicularis*)

- **Essentials of Diagnosis**
  - Nocturnal perianal and vulvar pruritus; insomnia, restlessness, and irritability
  - Children infected commonly
  - Vague gastrointestinal symptoms
  - Eggs of pinworms on skin or perianal area by cellulose tape test

- **Differential Diagnosis**
  - Perianal pruritus from other causes (mycotic infections, allergies, hemorrhoids, proctitis, fissures, strongyloidiasis)
  - Enuresis, insomnia, or restlessness in children due to other causes

- **Treatment**
  - Mebendazole drug of choice; do not give during pregnancy
  - Pyrantel pamoate also effective
  - Treat all household members

- **Pearl**

The nightmare—no pun intended—of any mother of a child with the problem.

Reference

Stermer E, Sukhotnic I, Shaoul R. Pruritus ani: an approach to an itching condition. J Pediatr Gastroenterol Nutr 2009;48:513. [PMID: 19412003]

Hookworm Disease

- ■ Essentials of Diagnosis
  - • Widespread in the moist tropics and subtropics; occurs sporadically in southern United States
  - • Weakness, fatigue, pallor, palpitations, dyspnea, diarrhea, abdominal discomfort, and weight loss
  - • Transient episodes of coughing or wheezing with sore throat sometimes seen
  - • Pruritic, erythematous, maculopapular or vesicular dermatitis; spoon-shaped nails
  - • Hypochromic microcytic anemia, eosinophilia
  - • Guaiac-positive stool
  - • Characteristic hookworm eggs in stool

- ■ Differential Diagnosis
  - • Iron deficiency due to other causes
  - • Recurrent pulmonary embolism
  - • Maculopapular or vesicular dermatitis due to other causes

- ■ Treatment
  - • Mebendazole drug of choice
  - • Pyrantel pamoate or albendazole are alternatives
  - • Iron supplementation for anemia

- ■ Pearl

Iron deficiency with eosinophilia in the rural southeast is hookworm until proven otherwise.

Reference

Keiser J, Utzinger J. Efficacy of current drugs against soil-transmitted helminth infections: systematic review and meta-analysis. JAMA 2008;299:1937. [PMID: 18430913]

Schistosomiasis (Bilharziasis; *Schistosoma* Species)

- ■ Essentials of Diagnosis
  - Endemic areas include parts of Africa, Asia, and South America
  - Acute: Katayama fever (fever, diarrhea, dry cough, urticaria; cercarial dermatitis, a transient erythematous pruritic skin rash in areas of contact with water)
  - Chronic: Depends on species, with *S. mansoni* producing severe portal hypertension and chronic portosystemic collateralization; terminal hematuria, urinary frequency, urethral and bladder pain in *S. haematobium*
  - Eggs in systemic circulation obstruct pulmonary resistance vessels, causing pulmonary hypertension and cor pulmonale, ischemia in other organs including spinal cord
  - Demonstration of schistosome ova in stools or urine or rectal biopsy diagnostic

- ■ Differential Diagnosis
  - Other causes of diarrhea (acute)
  - Cirrhosis
  - Hepatoma
  - Gastrointestinal neoplasm
  - Cystitis due to other causes
  - Genitourinary tumor
  - Transverse myelitis
  - Pulmonary hypertension due to other causes, especially mitral stenosis, primary pulmonary hypertension

- ■ Treatment
  - Praziquantel drug of choice
  - Steroids for Katayama fever or neurologic disease

- ■ Pearl

One of the few helminths that survives long after the patient has left the endemic area; learn these and you probably know enough parasitology for purposes of American practice.

Reference

Burke ML, Jones MK, Gobert GN, Li YS, Ellis MK, McManus DP. Immunopathogenesis of human schistosomiasis. Parasite Immunol 2009;31:163. [PMID: 19292768]

Strongyloidiasis (*Strongyloides stercoralis*)

■ **Essentials of Diagnosis**

- Endemic in many parts of the world, including the southeastern United States.
- Pruritic dermatitis at sites of larval penetration
- Diarrhea, epigastric pain, nausea, malaise, weight loss, cough, rales and wheezing with chronic infection
- Transient or fleeting pulmonary infiltrates
- Eosinophilia; characteristic larvae in stool, duodenal aspirate, or sputum; serology
- Parasite may live in intestine for years after patient leaves endemic area
- Hyperinfection syndrome: Severe diarrhea with malabsorption, bronchopneumonia, gram-negative sepsis, with meningitis, often after corticosteroids given for "asthma"

■ **Differential Diagnosis**

- Eosinophilia due to other causes
- Recurrent diarrhea due to other causes
- Duodenal ulcer
- Asthma
- Recurrent pulmonary emboli
- Cholecystitis or pancreatitis due to other causes
- Intestinal malabsorption due to other causes

■ **Treatment**

- Ivermectin or albendazole

■ **Pearl**

Apparent duodenal ulcer with eosinophilia is strongyloidiasis until proven otherwise; the organism lives in the upper small bowel.

Reference

Segarra-Newnham M. Manifestations, diagnosis, and treatment of *Strongyloides stercoralis* infection. Ann Pharmacother 2007;41:1992. [PMID: 17940124]

Tapeworm Infections
(See also Echinococcosis and Cysticercosis)

- ■ Essentials of Diagnosis
  - Six infect humans: *Taenia saginata* (beef tapeworm), *Taenia solium* (pork tapeworm), *Diphyllobothrium latum* (fish tapeworm), *Hymenolepis nana* (dwarf tapeworm), *Hymenolepis diminuta* (rodent tapeworm), *Dipylidium caninum* (dog tapeworm)
  - Usually asymptomatic but may cause nausea, diarrhea, abdominal cramps, malaise, weight loss
  - Segments of worm found in clothing or on bedding
  - Megaloblastic anemia (*D. latum*) due to competition for intestinal vitamin B_{12}
  - Characteristic eggs or proglottid segments of tapeworms in stool

- ■ Differential Diagnosis
  - Diarrhea due to other causes
  - Malabsorption states due to other causes
  - Pernicious anemia and folic acid deficiency

- ■ Treatment
  - Praziquantel for all infections

- ■ Pearl

Sushi and gefilte fish are rare but occasionally encountered causes of fish tapeworms in North America.

Reference

Scholz T, Garcia HH, Kuchta R, Wicht B. Update on the human broad tapeworm (genus diphyllobothrium), including clinical relevance. Clin Microbiol Rev 2009;22:146. [PMID: 19136438]

Trichinellosis (*Trichinella spiralis*)

- ## Essentials of Diagnosis
  - Vomiting, diarrhea, abdominal pain within first week of ingestion of inadequately cooked pork, boar, or bear; often in homemade sausage, but lean meat is most common cause in United States
  - Second week characterized by muscle pain and tenderness, fever, periorbital and facial edema, conjunctivitis; multiple splinter hemorrhages; symptoms due to dissemination of larvae
  - Eosinophilia and variably elevated serum creatine kinase, lactate dehydrogenase, and AST; erythrocyte sedimentation rate low
  - Positive serology
  - Diagnosis confirmed by finding larvae in muscle biopsy

- ## Differential Diagnosis
  - Dermatomyositis
  - Polyarteritis nodosa
  - Endocarditis
  - Diarrhea due to other infections

- ## Treatment
  - Mebendazole or albendazole for intestinal phase
  - Corticosteroids during larval invasion and for systemic sequelae; should not be used during the intestinal phase

- ## Pearl

The only cause of numerous splinter hemorrhages in all fingers and toes.

Reference

Gottstein B, Pozio E, Nöckler K. Epidemiology, diagnosis, treatment, and control of trichinellosis. Clin Microbiol Rev 2009;22:127. [PMID: 19136437]

PROTOZOAL INFECTIONS

Amebiasis (*Entamoeba histolytica*)

■ Essentials of Diagnosis
  - May occur sporadically or in epidemics
  - Infection of the large intestine; the parasite may be carried to the liver, lungs, brain, or other organs
  - Recurrent bouts of diarrhea and abdominal cramps, often alternating with constipation
  - In fulminant cases, frank bloody dysentery
  - Tenderness and enlargement of liver with abscess
  - Colonic ameboma or liver abscess may occur without dysentery
  - Leukocytosis in some, but eosinophilia uncommon; positive fecal leukocytes
  - Organism often not demonstrable in stools or aspirate of liver abscess; stool antigen testing more sensitive
  - Serologic tests very sensitive (99%) in invasive disease (liver abscess, ameboma), less so in intestinal disease (60%)
  - Ultrasound and CT scan useful to image hepatic abscesses

■ Differential Diagnosis
  - Other causes of acute or chronic diarrhea
  - Ulcerative colitis
  - Pyogenic liver abscess
  - Hepatoma
  - Echinococcal hepatic cyst
  - Carcinoma of sigmoid colon or cecum (ameboma)

■ Treatment
  - Metronidazole followed by luminal agent such as paromomycin or iodoquinol for invasive colitis or liver abscess
  - Paromomycin or iodoquinol alone for asymptomatic intestinal infection

■ Pearl

Do not give steroids for "inflammatory bowel disease" until this condition has been excluded; it is more endemic in America than most clinicians believe.

Reference

Pritt BS, Clark CG. Amebiasis. Mayo Clin Proc 2008;83:1154. [PMID: 18828976]

American Trypanosomiasis
(Chagas' Disease; *Trypanosoma cruzi*)

- ■ Essentials of Diagnosis

    - Transmitted by reduviid insects in endemic areas (Latin America and increasingly in the southwestern United States); most patients asymptomatic; some cases laboratory-acquired
    - Most asymptomatic during acute phase of infection although meningoencephalitis can occur in children; chronic phase of infection manifests many years later
    - Unilateral bipalpebral or facial edema, conjunctivitis (Romaña's sign)
    - Hard, edematous, erythematous, furuncle-like lesion with local lymphadenopathy (chagoma)
    - Cardiac disease with arrhythmias and right-sided congestive heart failure; gastrointestinal disease characterized by megacolon or megaesophagus
    - Trypanosomes in blood during acute phase of illness; serology or PCR during chronic phase of illness

- ■ Differential Diagnosis

    - Trichinosis
    - Kala-azar
    - Malaria
    - Congestive heart failure due to other causes
    - Meningoencephalitis due to other causes

- ■ Treatment

    - Nifurtimox effective acutely but less valuable in chronic stage
    - Benznidazole effective (not available in the United States)

- ■ Pearl

The most common cause of congestive heart failure in South and Central America, with recent cases now appearing in Arizona and New Mexico.

Reference

Dubner S, Schapachnik E, Riera AR, Valero E. Chagas disease: state-of-the-art of diagnosis and management. Cardiol J 2008;15:493. [PMID: 19039752]

Babesiosis

- **Essentials of Diagnosis**
  - Exposure to *Ixodes* ticks in endemic area
  - *Babesia microti* (United States): Irregular fever, chills, headache, diaphoresis, malaise without periodicity; hemolytic anemia and hepatosplenomegaly characteristic
  - *B. divergens* (Europe): High fever, toxic appearance, severe hemolytic anemia, liver and renal failure, with splenectomized patients particularly at risk
  - Intraerythrocytic parasite on blood smear diagnostic; serology or PCR helpful when organisms not seen on blood smear

- **Differential Diagnosis**
  - Malaria
  - Lyme disease (may coinfect)
  - Idiopathic autoimmune hemolytic anemia

- **Treatment**
  - *B. microti* infection usually benign and self-limited
  - *B. divergens* infection more severe
  - Quinine plus clindamycin; consider exchange transfusion for severe infection with high parasite burden

- **Pearl**

If you diagnose babesiosis, take a second look for Lyme disease.

Reference

Vannier E, Gewurz BE, Krause PJ. Human babesiosis. Infect Dis Clin North Am 2008;22:469. [PMID: 18755385]

Coccidiosis (*Isospora belli*; *Cryptosporidium*; *Cyclospora*)

■ **Essentials of Diagnosis**

- An intestinal infection caused by one of three genera: *Isospora, Cryptosporidium,* and *Cyclospora* most common in HIV disease
- Watery diarrhea, crampy abdominal pain, nausea, low-grade fever, malaise
- Fecal leukocytes absent
- Usually self-limited disease over weeks to months in immunocompetent, but may be catastrophic or life-threatening in AIDS patients
- Diagnosis with identification of parasite in feces or duodenal aspirate or biopsy (antigen test available for *Cryptosporidium*)

■ **Differential Diagnosis**

- Giardiasis
- Cholera
- Infectious colitis
- Ulcerative colitis or Crohn's disease
- Viral gastroenteritis

■ **Treatment**

- *Isospora* and *Cyclospora*: Trimethoprim-sulfamethoxazole; in AIDS patients, indefinite course
- *Cryptosporidium*: No consistently effective therapy available; paromomycin or nitazoxanide often tried

■ **Pearl**

Large outbreaks involving hundreds of thousands of people have occurred when sewage systems were overwhelmed by floods.

Reference

Karanis P, Kourenti C, Smith H. Waterborne transmission of protozoan parasites: a worldwide review of outbreaks and lessons learnt. J Water Health 2007;5:1. [PMID: 17402277]

8

Giardiasis (*Giardia lamblia*)

- **Essentials of Diagnosis**
  - Infection of the upper small intestine that occurs worldwide; most infections asymptomatic
  - Outbreaks common in day care centers, individual cases from contaminated water
  - Acute or chronic diarrhea with bulky, greasy stools
  - Upper abdominal discomfort, cramps, distention
  - No fecal leukocytes
  - Cysts and occasionally trophozoites in stools, especially in high-volume diarrhea; trophozoites in duodenal aspirate or biopsy; IgA deficiency predisposes, antigen test widely available
  - Malabsorption syndrome may be seen in chronic disease

- **Differential Diagnosis**
  - Gastroenteritis or diarrhea due to other causes
  - Mucosal small bowel disease such as sprue
  - Other causes of malabsorption, such as pancreatic insufficiency

- **Treatment**
  - Metronidazole
  - Tinidazole, quinacrine, or furazolidone also effective
  - Recheck stools to ensure success of therapy

- **Pearl**

Diarrhea and vague intestinal symptoms in spring and summer demand a history of recent camping; countless streams in American mountain ranges are contaminated with this parasite.

Reference

Buret AG. Pathophysiology of enteric infections with *Giardia duodenalis*. Parasite 2008;15:261. [PMID: 18814692]

Malaria (*Plasmodium* Species)

- ### Essentials of Diagnosis
  - History of exposure to mosquitoes in endemic area
  - Paroxysms of periodic chills, fever, headache, myalgias, and sweating with delirium; periodicity of fever determined by species
  - Jaundice, hepatosplenomegaly
  - Hemolytic anemia, leukopenia with relative monocytosis, thrombocytopenia, and nonspecific liver function test abnormalities
  - Characteristic plasmodia seen in erythrocytes in thick (experienced observers only) or thin blood smear
  - Rapid diagnostic tests based on antigen detection also available
  - Pulmonary edema, hepatic failure, hypoglycemia, acute tubular necrosis (blackwater fever) may complicate falciparum malaria
  - Recurrent attacks over months or years indicate *P. vivax* infection

- ### Differential Diagnosis
  - Influenza
  - Typhoid fever
  - Infectious hepatitis
  - Dengue
  - Kala-azar
  - Leptospirosis
  - Borreliosis
  - Lymphoma

- ### Treatment
  - Chemotherapy determined by species and drug sensitivities of endemic area
  - Chemoprophylaxis for travel to endemic area: Oral chloroquine with addition of primaquine after leaving endemic area; mefloquine, doxycycline, or proguanil and atovaquone if exposure to resistant falciparum malaria anticipated

- ### Pearl

Wright's stain of insufficiently dried blood smears shows a central ring artifact similar to plasmodia in red cells.

Reference

Wellems TE, Hayton K, Fairhurst RM. The impact of malaria parasitism: from corpuscles to communities. J Clin Invest 2009;119:2496. [PMID: 19729847]

Primary Amebic Meningoencephalitis (*Naegleria* Species; *Acanthamoeba* Species)

- **Essentials of Diagnosis**

  Naegleria:
  - Upper respiratory syndrome followed by rapidly progressing, usually fatal meningoencephalitis
  - Generally young, healthy persons with history of swimming in fresh water 3–7 days before onset of symptoms
  - Amebas with large, central karyosome in fresh wet mount of uncentrifuged cerebrospinal fluid; can be cultured

  Acanthamoeba:
  - Skin lesions and ulceration with multiple organ dissemination, chronic keratitis, or more insidious onset of severe meningoencephalitis
  - History of preexisting specific or nonspecific immunosuppression; trauma to skin, mucous membranes, or eye usually present

- **Differential Diagnosis**
  - Other causes of meningitis or encephalitis
  - Other causes of keratitis

- **Treatment**
  - Amphotericin B, miconazole, and rifampin with marginal success for *Naegleria* infections
  - Systemic ketoconazole, topical antifungals of uncertain benefit for *Acanthamoeba* infections

- **Pearl**

  One of medicine's few infectious diseases caused by free-living organisms with all cases rapidly fatal, save the more chronic granulomatous Acanthamoeba *infection.*

Reference

Marciano-Cabral F, Cabral GA. The immune response to *Naegleria fowleri* amebae and pathogenesis of infection. FEMS Immunol Med Microbiol 2007;51:243. [PMID: 17894804]

Toxoplasmosis (*Toxoplasma gondii*)

■ Essentials of Diagnosis

- Serious disease encountered extremely rarely in immunocompetent adults
- Fever, malaise, headache, sore throat, myalgias, blurred vision
- Rash, hepatosplenomegaly, cervical lymphadenopathy, chorioretinitis
- In immunocompromised patients, brain abscess with focal neurologic abnormalities most common; pneumonitis, myocarditis also occur, likewise lesions elsewhere including testes
- IgM diagnostic in nonimmunosuppressed population; negative IgG makes CNS disease unlikely in HIV patients
- PCR from bronchoalveolar lavage, cerebrospinal fluid, blood, or tissue biopsies diagnostic; resolution of brain abscess with empiric therapy highly suggestive

■ Differential Diagnosis

- Other causes of space-occupying brain lesions (primary or secondary malignancy, bacterial abscess, lymphoma)
- Other causes of encephalitis (herpes simplex, cytomegalovirus [CMV], viral encephalitis)
- CMV infection (may coexist in HIV disease)
- Epstein-Barr virus
- Other causes of myocarditis
- Other atypical pneumonias; *Pneumocystis*
- Other causes of lymphadenopathy (sarcoidosis, tuberculosis, lymphoma)

■ Treatment

- Pyrimethamine in combination with sulfadiazine or clindamycin effective
- Corticosteroids useful adjuvant in severe CNS disease
- Therapy in AIDS patients may be stopped if they are successfully treated with highly active antiretroviral therapy

■ Pearl

Seronegative heart transplant recipients of seropositive donors have a very high incidence of systemic disease; toxoplasma prophylaxis is essential in these individuals.

Reference

Petersen E. Toxoplasmosis. *Semin Fetal Neonatal Med* 2007;12:214. [PMID: 17321812]

Visceral Leishmaniasis
(Kala-Azar; *Leishmania donovani* Complex)

■ Essentials of Diagnosis

- A zoonotic disease transmitted by bites of sandflies; incubation period is 4–6 months
- Local, typically inapparent nonulcerating nodule at site of sandfly bite
- Irregular fever (often biquotidian) with progressive darkening of skin (especially on forehead and hands), diarrhea
- Cachexia, progressive and marked splenomegaly and hepatomegaly, generalized lymphadenopathy, petechiae
- Pancytopenia with relative lymphocytosis and monocytosis
- Leishman-Donovan bodies demonstrable in splenic, bone marrow, or lymph node smears or buffy coat blood smear; serologic tests helpful after second week of illness

■ Differential Diagnosis

- Malaria
- Lymphoma
- Brucellosis
- Schistosomiasis
- Infectious mononucleosis
- Myeloproliferative syndromes, especially myelofibrosis
- Anemia due to other causes
- Tuberculosis
- Leprosy
- African trypanosomiasis
- Subacute infective endocarditis
- Adult Still's disease

■ Treatment

- Sodium stibogluconate
- Pentamidine, liposomal amphotericin for treatment failures
- High fatality rate if not treated

■ Pearl

A biquotidian fever, massive splenomegaly, and wasting suggest the diagnosis in endemic regions.

Reference

Maltezou HC. Visceral leishmaniasis: advances in treatment. Recent Pat Antiinfect Drug Discov 2008;3:192. [PMID: 18991801]

RICKETTSIAL INFECTIONS

Epidemic Louse-Borne Typhus (*Rickettsia prowazekii*)

■ Essentials of Diagnosis

- Transmission of *R. prowazekii* favored by crowded living conditions, famine
- Headache, chills, fever, often severe or intractable
- Maculopapular rash appears on fourth to seventh days on trunk and axillae, then extremities; spares face, palms, and soles
- Conjunctivitis, rales, splenomegaly, hypotension, and delirium in some patients; renal insufficiency
- Serologic confirmation by second week of illness
- Brill's disease: Recrudescence of disease after apparent recovery

■ Differential Diagnosis

- Other viral syndromes
- Pneumonia
- Other exanthems
- Meningococcemia
- Sepsis
- Toxic shock syndrome

■ Treatment

- Prevention with louse control
- Tetracycline and chloramphenicol equally effective

■ Pearl

A more lethal enemy for armies than combat in endemic countries during World War II.

Reference

Bechah Y, Capo C, Mege JL, Raoult D. Epidemic typhus. Lancet Infect Dis 2008;8:417. [PMID: 18582834]

8

Q Fever (*Coxiella burnetii*)

■ **Essentials of Diagnosis**

- Infection after exposure to sheep, goats, cattle, or fowl
- Acute or chronic febrile illness with severe headache, cough, and abdominal discomfort
- Granulomatous hepatitis and culture-negative endocarditis in occasional cases
- Pulmonary infiltrates by chest x-ray; thrombocytopenia and elevated transaminases
- Serologic confirmation by second to fourth weeks of illness using phase I and II antibodies to determine chronicity

■ **Differential Diagnosis**

- Atypical pneumonia
- Granulomatous hepatitis due to other cause
- Brucellosis
- Other causes of culture-negative endocarditis

■ **Treatment**

- Tetracyclines suppressive but not always curative, especially with endocarditis; long-term combination therapy with hydroxychloroquine indicated for endocarditis
- Vaccine available outside United States

■ **Pearl**

The only rickettsial disease without a rash.

Reference

Tissot-Dupont H, Raoult D. Q fever. Infect Dis Clin North Am 2008;22:505. [PMID: 18755387]

Rocky Mountain Spotted Fever (*Rickettsia rickettsii*)

■ Essentials of Diagnosis

- Exposure to ticks in endemic area
- Influenzal prodrome followed by chills, fever, severe headache, myalgias, occasionally delirium and coma
- Red macular rash with onset between second and sixth days of fever; first on extremities, then centrally, may become petechial or purpuric
- Thrombocytopenia, proteinuria, hematuria
- Serologic tests positive by second week of illness, but diagnosis best made earlier by skin biopsy with immunologic staining

■ Differential Diagnosis

- Meningococcemia
- Endocarditis
- Gonococcemia
- Ehrlichiosis
- Measles

■ Treatment

- Tetracyclines or chloramphenicol

■ Pearl

The name notwithstanding, there are more cases in North Carolina than in Colorado.

Reference

Dantas-Torres F. Rocky Mountain spotted fever. Lancet Infect Dis 2007;7:724. [PMID: 17961858]

Scrub Typhus (Tsutsugamushi Disease)

■ Essentials of Diagnosis

- Caused by *Orientia tsutsugamushi,* transmitted by mites
- Exposure to mites in endemic area of Southeast Asia, western Pacific, Australia
- Black eschar at site of bite with regional or generalized lymphadenopathy, malaise, chills, headache, backache
- Fleeting macular rash in half of patients
- Pneumonitis, encephalitis, and cardiac failure may complicate
- Serologic confirmation by second week of illness

■ Differential Diagnosis

- Typhoid fever
- Dengue
- Malaria
- Leptospirosis
- Other rickettsial infections

■ Treatment

- Tetracyclines or chloramphenicol, though some resistance is being encountered
- Rifampin may also be effective

■ Pearl

Remember that the eschar may be on the scalp and the lymph node behind the ear, making diagnosis tricky at times.

Reference

Nachega JB, Bottieau E, Zech F, Van Gompel A. Travel-acquired scrub typhus: emphasis on the differential diagnosis, treatment, and prevention strategies. J Travel Med 2007;14:352. [PMID: 17883470]

VIRAL INFECTIONS

Colorado Tick Fever

■ Essentials of Diagnosis

- A self-limited acute viral (coltivirus) infection transmitted by *Dermacentor andersoni* tick bites
- Onset 3–6 days after bite
- Abrupt onset of fever, chills, myalgia, headache, photophobia
- Occasional faint rash
- Second phase of fever after remission of 2–3 days common
- Imbedded ticks, especially in children's scalps, may cause marked muscle weakness (tick paralysis) due to neurotoxin in tick saliva

■ Differential Diagnosis

- Borreliosis
- Influenza
- Adult Still's disease
- Other viral exanthems
- Guillain-Barré syndrome (if paralysis present)

■ Treatment

- Supportive for uncomplicated cases
- With paresis, removal of tick results in prompt resolution of symptoms

■ Pearl

In endemic areas, search the entire epidermis as well as accessible mucous membranes for ticks before treating supposed Guillain-Barré; removal results in prompt remission of paralysis.

Reference

Romero JR, Simonsen KA. Powassan encephalitis and Colorado tick fever. Infect Dis Clin North Am 2008;22:545. [PMID: 18755390]

Cytomegalovirus (CMV) Disease

■ Essentials of Diagnosis

- Neonatal infection: Hepatosplenomegaly, purpura, central nervous system abnormalities
- Immunocompetent adults: Mononucleosis-like illness characterized by fever, myalgias, hepatosplenomegaly, leukopenia with lymphocytic predominance; pharyngitis less common
- Immunocompromised adults: Pneumonia, meningoencephalitis, polyradiculopathy, chorioretinitis, chronic diarrhea; fever, occasionally prolonged
- In immunocompetent adults, IgM is diagnostic; PCR increasingly used for immunocompromised patients
- In AIDS patients with chorioretinitis, funduscopic examination establishes the diagnosis
- Contributes to organ rejection and other infections in transplant recipients

■ Differential Diagnosis

- Infectious mononucleosis (Epstein-Barr virus)
- Acute HIV infection
- Other causes of prolonged fever (eg, lymphoma, endocarditis)
- In immunocompromised patients: Other causes of atypical pneumonia, meningoencephalitis, or chronic diarrhea
- In infants: Toxoplasmosis, rubella, herpes simplex, syphilis

■ Treatment

- Appropriate supportive care
- Ganciclovir, foscarnet, or cidofovir intravenously in immunocompromised patients

■ Pearl

Think CMV in a patient with "mononucleosis" without pharyngitis—although the disorder is far more pleomorphic than that.

Reference

Britt W. Manifestations of human cytomegalovirus infection: proposed mechanisms of acute and chronic disease. Curr Top Microbiol Immunol 2008;325:417. [PMID: 18637519]

Dengue (Breakbone Fever, Dandy Fever)

■ Essentials of Diagnosis

- A viral (togavirus, flavivirus) illness transmitted by the bite of the *Aedes* mosquito
- Sudden onset of high fever, chills, severe myalgias, headache, sore throat; rare orchitis
- Biphasic fever curve with initial phase of 3–4 days, short remission, and second phase of 1–2 days
- Rash is biphasic—first evanescent, followed by maculopapular, scarlatiniform, morbilliform, or petechial changes during remission or second phase of fever; first in the extremities and spreads to torso
- Dengue hemorrhagic fever is a severe form in which gastrointestinal hemorrhage is prominent and patients often present with shock; occurs with repeat viral challenge with similar serotype

■ Differential Diagnosis

- Malaria
- Yellow fever
- Influenza
- Typhoid fever
- Borreliosis
- Other viral exanthems

■ Treatment

- Supportive care
- Vaccine has been developed but not commercially available

■ Pearl

This disorder has the synonym of breakbone fever for a reason; classical cases suffer severe myalgias, akin to a bad case of influenza.

Reference

Teixeira MG, Barreto ML. Diagnosis and management of dengue. BMJ 2009;339:b4338. [PMID: 19923152]

Herpes Simplex

■ **Essentials of Diagnosis**

- Recurrent grouped small vesicles on erythematous base, usually perioral or perigenital
- Primary infection more severe and often associated with fever, regional lymphadenopathy, and aseptic meningitis
- Recurrences precipitated by minor infections, trauma, stress, sun exposure
- Oral and genital lesions highly infectious
- Systemic infection may occur in immunosuppressed patients
- Proctitis, esophagitis, meningitis/encephalitis, and keratitis may complicate
- Direct fluorescent antibody or culture of ulcer can be diagnostic

■ **Differential Diagnosis**

- Herpangina, hand-foot-and-mouth disease
- Aphthous ulcers
- Stevens-Johnson syndrome
- Bacterial infection of the skin
- Syphilis and other sexually transmitted diseases
- Other causes of encephalitis, proctitis, or keratitis

■ **Treatment**

- Acyclovir, famciclovir, and valacyclovir may attenuate recurrent course of genital or oral lesions and are obligatory for systemic or central nervous system disease

■ **Pearl**

In unexplained heel pain with a normal exam in a young person, inquire about genital herpes; the virus lives in the sacral ganglia and radiates in the sacral nerve distribution.

Reference

Wilson SS, Fakioglu E, Herold BC. Novel approaches in fighting herpes simplex virus infections. Expert Rev Anti Infect Ther 2009;7:559. [PMID: 19485796]

HIV Infection

■ Essentials of Diagnosis

- Caused by a retrovirus slowly destroying CD4 lymphocytes
- At-risk populations include intravenous drug users and their partners, blood product recipients before 1984, health care workers injured with needles used for HIV-positive patients, homosexual men; heterosexual transmission most common in much of the world
- Coinfection with hepatitis C common
- Acute HIV infection characterized by nonspecific flulike syndrome and aseptic meningitis
- Later, opportunistic infections, certain malignancies, and AIDS wasting dictate the clinical picture, 2–15 years after primary infection
- Picture deteriorates as CD4 count falls below 200; certain opportunistic infections occur predictably at various levels (eg, P. jiroveci pneumonia < 200)

■ Differential Diagnosis

- Depends upon which infection is complicating
- Interstitial lung diseases of numerous types
- Non-AIDS lymphoma
- Tuberculosis
- Sarcoidosis
- Brain abscess
- Fever of unknown origin of other cause

■ Treatment

- Combination antiretroviral treatment can restore lost immunity and dramatically extend life expectancy
- Prophylaxis for *P. jiroveci* pneumonia when CD4 count reaches 200, and *Mycobacterium avium* complex when CD4 is < 50
- Otherwise, treatment for associated lymphoma, toxoplasmosis, mycobacteriosis, CMV, Kaposi's sarcoma as indicated

■ Pearl

Although a great success story in the United States, much of the world still cannot access adequate treatment with antiretrovirals.

Reference

Pham PA. Antiretroviral adherence and pharmacokinetics: review of their roles in sustained virologic suppression. AIDS Patient Care STDS 2009;23:803. [PMID: 19795999]

Infectious Mononucleosis (Epstein-Barr Virus Infection)

- ■ Essentials of Diagnosis
  - An acute illness due to Epstein-Barr virus, usually occurring up to age 35 but possible throughout life
  - Transmitted by saliva; incubation period is 5–15 days or longer
  - Fever, severe sore throat, striking malaise
  - Maculopapular rash, lymphadenopathy, splenomegaly common
  - Leukocytosis and lymphocytosis with atypical large lymphocytes by smear; positive heterophil agglutination test (Monospot) by fourth week of illness; false-positive rapid plasma reagin (RPR) test in 10%
  - Clinical picture much less typical in older patients
  - Complications include splenic rupture, hepatitis, myocarditis, any cytopenia in the blood, and encephalitis

- ■ Differential Diagnosis
  - Other causes of pharyngitis
  - Other causes of hepatitis
  - Toxoplasmosis
  - Rubella
  - Acute HIV, CMV, or rubella infections
  - Acute leukemia or lymphoma
  - Kawasaki's syndrome
  - Hypersensitivity reaction due to carbamazepine

- ■ Treatment
  - Supportive care only; fever usually disappears in 10 days, lymphadenopathy and splenomegaly in 4 weeks
  - Ampicillin apt to cause rash
  - Avoid vigorous abdominal activity or exercise

- ■ Pearl

Mononucleosis is the most commonly identified cause of anti-i hemolytic anemia.

Reference

Hurt C, Tammaro D. Diagnostic evaluation of mononucleosis-like illnesses. Am J Med 2007;120:911.e1. [PMID: 17904463]

Influenza

- ■ Essentials of Diagnosis
  - • Caused by an orthomyxovirus transmitted via the respiratory route
  - • Abrupt onset of fever, headache, chills, malaise, dry cough, coryza, and myalgias; constitutional signs out of proportion to catarrhal symptoms
  - • Epidemic outbreaks in fall or winter, with short incubation period
  - • Rapid tests on nasopharyngeal swabs widely available, confirmed by viral culture or PCR
  - • Complications include pneumonia and encephalitis
  - • Myalgias occur early in course, rhabdomyolysis late

- ■ Differential Diagnosis
  - • Other viral syndromes
  - • Primary bacterial pneumonia
  - • Meningitis
  - • Dengue in returned travelers
  - • Rhabdomyolysis of other cause

- ■ Treatment
  - • Yearly active immunization of persons at high risk (eg, chronic respiratory disease, pregnant women, cardiac disease, health care workers, immunosuppressed); also for all older than 50 years
  - • Chemoprophylaxis for epidemic influenza A or B with zanamivir or oseltamivir
  - • Antivirals reduce duration of symptoms and infectivity if given within 48 hours
  - • Avoid salicylates in children because of association with Reye's syndrome

- ■ Pearl

The 1918 worldwide epidemic caused as many as 50 million fatalities over 2 years; thus the justified concern for widespread immunization on a yearly basis, and the similar worry about avian influenza.

Reference

Jefferson T, Jones M, Doshi P, Del Mar C. Neuraminidase inhibitors for preventing and treating influenza in healthy adults: systematic review and meta-analysis. BMJ 2009;339:b5106. [PMID: 19995812]

Lymphocytic Choriomeningitis

■ Essentials of Diagnosis
- History of exposure to mice or hamsters
- Influenza-like prodrome with fever, chills, headache, malaise, and cough followed by headache, photophobia, or neck pain
- Kernig's and Brudzinski's signs positive
- Cerebrospinal fluid with lymphocytic pleocytosis and slight increase in protein
- Serology for arenavirus positive 2 weeks after onset of symptoms
- Illness usually lasts 1–2 weeks

■ Differential Diagnosis
- Other aseptic meningitides
- Bacterial or granulomatous meningitis

■ Treatment
- Supportive care

■ Pearl

One of the few causes of hypoglycorrhachia in a patient who appears to be well.

Reference

Kang SS, McGavern DB. Lymphocytic choriomeningitis infection of the central nervous system. Front Biosci 2008;13:4529. [PMID: 18508527]

Measles (Rubeola)

- **Essentials of Diagnosis**
  - An acute systemic viral illness transmitted by inhalation of infective droplets; 800,000 deaths yearly worldwide
  - Incubation period 10–14 days
  - Prodrome of fever, coryza, cough, conjunctivitis, photophobia
  - Progression of brick-red, irregular maculopapular rash 3 days after prodrome from face to trunk to extremities; patients appear quite ill
  - Koplik's spots (tiny "table salt crystals") on the buccal mucosa are pathognomonic but appear and disappear rapidly
  - Leukopenia
  - Encephalitis in 1–3%; pneumonia and hepatitis can also occur

- **Differential Diagnosis**
  - Other acute exanthems (eg, rubella, enterovirus, Epstein-Barr virus infection, varicella, roseola)
  - Drug allergy
  - Pneumonia or encephalitis due to other cause
  - Toxic shock syndrome

- **Treatment**
  - Primary immunization preventive after age 15 months; revaccination of adults born after 1956 without documented immunity recommended
  - Isolation for 1 week after onset of rash
  - Specific treatment of secondary bacterial complications

- **Pearl**

Becoming more common, along with pertussis, in under-vaccinated societies, whether by volition or poverty.

Reference

Moss WJ. Measles control and the prospect of eradication. Curr Top Microbiol Immunol 2009;330:173. [PMID: 19203110]

Mumps (Epidemic Parotitis)

- ■ Essentials of Diagnosis
  - Incubation period 14–24 days
  - Painful, swollen salivary glands, usually parotid; may be unilateral; systemic symptoms of infection
  - Orchitis or oophoritis, meningoencephalitis, or pancreatitis may occur
  - Cerebrospinal fluid shows lymphocytic pleocytosis in meningoencephalitis with hypoglycorrhachia
  - Diagnosis confirmed by isolation of virus in saliva or appearance of antibodies after second week

- ■ Differential Diagnosis
  - Parotitis or enlarged parotids due to other causes (eg, bacteria, sialolithiasis with sialadenitis, cirrhosis, diabetes, starch ingestion, Sjögren's syndrome, sarcoidosis, tumor)
  - Aseptic meningitis, pancreatitis, or orchitis due to other causes

- ■ Treatment
  - Immunization is preventive
  - Supportive care with surveillance for complications

- ■ Pearl

Mumps orchitis is a potentially treatable cause of sterility, associated with high blood FSH and low plasma testosterone levels.

Reference

Cascarini L, McGurk M. Epidemiology of salivary gland infections. Oral Maxillofac Surg Clin North Am 2009;21:353. [PMID: 19608052]

Poliomyelitis

- Essentials of Diagnosis

  - Enterovirus acquired via fecal-oral route; many cases asymptomatic, majority of symptomatic cases are not neurologic
  - Muscle weakness, malaise, headache, fever, nausea, abdominal pain, sore throat
  - Signs of lower motor neuron lesions: Asymmetric, flaccid paralysis with decreased deep tendon reflexes, muscle atrophy; may include cranial nerve abnormalities (bulbar form)
  - Cerebrospinal fluid lymphocytic pleocytosis with slight elevation of protein
  - Virus recovered from throat washings or stool

- Differential Diagnosis

  - Other aseptic meningitides
  - Postinfectious polyneuropathy (Guillain-Barré syndrome)
  - Amyotrophic lateral sclerosis
  - Myopathy

- Treatment

  - Vaccination is preventive and has eliminated the disease in the United States
  - Supportive care with particular attention to respiratory function, skin care, and bowel and bladder function

- Pearl

In North America, post-polio neurologic syndrome is more a concern than the acute polio still encountered in various parts of the developing world.

Reference

De Jesus NH. Epidemics to eradication: the modern history of poliomyelitis. Virol J 2007;4:70. [PMID: 17623069]

Rabies

■ Essentials of Diagnosis

- A rhabdovirus encephalitis transmitted by infected saliva
- History of animal bite (bats, skunks, foxes, raccoons; dogs and cats in developing countries)
- Paresthesias, hydrophobia, rage alternating with calm
- Convulsions, paralysis, thick tenacious saliva, and muscle spasms

■ Differential Diagnosis

- Tetanus
- Encephalitis due to other causes

■ Treatment

- Active immunization of household pets and persons at risk (eg, veterinarians)
- Thorough, repeated washing of bite and scratch wounds
- Postexposure immunization, both passive and active
- Observation of healthy biting animals, examination of brains of sick or dead biting animals
- Treatment is supportive only; disease is almost uniformly fatal

■ Pearl

Bats are the most common vector for rabies in the United States, and even absent history of a bite, children exposed to bats indoors should be immunized.

Reference

Nigg AJ, Walker PL. Overview, prevention, and treatment of rabies. Pharmacotherapy 2009;29:1182. [PMID: 19792992]

Rubella

■ **Essentials of Diagnosis**

- A systemic illness transmitted by inhalation of infected droplets, with incubation period of 14–21 days
- No prodrome in children (mild in adults); fever, malaise, coryza coincide with eruption of fine maculopapular rash on face to trunk to extremities, which fades after 3–5 days
- Arthralgias common, particularly in young women
- Posterior cervical, suboccipital, and posterior auricular lymphadenopathy 5–10 days before rash
- Leukopenia, thrombocytopenia
- In one of 6000 cases, postinfectious encephalopathy develops 1–6 days after the rash; mortality rate is 20%

■ **Differential Diagnosis**

- Other acute exanthems (eg, rubeola, enterovirus, Epstein-Barr virus infection, varicella)
- Drug allergy

■ **Treatment**

- Active immunization after age 15 months; girls should be immunized before menarche though not during pregnancy
- Symptomatic therapy only

■ **Pearl**

Rubella-associated arthritis is more symptomatic after vaccination than with natural infection.

Reference

Morice A, Ulloa-Gutierrez R, Avila-Agüero ML. Congenital rubella syndrome: progress and future challenges. Expert Rev Vaccines 2009;8:323. [PMID: 19249974]

Smallpox (Variola)

■ Diagnosis

- Generally requires prolonged close contact for transmission
- Incubation period 1–2 weeks
- Initial symptoms include fever, malaise, headache
- Rash progresses rapidly from mouth sores to macules then papules and pustules
- Central umbilication characteristic
- Unlike most other viral vesicular diseases, lesions in any part of the body are all at the same stage at the same time
- Suspected cases should be reported to public health authorities; confirmation requires PCR or culture

■ Differential Diagnosis

- Varicella
- Herpes simplex virus
- Other viral exanthema
- Drug reaction
- Other pox viruses (eg, monkey pox)

■ Treatment

- Contact and airborne isolation critical
- Supportive care as no specific treatment is available

■ Pearl

The last known case in the world was in the late 1970s; the virus is still propagated, in situ, a source of ongoing debate in the scientific community.

Reference

Metzger W, Mordmueller BG. Vaccines for preventing smallpox. Cochrane Database Syst Rev 2007:CD004913. [PMID: 17636779]

Varicella (Acute Chickenpox, Zoster [Shingles])

- **Essentials of Diagnosis**
  - Incubation period 10–21 days
  - Acute varicella: Fever, malaise with eruption of pruritic, centripetal, papular rash, becoming vesicular and pustular before crusting; lesions in all stages at any given time; "drop on rose petal" is the first lesion
  - Bacterial infection, pneumonia, and encephalitis may complicate
  - Reactivation varicella (herpes zoster): Dermatomal distribution, vesicular rash with pain often preceding eruption; thoracic and cranial nerve V most commonly involved

- **Differential Diagnosis**
  - Other viral infections
  - Drug allergy
  - Dermatitis herpetiformis
  - Pemphigus

- **Treatment**
  - Supportive measures with topical lotions and antihistamines; antivirals (acyclovir, valacyclovir, famciclovir) for all adults with varicella
  - Immune globulin or antivirals for exposed susceptible immunosuppressed or pregnant patients
  - Acyclovir early for immunocompromised or pregnant patients, severe disease (eg, pneumonitis, encephalitis), or ophthalmic division of trigeminal nerve involvement with zoster signaled by vesicle on tip of nose
  - Treatment with antiviral agent may diminish postherpetic neuralgia in older patients with zoster

- **Pearl**

Better prevented by vaccination than treated–like many diseases.

Reference

Bennett GJ, Watson CP. Herpes zoster and postherpetic neuralgia: past, present and future. Pain Res Manag 2009;14:275. [PMID: 19714266]

8

Viral Encephalitis

■ Essentials of Diagnosis

- Most common agents include enterovirus, Epstein-Barr virus, herpes simplex, measles, rubella, varicella, West Nile, St. Louis, Western and Eastern equine
- Some sporadic, some epidemic
- Fever, malaise, stiff neck, nausea, altered mentation
- Signs of upper motor neuron lesion: Exaggerated deep tendon reflexes, absent superficial reflexes, spastic paralysis
- Increased cerebrospinal fluid protein with lymphocytic pleocytosis, occasional hypoglycorrhachia
- PCR for HSV is sensitive and specific
- Isolation of virus from blood or cerebrospinal fluid; serology positive in paired specimens 3–4 weeks apart
- Brain imaging shows temporal lobe abnormalities in herpetic encephalitis

■ Differential Diagnosis

- Other noninfectious encephalitides (postvaccination, Reye's syndrome, toxins)
- Lymphocytic choriomeningitis
- Primary or secondary neoplasm
- Brain abscess or partially treated bacterial meningitis
- Fungal meningitis, especially coccidioidomycosis

■ Treatment

- Vigorous supportive measures with attention to elevated central nervous system pressures
- Mannitol in selected patients
- Acyclovir for suspected herpes simplex encephalitis; other specific antiviral therapy is under study

■ Pearl

In patients with suspected meningoencephalitis, acyclovir is given immediately and continued until herpes is excluded; few other viruses are susceptible to treatment.

References

Tyler KL. Emerging viral infections of the central nervous system: part 1. Arch Neurol 2009;66:939. [PMID: 19667214]

Tyler KL. Emerging viral infections of the central nervous system: part 2. Arch Neurol 2009;66:1065. [PMID: 19752295]

Yellow Fever

- ## Essentials of Diagnosis
  - Flavivirus transmitted by mosquito bites
  - Endemic only in Africa and South America
  - Sudden onset of severe headache, photophobia, myalgias, and palpitations
  - Early tachycardia with late bradycardia and hypotension, jaundice, hemorrhagic phenomena (gastrointestinal bleeding, mucosal lesions) in the severe form
  - Proteinuria, leukopenia, hyperbilirubinemia
  - Virus isolated from blood; serologic tests positive after second week of illness

- ## Differential Diagnosis
  - Leptospirosis
  - Viral hepatitis
  - Typhoid fever
  - Biliary tract disease
  - Malaria
  - Dengue

- ## Treatment
  - Active immunization of persons living in or traveling to endemic areas
  - Supportive care

- ## Pearl

A yearly urban epidemic occurrence treated by phlebotomy by the most distinguished physicians (eg, Benjamin Rush) in 18th- and 19th-century urban America.

Reference

Monath TP. Treatment of yellow fever. Antiviral Res 2008;78:116. [PMID: 18061688]

9

Oncologic Diseases

Biliary Tract Malignant Tumors

■ Essentials of Diagnosis

- Predisposing factors include choledochal cysts, primary sclerosing cholangitis, ulcerative colitis with sclerosing cholangitis, *Clonorchis sinensis* infection
- Jaundice, pruritus, anorexia, right upper quadrant pain
- Hepatomegaly, ascites, right upper quadrant tenderness
- Dilated intrahepatic bile ducts by ultrasound or CT scan
- Retrograde endoscopic cholangiogram characteristic; tissue biopsy is diagnostic
- Hyperbilirubinemia (conjugated), markedly elevated alkaline phosphatase and cholesterol

■ Differential Diagnosis

- Choledocholithiasis
- Drug-induced cholestasis
- Cirrhosis
- Chronic hepatitis
- Metastatic hepatic malignancy
- Pancreatic or ampullary carcinoma
- Biliary stricture

■ Treatment

- Palliative surgical bypass of biliary flow
- Stent bypass of biliary flow in selected patients
- Pancreaticoduodenectomy for resectable distal duct tumors curative in minority
- Chemoradiation or chemotherapy alone is offered for unresectable locally advanced disease, and palliative chemotherapy may provide survival benefit for metastatic disease

■ Pearl

Sclerosing cholangitis, and thus the risk of cholangiocarcinoma, does not abate after colectomy in the commonly associated ulcerative colitis.

Reference

Valle JW, Wasan H, Johnson P, et al. Gemcitabine alone or in combination with cisplatin in patients with advanced or metastatic cholangiocarcinomas or other biliary tract tumours: a multicentre randomised phase II study—The UK ABC-01 Study. Br J Cancer 2009;101:621. [PMID: 19672264]

Bladder Cancer (Transitional Cell Carcinoma)

- ■ Essentials of Diagnosis
  - More common in men over 40 years of age; predisposing factors include smoking, alcohol, occupational exposure to aromatic amines, aniline dyes or previous cyclophosphamide therapy; in the Middle East and Egypt, chronic *Schistosoma haematobium* infection can lead to squamous cell carcinomas of the bladder
  - Microscopic or gross hematuria with no other symptoms is the most common presentation
  - Suprapubic pain, urgency, and frequency when concurrent infection present
  - Occasional uremia if both ureterovesical orifices obstructed
  - Tumor visible by cystoscopy

- ■ Differential Diagnosis
  - Other urinary tract tumor
  - Acute cystitis
  - Renal tuberculosis
  - Urinary calculi
  - Glomerulonephritis or interstitial nephritis

- ■ Treatment
  - Endoscopic transurethral resection for superficial or submucosal tumors; intravesical chemotherapy reduces the likelihood of recurrence
  - Radical cystectomy standard with muscle-invasive tumors with increasing use of neoadjuvant cisplatin-based chemotherapy; bladder-sparing approaches can be applied to select cases or patients unfit for surgery
  - Adjuvant chemotherapy or radiation for completely resected patients is generally offered to those at high risk of recurrence, though data is conflicting on clinical benefit
  - Combination cisplatin-based chemotherapy for metastatic disease has a high response rate and may be curative in a small percentage of patients

- ■ Pearl

Remember Kaposi's sarcoma of the bladder in an AIDS patient with a urinary catheter and gross hematuria; cutaneous disease is not invariably present or obvious.

Reference

Vikram R, Sandler CM, Ng CS. Imaging and staging of transitional cell carcinoma: part 1, lower urinary tract. AJR Am J Roentgenol 2009;192:1481. [PMID: 19457808]

Breast Cancer in Men

■ Essentials of Diagnosis

- Rare disease but incidence is rising
- Men with Klinefelter's syndrome, family history of breast cancer in a female relative, or chest wall irradiation have an increased risk for breast cancer
- Painless lump or skin changes of breast
- Nipple discharge, bleeding, retraction or ulceration, palpable mass, gynecomastia
- Staging as in women
- 90% express estrogen receptor, and 80% express progesterone receptor; higher rates than in women; but fewer overexpress her2/neu oncogene

■ Differential Diagnosis

- Gynecomastia due to other causes (seen in up to 30% of healthy men)
- Benign tumor

■ Treatment

- Modified radical mastectomy with staging as in women, as well as axillary lymph node dissection or sentinel lymph node biopsy (for clinically negative nodal disease)
- As in female breast cancer, adjuvant hormonal therapy is recommended for many with completely resected disease; adjuvant chemotherapy is added for higher-risk disease, including node-positive disease
- For metastatic disease, endocrine manipulation (physical or chemical castration) with tamoxifen or related compounds, aminoglutethimide, or corticosteroids often quite effective

■ Pearl

This constitutes less than 1% of all breast cancer, but it is invariably diagnosed later in its course because men are neither suspected nor screened.

Reference

Niewoehner CB, Schorer AE. Gynaecomastia and breast cancer in men. BMJ 2008;336:709. [PMID: 18369226]

Breast Cancer in Women

- ■ Essentials of Diagnosis
  - Increased incidence in those with a family history of breast cancer and in nulliparous or late-childbearing women
  - Painless lump, often found by the patient; nipple or skin changes over breast (peau d'orange, redness, ulceration) later findings; axillary mass, malaise, or weight loss even later findings
  - Minority found by mammography
  - Metastatic disease to lung, bone, or central nervous system may dominate clinical picture
  - Staging based on size of tumor, involvement of lymph nodes, and presence of metastases
  - Extent of involvement of axillary lymph nodes is most powerful prognostic indicator in localized disease

- ■ Differential Diagnosis
  - Mammary dysplasia (fibrocystic disease)
  - Benign tumor (fibroadenoma, ductal papilloma)
  - Fat necrosis
  - Mastitis
  - Thrombophlebitis (Mondor's disease) of superficial chest vein

- ■ Treatment
  - Resection (lumpectomy plus radiation therapy versus modified radical mastectomy) in early-stage disease
  - Sentinel lymph node biopsy is preferred over axillary lymph node dissection if no clinically positive nodes
  - Menopausal status, hormone receptor (estrogen and progesterone) status, and human epidermal growth factor receptor (HER2) status dictate best adjuvant therapy
  - Adjuvant hormonal therapy is recommended for many with completely resected disease except those at very low risk for recurrence; adjuvant chemotherapy is recommended for node-positive disease and subset of node-negative disease with high-risk features
  - Metastatic disease is incurable, but treatment with hormonal manipulation, chemotherapy, radiation, and monoclonal antibody therapy (trastuzumab for HER2-positive disease) may provide long-term remission or stabilization

- ■ Pearl

Denial is common in this disease; it should be addressed by all primary care providers.

Reference

Gøtzsche PC, Nielsen M. Screening for breast cancer with mammography. Cochrane Database Syst Rev 2009:CD001877. [PMID: 19821284]

Central Nervous System Tumors (Intracranial Tumors)

■ Essentials of Diagnosis

- Prognosis depends on histology; half are gliomas
- Most present with generalized or focal disturbances of cerebral function: Generalized symptoms include nocturnal headache, seizures, and projectile vomiting; focal deficits relate to location of the tumor
- CT or MRI with gadolinium enhancement defines the lesion; posterior fossa tumors are better visualized by MRI
- Biopsy is the definitive diagnostic procedure, distinguishes primary brain tumors from brain abscess or metastasis
- Glioblastoma multiforme: In strictest sense an astrocytoma, but rapidly progressive with a poor prognosis
- Astrocytoma: More chronic course than glioblastoma, with a variable prognosis
- Medulloblastoma: Seen primarily in children and arises from roof of fourth ventricle
- Cerebellar hemangioblastoma: Patients usually present with disequilibrium and ataxia and occasional erythrocytosis
- Meningioma: Compresses rather than invades; benign
- CNS lymphoma: Usually in HIV/AIDS, though may occur rarely in immunocompetent individuals

■ Treatment

- Treatment depends on the type and site of the tumor and the condition of the patient
- Maximal resection predicts outcome in most
- Radiation postsurgery is mainstay of therapy; newer conformal radiation techniques decrease toxicity to normal brain; temozolomide can be given concurrently
- Combination chemotherapy or single-agent temozolomide active in some cases
- Herniation treated with intravenous corticosteroids, mannitol, and surgical decompression if possible
- Prophylactic anticonvulsants are also commonly given, but their role is uncertain in patients without history of seizure

■ Pearl

A headache that awakens a patient from sleep, though not diagnostic, is highly suggestive; take the complaint seriously.

Reference

Schor NF. Pharmacotherapy for adults with tumors of the central nervous system. Pharmacol Ther 2009;121:253. [PMID: 19091301]

Cervical Cancer

■ Essentials of Diagnosis

- Associated with human papillomavirus (HPV) infection in almost all cases
- Abnormal uterine bleeding, vaginal discharge, pelvic or abdominal pain
- Cervical lesion may be visible on inspection as tumor or ulceration
- Vaginal cytology is usually positive; must be confirmed by biopsy
- CT or MRI of abdomen and pelvis, examination under anesthesia useful for staging disease

■ Differential Diagnosis

- Cervicitis
- Chronic vaginitis or infection (tuberculosis, actinomycosis)
- Sexually transmitted diseases (syphilis, lymphogranuloma venereum, chancroid, granuloma inguinale)
- Aborted cervical pregnancy

■ Treatment

- Stage-dependent and requires input of surgeons, medical oncologists, and radiation oncologists
- Radical or extended hysterectomy curative in patients with early-stage disease
- For young patients who wish to preserve their fertility, newer fertility-sparing surgical approaches are acceptable alternatives
- Combination of radiation therapy and radiosensitizing chemotherapy is curative in majority of patients with localized disease not amenable to primary resection
- Role of surgery after chemotherapy and radiotherapy still being defined
- Combination chemotherapy for metastatic disease has significant response rate, but unclear magnitude of benefit on survival

■ Pearl

Vaccination to HPV and adherence to screening guidelines prevent invasive cervical carcinoma.

Reference

Widdice LE, Moscicki AB. Updated guidelines for Papanicolaou tests, colposcopy, and human papillomavirus testing in adolescents. J Adolesc Health 2008;43(suppl):S41. [PMID: 18809144]

Cervical Intraepithelial Neoplasia (CIN; Dysplasia or Carcinoma in Situ of the Cervix)

- ■ Essentials of Diagnosis
  - Associated with human papillomavirus (HPV) infection in up to 90% of advanced CIN (almost 100% of invasive cervical cancers)
  - Other risk factors include multiple sexual partners, HIV, cigarette smoking, other sexually transmitted diseases
  - Asymptomatic in many
  - Cervix appears grossly normal with dysplastic or carcinoma in situ cells by cytologic smear preparation
  - Culdoscopic examination with coarse punctate or mosaic pattern of surface capillaries, atypical transformation zone, and thickened white epithelium
  - Iodine-nonstaining (Schiller-positive) squamous epithelium is typical

- ■ Differential Diagnosis
  - Cervicitis

- ■ Treatment
  - Varies depending upon degree and extent of cervical or intraepithelial neoplasia; thus staging is crucial
  - Observation for mild dysplasia
  - Cryosurgery or CO_2 laser vaporization for moderate dysplasia
  - Cone biopsy or hysterectomy for severe dysplasia or carcinoma in situ
  - Repeat examinations to detect recurrence
  - HPV vaccination may prevent CIN or recurrence in at-risk individuals

- ■ Pearl

One of the relatively few cancers or precancerous conditions for which screening has made an important difference.

Reference

Dunton CJ. Management of atypical glandular cells and adenocarcinoma in situ. Obstet Gynecol Clin North Am 2008;35:623. [PMID: 19061821]

Colorectal Carcinoma

■ Essentials of Diagnosis

- Risk factors include colonic polyposis, Lynch syndrome (hereditary nonpolyposis colon cancer), and ulcerative colitis
- Altered bowel habits, rectal bleeding from left-sided carcinoma; occult blood in bowel movements; iron deficiency anemia in right-sided lesions
- Palpable abdominal or rectal mass in minority
- Characteristic barium enema or colonoscopic appearance; tissue biopsy is diagnostic
- Elevated carcinoembryonic antigen (CEA) useful as marker of disease recurrence in patients with elevated CEA at diagnosis but is not useful as a diagnostic tool

■ Differential Diagnosis

- Hemorrhoids
- Diverticular disease
- Benign colonic polyps
- Peptic ulcer disease
- Ameboma
- Functional bowel disease
- Iron deficiency anemia due to other causes

■ Treatment

- Surgical resection for cure; can also be done for palliation
- Adjuvant chemotherapy recommended for those with significant risk of recurrence, mainly lymph node positive disease, after surgery
- Combination chemotherapy is palliative for distant metastatic disease; adding novel agents targeting angiogenesis and growth factor pathways has improved response and survival rates
- If only limited liver or lung metastasis, resection is recommended if feasible, followed by combination chemotherapy
- For patients with rectal cancer with high risk features, radiation with chemotherapy is given before, and chemotherapy alone is given after, surgery
- Concurrent chemotherapy and radiotherapy curative in majority of localized anal cancers without need for surgery
- The American Gastroenterological Association and US Preventive Services Task Force strongly recommend colonoscopy for screening due to increasing incidence of right-sided tumors

■ Pearl

Streptococcus bovis endocarditis obligates a search for colonic neoplasm, both polyps and adenocarcinoma; there is an extremely common association between the two.

Reference

Lieberman DA. Clinical practice. Screening for colorectal cancer. N Engl J Med 2009;361:1179. [PMID: 19759380]

Endometrial Carcinoma

- **Essentials of Diagnosis**
  - Higher incidence in obesity, diabetes, nulliparity, polycystic ovaries, and women receiving tamoxifen as adjuvant therapy for breast cancer
  - Abnormal uterine bleeding, pelvic or abdominal pain
  - Uterus frequently not enlarged on palpation
  - Endometrial biopsy or curettage is required to confirm diagnosis after negative pregnancy test; vaginal cytologic examination is negative in high percentage of cases
  - Examination under anesthesia, chest x-ray, CT, or MRI required in staging

- **Differential Diagnosis**
  - Pregnancy, especially ectopic
  - Atrophic vaginitis
  - Exogenous estrogens
  - Endometrial hyperplasia or polyps
  - Other pelvic or abdominal neoplasms

- **Treatment**
  - Hysterectomy and salpingo-oophorectomy for well-differentiated or localized tumors
  - Combined surgery and radiation for poorly differentiated tumors, cervical extension, deep myometrial penetration, and regional lymph node involvement
  - Radiotherapy for unresectable localized malignancies
  - Palliative cisplatin-based chemotherapy may benefit those with metastatic disease
  - Progestational agents may help some women with metastatic disease

- **Pearl**

Not really a screenable cancer; a high index of suspicion is the most important aspect of diagnosis.

Reference

Linkov F, Edwards R, Balk J, Yurkovetsky Z, Stadterman B, Lokshin A, Taioli E. Endometrial hyperplasia, endometrial cancer and prevention: gaps in existing research of modifiable risk factors. Eur J Cancer 2008;44:1632. [PMID: 18514507]

Esophageal Cancer (Squamous Carcinoma and Adenocarcinoma)

■ Essentials of Diagnosis

- Progressive dysphagia initially during ingestion of solid foods, later with liquids; progressive weight loss and inanition ominous
- Smoking, alcoholism, chronic esophageal reflux with Barrett's esophagus, achalasia, caustic injury, and asbestos are risk factors
- Noninvasive imaging (barium swallow, CT scan) suggestive, diagnosis confirmed by endoscopy and biopsy
- Staging of disease aided by endoscopic ultrasound
- Squamous histology more common, though incidence of adenocarcinoma increasing rapidly in Western countries for unclear reasons

■ Differential Diagnosis

- Benign tumors of the esophagus
- Benign esophageal stricture or achalasia
- Esophageal diverticulum
- Esophageal webs
- Achalasia (may be associated)
- Globus hystericus

■ Treatment

- Combination chemotherapy and radiotherapy or surgery for localized disease, though long-term remission or cure is achieved in only 10–15%
- Dilation or esophageal stenting may palliate advanced disease; chemotherapy or radiation may help palliate advanced or metastatic disease

■ Pearl

Dysphagia is one of the few symptoms in medicine for which anatomic correlation always exists—too often it represents carcinoma.

Reference

Dubecz A, Molena D, Peters JH. Modern surgery for esophageal cancer. Gastroenterol Clin North Am. 2008;37:965. [PMID: 19028327]

Gastric Carcinoma

- ■ Essentials of Diagnosis
  - • Few early symptoms, but abdominal pain not unusual; late complaints include dyspepsia, anorexia, nausea, early satiety, weight loss
  - • Palpable abdominal mass (late)
  - • Iron deficiency anemia, fecal occult blood positive; achlorhydria present in minority of patients
  - • Mass or ulcer visualized radiographically; endoscopic biopsy and cytologic examination diagnostic
  - • Associated with atrophic gastritis, *Helicobacter pylori*; role of diet, previous partial gastrectomy controversial

- ■ Differential Diagnosis
  - • Benign gastric ulcer
  - • Gastritis
  - • Functional or irritable bowel syndrome
  - • Other gastric tumors (eg, leiomyosarcoma, lymphoma)

- ■ Treatment
  - • Resection for cure; palliative resection with gastroenterostomy in selected cases
  - • Perioperative chemotherapy or adjuvant chemoradiotherapy in addition to surgery improves long-term survival in high-risk patients
  - • For patients with metastatic disease, combination chemotherapy has significant response rate and may prolong survival; endoscopic laser ablation, venting gastrostomy, and stenting may palliate symptoms

- ■ Pearl

No acid, no ulcer: a gastric ulcer in an achlorhydric patient after histamine stimulation is carcinoma in 100% of cases.

Reference

Magnusson J. Stomach cancer. Curr Surg 2006;63:96. [PMID: 16520108]

Gestational Trophoblastic Neoplasia (Hydatidiform Mole and Choriocarcinoma)

- **Essentials of Diagnosis**
  - Uterine bleeding in first trimester
  - Uterus larger than expected for duration of pregnancy
  - No fetus demonstrated by ultrasound with sometimes characteristic findings of mole; excessively elevated levels of serum beta human chorionic gonadotropin (β-hCG) for gestational duration of pregnancy
  - Vesicles may be passed from vagina
  - Preeclampsia seen in first trimester

- **Differential Diagnosis**
  - Multiple pregnancy
  - Threatened abortion
  - Ectopic pregnancy

- **Treatment**
  - Suction curettage for hydatidiform mole
  - For nonmetastatic malignant disease, single-agent chemotherapy (eg, methotrexate or dactinomycin) very effective, but the role of hysterectomy is uncertain
  - For metastatic disease, single-agent or combination chemotherapy depending on clinical setting
  - Follow quantitative β-hCG until negative and then frequently for surveillance of tumor recurrence

- **Pearl**

Remember a mole in a hyperthyroid woman with severe hyperemesis gravidarum; β-hCG has the capability of activating thyroid hormone receptors.

Reference

Ben-Arie A, Deutsch H, Volach V, Peer G, Husar M, Lavie O, Gemer O. Reduction of postmolar gestational trophoblastic neoplasia by early diagnosis and treatment. J Reprod Med 2009;54:151. [PMID: 19370899]

Head and Neck Cancer (Squamous Cell Carcinoma)

■ Essentials of Diagnosis

- Most common between ages 50 and 70; occurs in heavy smokers, with alcohol as a co-carcinogen
- Early hoarseness in true cord lesions; sore throat, otalgia fairly common; odynophagia, hemoptysis indicate more advanced disease
- Comorbid lung cancer in some patients, which may not appear clinically until several years later
- Lesions found by physical examination or direct or indirect laryngoscopy; regional lymphadenopathy common at presentation

■ Differential Diagnosis

- Chronic laryngitis, including reflux laryngitis
- Laryngeal tuberculosis
- Myxedema
- Vocal cord paralysis due to laryngeal nerve palsy caused by left hilar lesion
- Serous otitis media
- Herpes simplex

■ Treatment

- Treatment varies by stage and tumor location and may include surgery, radiation, concurrent chemotherapy (cisplatin-based) and radiation, or combinations of above
- Cetuximab (monoclonal antibody to epidermal growth factor receptor) is an alternative to cisplatin therapy for definitive concurrent chemoradiation and is used alone or in combination with chemotherapy for metastatic disease
- Chemotherapy may provide palliative benefit for metastatic or recurrent disease
- Smoking cessation crucial for increasing treatment efficacy and preventing second malignancies

■ Pearl

A typical head-neck squamous carcinoma escapes diagnosis for many months after the patient's initial awareness of the first symptom or sign.

Reference

Argiris A, Karamouzis MV, Raben D, Ferris RL. Head and neck cancer. Lancet 2008;371:1695. [PMID: 18486742]

Hepatocellular Carcinoma

- **Essentials of Diagnosis**

  - Most common visceral malignancy worldwide; usually asymptomatic until disease advanced
  - Alcoholic cirrhosis, chronic hepatitis B or C, and hemochromatosis are risk factors
  - Abdominal enlargement, pain, jaundice, weight loss
  - Hepatomegaly, abdominal mass; rub or bruit heard over right upper quadrant in some
  - Anemia or erythrocytosis; liver function test abnormalities
  - Dramatic elevation in alpha-fetoprotein (AFP) helpful in diagnosis, though significant percentage have normal AFPs
  - Tendency to ascend hepatic vein and inferior vena cava
  - Angiography (though rarely performed) with characteristic abnormality; CT or MRI suggests diagnosis; tissue biopsy for confirmation

- **Differential Diagnosis**

  - Benign liver tumors: hemangioma, adenoma, focal nodular hyperplasia
  - Bacterial hepatic abscess
  - Amebic liver cyst
  - Metastatic tumor

- **Treatment**

  - Therapeutic options often limited by severe underlying liver disease; no surgical option if cirrhosis is present in remainder of liver
  - Surgical resection thought best curative option if lesions are resectable and patient is operative candidate
  - Liver transplant may be curative in small percentage of highly selected patients
  - For unresectable but localized disease, various approaches are applied, including radiofrequency ablation, percutaneous ethanol ablation, transarterial chemoembolization and cryoablation
  - Sorafenib (multitargeted tyrosine kinase inhibitor) has shown modest survival benefit in advanced disease

- **Pearl**

Merely carrying surface antigen for hepatitis B is a risk factor; in hepatitis C, it is the cirrhosis that predisposes malignant tumors of the biliary tract.

Reference

Shariff MI, Cox IJ, Gomaa AI, Khan SA, Gedroyc W, Taylor-Robinson SD. Hepatocellular carcinoma: current trends in worldwide epidemiology, risk factors, diagnosis and therapeutics. Expert Rev Gastroenterol Hepatol 2009;3:353. [PMID: 19673623]

Lung Cancer (Non–Small-Cell and Small-Cell Lung Carcinoma)

■ Essentials of Diagnosis

- Smoking most important cause, asbestos exposure synergistic
- Chronic cough, dyspnea; chest pain, hoarseness, hemoptysis, weight loss; may be asymptomatic, however
- Localized wheezing, clubbing, superior vena cava syndrome, decreased breath sounds due to effusion
- Mass, infiltrate, pleural effusion, or cavitation by chest x-ray
- Adenocarcinomas usually present peripherally, whereas squamous cell and small-cell lung carcinoma usually present centrally
- Diagnostic: Presence of malignant cells by sputum or pleural fluid cytology or on histologic examination of tissue biopsy
- Metastases or paraneoplastic effects may dominate
- PET-CT scanning before resection

■ Differential Diagnosis

- Tuberculosis
- Pulmonary mycoses, lung abscess
- Metastasis from extrapulmonary primary tumor
- Benign lung tumor (eg, hamartoma)
- Noninfectious granulomatous disease

■ Treatment

- Resection for early-stage non–small-cell carcinomas, assuming no evidence of spread or other primary; adjuvant chemotherapy recommended for pathologic lymph node–positive disease
- Concurrent chemotherapy and radiation for limited-stage small-cell carcinoma and for advanced-stage non–small-cell carcinomas that are unresectable but without distant metastasis (stage III); may be curative
- Prophylactic cranial radiation is beneficial for those patients with limited-stage and select cases of extensive-stage small-cell carcinoma
- Palliative therapy for metastatic non–small-cell carcinoma
- Extensive-stage small-cell carcinoma has excellent response rate to combination chemotherapy, but responses seldom durable

■ Pearl

Although digital clubbing is common in lung cancer, generally, it is not encountered in small-cell tumors, which have most other paraneoplastic manifestations.

Reference

Harichand-Herdt S, Ramalingam SS. Gender-associated differences in lung cancer: clinical characteristics and treatment outcomes in women. Semin Oncol 2009;36:572. [PMID: 19995649]

Ovarian Cancer (Epithelial Carcinoma)

■ Essentials of Diagnosis

- Family history, *BRCA1* or *BRCA2* mutations, nulliparity, long total duration of ovulation are risk factors
- Abdominal distention, pelvic pain, vaginal bleeding
- Ascites, abdominal or pelvic mass
- Ultrasonography, CT scan, or MRI delineates extent
- Laparoscopy or laparotomy to obtain tissue from mass or ascites for cytologic examination
- CA 125 useful for recurrence, not screening

■ Differential Diagnosis

- Uterine leiomyoma
- Endometriosis
- Tubal pregnancy
- Pelvic kidney
- Chronic pelvic inflammatory disease (especially tuberculosis)
- Benign ovarian masses

■ Treatment

- Premenopausal women with small ovarian masses can be observed with a trial of ovulation suppression for two cycles followed by repeat examination to exclude physiologic cysts
- Simple excision with ovarian preservation for benign cell types
- Unilateral salpingo-oophorectomy for certain cell types in younger women
- Hysterectomy with bilateral salpingo-oophorectomy in post-menopausal women, or premenopausal women with resectable disease not candidates for more conservative surgery
- Adjuvant chemotherapy for most patients with resected disease
- Cytoreductive surgery followed by combination chemotherapy for women with advanced disease without distant metastases; intraperitoneal and intravenous chemotherapy for patients with small-volume residual disease after surgery
- Combination chemotherapy with platinum-based regimen has high response rate and may provide durable remissions in women with metastatic disease

■ Pearl

A woman with a personal history of breast cancer, or a family history of breast or ovarian cancer, has a two- to sixfold increase in the risk of ovarian cancer.

Reference

Clarke-Pearson DL. Clinical practice. Screening for ovarian cancer. N Engl J Med 2009;361:170. [PMID: 19587342]

Pancreatic Cancer

- **Essentials of Diagnosis**
  - Peak incidence in seventh decade; more common in blacks, patients with chronic pancreatitis, and debatably, diabetes mellitus
  - Upper abdominal pain with radiation to back, weight loss, diarrhea, pruritus, thrombophlebitis; painless jaundice, with symptoms depending on where tumor is located, most being in the head of the pancreas
  - Palpable gallbladder or abdominal mass in some
  - Elevated amylase with liver function abnormalities; anemia, hyperglycemia, or frank diabetes in minority
  - Dilated common hepatic ducts by ultrasound or endoscopic retrograde cholangiogram
  - CT, MRI, and endoscopic ultrasound may delineate extent of disease and guide biopsy
  - Often, true extent of disease not appreciated before exploratory laparotomy

- **Differential Diagnosis**
  - Choledocholithiasis
  - Drug-induced cholestasis
  - Hepatitis
  - Cirrhosis
  - Carcinoma of ampulla of Vater

- **Treatment**
  - Surgical diversion for palliation in most cases
  - Radical pancreaticoduodenal resection for disease limited to head of pancreas or periampullary zone (Whipple resection) curative in rare cases, but more so in ampullary tumors
  - Chemotherapy, radiation, or combination in patients with advanced local disease may improve outcomes
  - Chemotherapy for metastatic disease may improve quality of life and prolong survival

- **Pearl**

Remember that cystadenocarcinoma, comprising 5% of pancreatic malignancies, has a much better prognosis than the related adenocarcinoma.

Reference

Freitas D, Fernandes Gdos S, Hoff PM, Cunha JE. Medical management of pancreatic adenocarcinoma. Pancreatology 2009;9:223. [PMID: 19420981]

Pleural Mesothelioma

- ■ Essentials of Diagnosis
  - Insidious dyspnea, nonpleuritic chest pain, weight loss
  - Dullness to percussion, diminished breath sounds, pleural friction rub, clubbing
  - Nodular or irregular unilateral pleural thickening, often with effusion by chest radiograph; CT scan often helpful
  - Pleural biopsy usually necessary for diagnosis, though malignant nature of tumor only confirmed by natural history; pleural fluid exudative and usually hemorrhagic
  - Strong association with asbestos exposure, with usual latency from time of exposure of 20 years or more

- ■ Differential Diagnosis
  - Primary pulmonary parenchymal malignancy
  - Empyema
  - Benign pleural inflammatory conditions (posttraumatic, asbestosis)

- ■ Treatment
  - Surgical approaches for localized disease range from palliative pleurodesis to attempted curative resection of involved lung and pleura
  - For highly select patients, extrapleural pneumonectomy (involving en-bloc resection of lung, pleura, ipsilateral diaphragm, and pericardium) can be considered along with adjuvant radiation and chemotherapy, but entails significant risk for complications and toxicity
  - Combination chemotherapy with pemetrexed and cisplatin has significant response rate and improvement in survival time, but response duration still short
  - One-year mortality rate > 75%

- ■ Pearl

Consider this when pleural thickening develops years after radiation, for lymphoma: it is a rare complication, commonly assumed to be an indolent infection.

Reference

Buduhan G, Menon S, Aye R, Louie B, Mehta V, Vallières E. Trimodality therapy for malignant pleural mesothelioma. Ann Thorac Surg 2009;88:870. [PMID: 19699914]

Prostate Cancer (Adenocarcinoma)

■ Essentials of Diagnosis

- Family history and African-American race are risk factors; African Americans tend to have more aggressive disease
- Routine screening with serum prostate-specific antigen (PSA) remains controversial; likely to be of greatest benefit in men > age 50 (especially blacks) with life expectancy > 10 years
- Symptoms of prostatism more often absent than present; bone pain if metastases present; asymptomatic in many
- Stony, hard, irregular prostate palpable
- Osteoblastic osseous metastases visible by plain radiograph
- PSA is age-dependent and is elevated in older patients with benign prostatic hyperplasia and also acute prostatitis; reliably predicts extent of neoplastic disease and recurrence after prostatectomy

■ Differential Diagnosis

- Benign prostatic hyperplasia (may be associated)
- Scarring secondary due to tuberculosis or calculi
- Urethral stricture
- Neurogenic bladder

■ Treatment

- Radiation therapy (external beam, brachytherapy, or combination) or radical prostatectomy, nerve-sparing for localized disease
- There is significant risk of erectile dysfunction and urinary incontinence complicating treatments for localized prostate cancer
- Adjuvant androgen deprivation therapy for lymph node–positive disease after radical prostatectomy, or for patients with high-risk disease receiving definitive radiation therapy
- Androgen ablation (chemical or surgical) for metastatic disease
- Combination chemotherapy may benefit selected patients with hormone-refractory metastatic disease
- Radiation therapy for symptomatic bony metastasis; bisphosphonates can help relieve pain and prevent further skeletal-related injury in metastatic hormone-refractory prostate cancer

■ Pearl

Approximately 1% of prostate tumors—most of these are highly aggressive small-cell carcinomas—are not adenocarcinoma and thus do not express PSA.

Reference

Cooperberg MR, Konety BR. Management of localized prostate cancer in men over 65 years. Curr Opin Urol 2009;19:309. [PMID: 19357512]

Renal Cell Carcinoma (Clear Cell Type)

- ■ Essentials of Diagnosis
  - Pleomorphic clinical manifestations: The internist's tumor
  - Gross or microscopic hematuria, back pain, fever, weight loss, night sweats
  - Flank or abdominal mass may be palpable
  - With increased utilization of CT and ultrasound (US), now commonly an incidental finding
  - Anemia in 30%, erythrocytosis in 3%; hypercalcemia, liver function test abnormalities, hypoglycemia sometimes seen
  - Tumor invasion of renal vein and inferior vena cava on occasion causes superior vena cava syndrome
  - Renal ultrasound, CT, or MRI reveals characteristic lesion

- ■ Differential Diagnosis
  - Polycystic kidney disease; simple cyst
  - Single complex renal cyst; 70% of these are malignant
  - Renal tuberculosis, calculi, or infarction
  - Endocarditis

- ■ Treatment
  - Nephrectomy curative for patients with early-stage lesions
  - Poor response to traditional chemotherapy or radiation in metastatic disease
  - Low response rate to high-dose interleukin 2, but if achieve complete response, long duration of remission; however, toxic and only for select good performance status patients
  - Novel agents, such as antiangiogenesis agents and mammalian target of rapamycin (mTOR) inhibitors, have improved response rate and survival times for metastatic cases
  - Resection of primary lesion has been documented to result in regression of metastases on rare occasions and may improve response to subsequent immunotherapy

- ■ Pearl

A small proportion of patients have a nonmetastatic hepatopathy (Stauffer's syndrome), with elevation of alkaline phosphatase; this abnormality does not imply inoperability and disappears with resection of the tumor.

Reference

Bellmunt J, Guix M. The medical management of metastatic renal cell carcinoma: integrating new guidelines and recommendations. BJU Int 2009;103:572. [PMID: 19154471]

Testicular Cancer (Seminomatous and Nonseminomatous Germ Cell Tumors)

■ Essentials of Diagnosis

- Painless testicular nodule; peak incidence at age 20–35 years
- Testis does not transilluminate
- Gynecomastia, premature virilization in occasional patients
- Tumor markers (AFP, lactate dehydrogenase, β-hCG) useful in diagnosis, prognosis/treatment planning, monitoring response to therapy, and surveillance for relapse
- Pure seminoma may produce β-hCG only, whereas nonseminomatous germ cell tumors may produce β-hCG and AFP; elevated AFP is pathognomonic for nonseminomatous germ cell tumor, even if not evident on histopathology

■ Differential Diagnosis

- Genitourinary tuberculosis
- Syphilitic orchitis
- Hydrocele
- Spermatocele
- Epididymitis

■ Treatment

- Orchiectomy, with lumbar and inguinal lymph nodes examined for staging
- Retroperitoneal lymph node dissection useful for accurate staging and prevention of relapse in nonseminomatous disease, but may be deferred in early-stage tumors in favor of close clinical follow-up
- Adjuvant retroperitoneal radiation for early-stage seminomatous germ cell tumors
- Platinum-based chemotherapy for higher-stage tumors and persistent tumor markers; curative in appreciable majority of patients with advanced or metastatic disease
- Chemotherapy regimen and intensity based on risk factors that include primary site, tumor marker elevation, and site of metastatic disease
- Late relapses possible, especially with seminoma, requiring long-term surveillance posttherapy

■ Pearl

A painless testicular nodule in a man between 20 and 40 is carcinoma until proven otherwise; the stakes are high, as the cure rate now approaches 95%.

Reference

Hayes-Lattin B, Nichols CR. Testicular cancer: a prototypic tumor of young adults. Semin Oncol 2009;36:432. [PMID: 19835738]

Thyroid Cancer

- **Essentials of Diagnosis**
  - History of irradiation to neck in some patients
  - Often hard, painless nodule; dysphagia or hoarseness occasionally
  - Cervical lymphadenopathy when local metastases present
  - Thyroid function tests normal; nodule is characteristically stippled with calcium on x-ray, cold by radioiodine scan, and solid by ultrasound; does not regress with thyroid hormone administration

- **Differential Diagnosis**
  - Thyroiditis
  - Other neck masses and other causes of lymphadenopathy
  - Thyroglossal duct cyst
  - Benign thyroid nodules

- **Treatment**
  - Fine-needle aspiration biopsy best differentiates benign from malignant nodules
  - Total thyroidectomy for carcinoma; radioactive iodine postoperatively for selected patients with iodine-avid metastases; combination chemotherapy in anaplastic tumors
  - Sorafenib (multitargeted tyrosine kinase inhibitor) showing promise in relapsed or refractory metastatic cases
  - Prognosis related to cell type and histology; papillary carcinoma offers excellent outlook, anaplastic the worst
  - Medullary thyroid cancer is typically refractory to chemotherapy and radiation; associated with multiple endocrine neoplasia (MEN) syndromes; diagnosable by calcitonin elevation

- **Pearl**

In patients who had thymus radiation during childhood—a common practice years ago for physiologic prominence on chest X-ray of the gland in childhood—a thyroid nodule is malignant until proved otherwise.

Reference

Ying AK, Huh W, Bottomley S, Evans DB, Waguespack SG. Thyroid cancer in young adults. Semin Oncol 2009;36:258. [PMID: 19460583]

Vulvar Cancer (Squamous Cell Carcinoma)

- **Essentials of Diagnosis**
  - Prolonged vulvar irritation, pruritus, local discomfort, slight bloody discharge
  - History of genital warts common; association with human papillomavirus established
  - Early lesions may suggest chronic vulvitis
  - Late lesions may present as a mass, exophytic growth, or firm ulcerated area in vulva
  - Biopsy makes diagnosis

- **Differential Diagnosis**
  - Sexually transmitted diseases (syphilis, lymphogranuloma venereum, chancroid, granuloma inguinale)
  - Crohn's disease
  - Benign tumors (granular cell myoblastoma)
  - Reactive or eczematoid dermatitis
  - Vulvar dystrophy

- **Treatment**
  - Local resection for cases of in situ squamous cell carcinoma
  - Wide surgical excision with lymph node dissection for invasive carcinoma
  - Radiation or radiation plus radiosensitizing chemotherapy in addition to surgery may improve outcomes in patients with locally advanced disease

- **Pearl**

This tumor's diagnosis may be needlessly delayed; think of it in all indolent venereal disease.

Reference

Woelber L, Mahner S, Voelker K, et al. Clinicopathological prognostic factors and patterns of recurrence in vulvar cancer. Anticancer Res 2009;29:545. [PMID: 19331201]

10

Fluid, Acid–Base, and Electrolyte Disorders

Dehydration

- **Essentials of Diagnosis**
  - Thirst, oliguria
  - Decreased skin turgor, especially on anterior thigh; dry mucous membranes, postural hypotension, tachycardia; none sensitive or specific
  - Impaired renal function (blood urea nitrogen:creatinine ratio > 20), elevated urinary osmolality and specific gravity, decreased urinary sodium, fractional excretion of sodium < 1% (for most causes)

- **Differential Diagnosis**
  - Hemorrhage
  - Sepsis
  - Gastrointestinal fluid losses
  - Skin sodium losses associated with burns or sweating
  - Renal sodium loss
  - Adrenal insufficiency
  - Nonketotic hyperosmolar state in type 2 diabetics

- **Treatment**
  - Identify source of volume loss if present
  - Replete with normal saline, blood, or colloid as indicated
  - Half-normal saline may be substituted when blood pressure normalizes

- **Pearl**

Tenting of the skin of the thigh is the most useful cutaneous sign of dehydration.

Reference

Bianchetti MG, Simonetti GD, Bettinelli A. Body fluids and salt metabolism: part I. Ital J Pediatr 2009;35:36. [PMID: 19925659]

Hypercalcemia

- **Essentials of Diagnosis**
  - Polyuria and constipation; bony and abdominal pain in some
  - Thirst and dehydration
  - Mild hypertension
  - Altered mentation, hyporeflexia, stupor, coma all possible
  - Serum calcium > 10.2 mg/dL (corrected with concurrent serum albumin)
  - Renal insufficiency or azotemia
  - Shortened QT interval due to short ST segment; ventricular extrasystoles

- **Differential Diagnosis**
  - Primary hyperparathyroidism
  - Adrenal insufficiency (rare)
  - Malignancy (multiple myeloma with osteoclast-activating factor; lymphoma secreting 1,25-vitamin D; other primary tumor or metastasis releasing parathyroid hormone–related peptide)
  - Vitamin D intoxication
  - Milk-alkali syndrome
  - Sarcoidosis
  - Tuberculosis
  - Paget's disease of bone, especially with immobilization
  - Familial hypocalciuric hypercalcemia
  - Hyperthyroidism
  - Thiazide diuretics

- **Treatment**
  - Identify and treat underlying disorder
  - Volume expansion, loop diuretics (once euvolemic)
  - Bisphosphonates, calcitonin, dialysis, and glucocorticoids all useful in certain instances
  - Resection of parathyroid adenoma, if present

- **Pearl**

Hypercalcemia begets hypercalcemia; polyuria causes hypovolemia and consequent increased proximal tubular calcium reabsorption.

Reference

Makras P, Papapoulos SE. Medical treatment of hypercalcaemia. Hormones (Athens) 2009;8:83. [PMID: 19570736]

Hyperkalemia

- ■ Essentials of Diagnosis
    - Weakness or flaccid paralysis, abdominal distention, diarrhea
    - Serum potassium > 5 mEq/L
    - Electrocardiographic changes: Peaked T waves, loss of P wave with sinoventricular rhythm, QRS widening, ventricular asystole, cardiac arrest

- ■ Differential Diagnosis
    - Renal failure with oliguria
    - Hypoaldosteronism (hyporeninism, potassium-sparing diuretics, angiotensin-converting enzyme inhibitors, adrenal insufficiency, interstitial renal disease)
    - Acidemia; type IV renal tubular acidosis
    - Burns, hemolysis, tumor lysis syndrome
    - Digitalis overdose, beta-blockers (rare), heparin
    - Spurious in patients with thrombocytosis; clot releases potassium into serum before laboratory determination

- ■ Treatment
    - Emergency (cardiac toxicity, paralysis): Calcium gluconate, intravenous bicarbonate, glucose, and insulin
    - Dietary potassium restriction and sodium polystyrene sulfonate or loop diuretic to lower potassium subacutely
    - Dialysis if oliguric renal failure or severe acidosis complicates
    - Anti-digitalis Tc antibodies in patients receiving digitalis

- ■ Pearl

As atrial muscle is more sensitive to hyperkalemia, a "junctional rhythm" may in fact be sinus; the SA node impulse fails to depolarize the atria, and thus no P waves are seen on the surface ECG.

Reference

Nyirenda MJ, Tang JI, Padfield PL, Seckl JR. Hyperkalaemia. BMJ 2009;339:b4114. [PMID: 19854840]

Hypermagnesemia

- **Essentials of Diagnosis**
  - Weakness, hyporeflexia, respiratory muscle paralysis
  - Confusion, altered mentation
  - Serum magnesium > 3 mg/dL; renal insufficiency the rule; increased uric acid, phosphate, potassium, and decreased calcium may be seen
  - Increased PR interval → heart block → cardiac arrest when marked

- **Differential Diagnosis**
  - Renal insufficiency
  - Excessive magnesium intake (food, antacids, laxatives, intravenous administration)

- **Treatment**
  - Correct renal insufficiency, if possible (volume expansion)
  - Intravenous calcium chloride for severe manifestations (eg, electrocardiographic changes, respiratory embarrassment)
  - Dialysis

- **Pearl**

  Be cautious about magnesium-containing antacids—available OTC—in patients with renal insufficiency; little is needed to elevate this cation.

Reference

Musso CG. Magnesium metabolism in health and disease. Int Urol Nephrol 2009;41:357. [PMID: 19274487]

Hypernatremia

■ Essentials of Diagnosis

- Severe thirst unless mentation altered; oliguria
- In severe cases, altered mental status, delirium, seizures, coma
- If hypovolemic, loose skin with poor turgor, tachycardia, hypotension
- Serum sodium > 145 mEq/L, serum osmolality > 300 mEq/L caused by free water loss
- Affected patients usually include the very old, very young, critically ill, or neurologically impaired

■ Differential Diagnosis

- Diabetes insipidus, either neurogenic or nephrogenic
- Loss of hypotonic fluid (insensible, diuretics, vomiting, diarrhea, nasogastric suctioning, osmotic diuresis due to hyperglycemia)
- Salt intoxication
- Volume resuscitation and continuation of normal saline (155 mEq/L) after euvolemia achieved
- Mineralocorticoid excess

■ Treatment

- Relatively rapid volume replacement (if hypovolemic) followed by free water replacement over 48–72 hours (beware of cerebral edema; correct sodium by no more than 0.5 mEq/L per hour)
- Desmopressin acetate for central diabetes insipidus

■ Pearl

A serum sodium in excess of 150 mEq/L indicates inability to access free water, such is the power of thirst; such patients are invariably seriously ill.

Reference

Agrawal V, Agarwal M, Joshi SR, Ghosh AK. Hyponatremia and hypernatremia: disorders of water balance. J Assoc Physicians India 2008;56:956. [PMID: 19322975]

Hyperphosphatemia

- **Essentials of Diagnosis**
  - Few distinct symptoms
  - Cataracts, basal ganglion calcifications in hypoparathyroidism
  - Serum phosphate > 5 mg/dL; renal failure, hypocalcemia occasionally seen

- **Differential Diagnosis**
  - Renal failure
  - Hypoparathyroidism
  - Excess phosphate intake, vitamin D toxicity
  - Phosphate-containing laxative use (cause of acute phosphate nephropathy)
  - Cell destruction (tumor lysis syndrome, rhabdomyolysis), respiratory or metabolic acidosis
  - Multiple myeloma

- **Treatment**
  - Treat underlying disease when possible
  - Oral calcium carbonate (use noncalcium binder in concomitant hypercalcemia) to reduce phosphate absorption
  - Hemodialysis if refractory

- **Pearl**

Overshoot hyperphosphatemia from therapy of hypophosphatemia may precipitate tetany.

Reference

Moe SM. Disorders involving calcium, phosphorus, and magnesium. Prim Care 2008;35:215. [PMID: 18486714]

Hypocalcemia

- ### Essentials of Diagnosis
  - Abdominal and muscle cramps, stridor; tetany and seizures
  - Diplopia, facial paresthesias, papilledema
  - Positive Chvostek's and Trousseau's signs
  - Cataracts if chronic, likewise basal ganglion calcifications
  - Serum calcium < 8.5 mg/dL (corrected with concurrent serum albumin); phosphate usually elevated; hypomagnesemia may cause or complicate
  - Electrocardiographic changes: Prolonged QT interval; ventricular arrhythmias, including ventricular tachycardia

- ### Differential Diagnosis
  - Vitamin D deficiency and osteomalacia
  - Malabsorption
  - Hypoparathyroidism
  - Hyperphosphatemia
  - Hypomagnesemia
  - Chronic renal failure
  - Pancreatitis
  - Drugs (loop diuretics, aminoglycosides, foscarnet)
  - Citrate excess due to massive blood transfusions

- ### Treatment
  - Identify and treat underlying disorder
  - For tetany, seizures, or arrhythmias, give calcium gluconate intravenously
  - Magnesium replacement if renal function normal
  - Oral calcium and vitamin D supplements (calcitriol in renal failure)
  - Phosphate binders in chronic hypocalcemia with hyperphosphatemia

- ### Pearl

Hypomagnesemia causes resistance to the action of parathyroid hormone, causing this problem; replete Mg^{++} first, then Ca^{++}.

Reference

Bosworth M, Mouw D, Skolnik DC, Hoekzema G. Clinical inquiries: what is the best workup for hypocalcemia? J Fam Pract 2008;57:677. [PMID: 18842196]

Hypokalemia

- **Essentials of Diagnosis**
  - Usually asymptomatic
  - Muscle weakness, lethargy, paresthesias, polyuria, anorexia, constipation, nausea, vomiting
  - Electrocardiographic changes: Ventricular ectopy; T-wave flattening and ST-segment depression → development of prominent U waves → AV block → cardiac arrest
  - Serum potassium < 3.5 mEq/L and metabolic alkalosis sometimes concurrent

- **Differential Diagnosis/Causes**
  - Diuretic use
  - Alkalemia
  - Beta-agonists (eg, albuterol)
  - Hyperaldosteronism (adrenal adenoma, primary hyperreninism, mineralocorticoid use, and European licorice ingestion)
  - Magnesium depletion
  - Hyperthyroidism
  - Diarrhea
  - Renal tubular acidosis (types I, II)
  - Bartter's, Gitelman's, and Liddle's syndromes
  - Familial hypokalemic periodic paralysis
  - Severe dietary potassium restriction
  - Hemodialysis and peritoneal dialysis

- **Treatment**
  - Identify and treat underlying cause
  - Oral or intravenous potassium supplementation
  - Magnesium repletion if indicated

- **Pearl**

Think of hypokalemia in unexplained orthostatic hypotension.

Reference

Greenlee M, Wingo CS, McDonough AA, Youn JH, Kone BC. Narrative review: evolving concepts in potassium homeostasis and hypokalemia. Ann Intern Med 2009;150:619. [PMID: 19414841]

Hypomagnesemia

- ### Essentials of Diagnosis
  - Muscle restlessness or cramps, weakness, athetoid movements, twitching or tremor, delirium, seizures
  - Muscle wasting, hyperreflexia, Babinski's sign, nystagmus, hypertension
  - Serum magnesium < 1.5 mEq/L; decreased calcium, potassium often associated
  - Electrocardiographic changes: Tachycardia, premature atrial or ventricular beats, increased QT interval, ventricular tachycardia or fibrillation

- ### Differential Diagnosis
  - Inadequate dietary intake
  - Hypervolemia
  - Diuretics, cisplatin, aminoglycosides, amphotericin B
  - Malabsorption or diarrhea
  - Alcoholism
  - Hyperaldosteronism, hyperthyroidism, hyperparathyroidism
  - Respiratory alkalosis
  - Gitelman's and Bartter's syndromes

- ### Treatment
  - Identify and treat underlying cause
  - Intravenous magnesium replacement followed by oral maintenance
  - Calcium and potassium supplements if needed

- ### Pearl

Many cardiologists believe in the antiarrhythmic effect of magnesium; consider repleting magnesium in patients with ventricular arrhythmias.

Reference

Soave PM, Conti G, Costa R, Arcangeli A. Magnesium and anaesthesia. Curr Drug Targets 2009;10:734. [PMID: 19702521]

Hyponatremia

■ Essentials of Diagnosis

- Nausea, headache, weakness, irritability, mental confusion (especially with serum sodium < 120 mEq/L, developing rapidly)
- Generalized seizures, lethargy, coma, respiratory arrest, and death may result, yet slowly developing cases may be asymptomatic
- Serum sodium < 135 mEq/L; osmolality < 280 mEq/L (hypotonic hyponatremia); hypouricemia if syndrome of inappropriate antidiuretic hormone hypersecretion (SIADH) or primary polydipsia is the cause

■ Differential Diagnosis

- Hypovolemic causes (thiazides, osmotic diuresis, adrenal insufficiency, vomiting, diarrhea, fluid sequestration)
- Hypervolemic causes (congestive heart failure, cirrhosis, nephrotic syndrome, advanced renal failure, pregnancy)
- Euvolemic causes (hypothyroidism, SIADH, glucocorticoid insufficiency, reset osmostat, primary polydipsia)
- Hypertonic or isotonic hyponatremia (hyperglycemia, intravenous mannitol)
- Pseudohyponatremia (hypertriglyceridemia, paraproteinemia) caused by laboratory artifact

■ Treatment

- Treat underlying disorder
- Corticosteroids empirically if adrenal insufficiency suspected
- Gradual correction (serum sodium change of no more than 0.5 mEq/L per hour) unless severe central nervous system signs present; central pontine myelinolysis may result from rapid overcorrection
- If hypovolemic, use normal saline
- If hypervolemic, use water restriction, loop diuretics, and normal saline volume replacement of urine output
- Vasopressin receptor antagonists or demeclocycline in selected patients with SIADH

■ Pearl

A sodium level less than 130, blood urea nitrogen less than 10, and hypouricemia in a patient without liver, heart, or kidney disease are virtually diagnostic of SIADH.

Reference

Agrawal V, Agarwal M, Joshi SR, Ghosh AK. Hyponatremia and hypernatremia: disorders of water balance. J Assoc Physicians India 2008;56:956. [PMID: 19322975]

Hypophosphatemia

■ Essentials of Diagnosis

- Seldom an isolated abnormality
- Anorexia, myopathy, arthralgias
- Irritability, confusion, seizures
- Rhabdomyolysis, if severe
- Serum phosphate < 2.5 mg/dL, severe < 1 mg/dL; elevated creatine kinase if rhabdomyolysis
- Hemolysis in severe cases

■ Differential Diagnosis

- Hyperparathyroidism, hyperthyroidism
- Alcoholism
- Hereditary hypophosphatemic rickets
- Tumor-induced osteomalacia
- Malabsorption, starvation
- Hypercalcemia, hypomagnesemia
- Correction of hyperglycemia
- Recovery from catabolic state

■ Treatment

- Intravenous phosphate replacement when severe
- Oral phosphate supplements (unless hypercalcemic); be cautious about overshooting
- Correct magnesium deficit, if present

■ Pearl

Phosphate levels even as low as 0–0.1 mg/dL are possible without clinical manifestations—in the rare instance of it being an isolated disorder.

Reference

Rastegar A. New concepts in pathogenesis of renal hypophosphatemic syndromes. Iran J Kidney Dis 2009;3:1. [PMID: 19377250]

10

Metabolic Acidosis

- **Essentials of Diagnosis**
  - Dyspnea, hyperventilation, respiratory fatigue
  - Tachycardia, tachypnea, hypotension, shock (depending on cause)
  - Acetone on breath (in ketoacidosis)
  - Arterial pH < 7.35, serum bicarbonate decreased; anion gap may be normal or high; ketonuria

- **Differential Diagnosis**
  - Ketoacidosis (diabetic, alcoholic, starvation)
  - Lactic acidosis
  - Poisons (methyl alcohol, ethylene glycol, salicylates)
  - Uremia
  - With normal anion gap, diarrhea, renal tubular acidosis
  - Post-hyperventilation

- **Treatment**
  - Identify and treat underlying cause
  - Correct volume, electrolyte status
  - Bicarbonate therapy indicated in ethylene glycol or methanol toxicity, renal tubular acidosis; debated for other causes
  - Hemodialysis, mechanical ventilation if necessary

- **Pearl**

A low pH in diabetic ketoacidosis is not the cause of an altered mental status—hyperosmolality or a systemic process like septicemia is.

Reference

Fidkowski C, Helstrom J. Diagnosing metabolic acidosis in the critically ill: bridging the anion gap, Stewart, and base excess methods. Can J Anaesth 2009;56:247. [PMID: 19247746]

Metabolic Alkalosis

■ Essentials of Diagnosis

- Weakness, malaise, lethargy; other symptoms depend on cause
- Hyporeflexia, tetany, ileus, muscle weakness
- Arterial pH > 7.45, P_{CO_2} up to 45 mm Hg, serum bicarbonate > 30 mEq/L; potassium and chloride usually low; hypoventilation is seldom prominent regardless of pH

■ Differential Diagnosis

- Loss of acid (vomiting or nasogastric aspiration)
- Diuretic overuse or other volume contraction
- Exogenous bicarbonate load
- Aldosterone excess: Hyperreninemia, ingestion of some types of licorice, adrenal tumor or hyperplasia, Bartter's or Gitelman's syndrome

■ Treatment

- Identify and correct underlying cause
- Replenish volume and electrolytes (use 0.9% sodium chloride)
- Hydrochloric acid rarely if ever needed
- Supplemental KCl in most

■ Pearl

Vomiting causes mild metabolic alkalosis from volume contraction; most severe cases are seen in gastric outlet obstruction, when the regurgitated contents from the stomach are pure HCl.

Reference

Pahari DK, Kazmi W, Raman G, Biswas S. Diagnosis and management of metabolic alkalosis. J Indian Med Assoc 2006;104:630. [PMID: 17444063]

10

Respiratory Acidosis

- ### Essentials of Diagnosis
  - Central to all is alveolar hypoventilation
  - Confusion, altered mentation, somnolence in many
  - Cyanosis and asterixis may or may not be present
  - Arterial P_{CO_2} increased; arterial pH decreased
  - Lung disease may be acute (pneumonia, asthma) or chronic (chronic obstructive pulmonary disorder)
  - Lung disease not present in all

- ### Differential Diagnosis
  - Chronic obstructive lung disease
  - Central nervous system depressants
  - Structural disorders of the thorax
  - Myxedema
  - Neurologic disorders (eg, Guillain-Barré syndrome, amyotrophic lateral sclerosis, myasthenia gravis)

- ### Treatment
  - Address underlying cause
  - Artificial ventilation if necessary to oxygenate, invasive or non-invasive

- ### Pearl

Hypoxemia must be considered before ascribing mental status changes to an elevated P_{CO_2}; it's the case in most chronically hypercapnic patients.

Reference

Ozsancak A, D'Ambrosio C, Hill NS. Nocturnal noninvasive ventilation. Chest 2008;133:1275. [PMID: 18460530]

Respiratory Alkalosis

- **Essentials of Diagnosis**
  - Lightheadedness, numbness or tingling of extremities, perioral paresthesias
  - Tachypnea; positive Chvostek's and Trousseau's signs in acute hyperventilation; carpopedal spasm and tetany
  - Arterial pH > 7.45, P_{CO_2} < 30 mm Hg

- **Differential Diagnosis**
  - Restrictive lung disease or hypoxemia
  - Pulmonary embolism
  - Salicylate toxicity
  - Anxiety or pain
  - End-stage cirrhosis
  - Sepsis
  - Pregnancy
  - High-altitude residence

- **Treatment**
  - Correct hypoxemia or underlying ventilatory stimulant
  - Increase ventilatory dead space (eg, breathe into paper bag, but only in anxiety-induced hyperventilation)

10

- **Pearl**

There are few causes of chronic respiratory alkalosis; cirrhosis is the bad one, pregnancy is the good one.

Reference

Wise RA, Polito AJ, Krishnan V. Respiratory physiologic changes in pregnancy. Immunol Allergy Clin North Am 2006;26:1. [PMID: 16443140]

Shock

- ■ Essentials of Diagnosis
  - • History of hemorrhage, myocardial infarction, sepsis, trauma, or anaphylaxis
  - • Tachycardia, hypotension, hypothermia, tachypnea
  - • Cool, sweaty skin with pallor; however, may be warm or flushed with early sepsis; altered level of consciousness
  - • Oliguria, acute tubular necrosis (if hypoperfusion prolonged), anemia, disseminated intravascular coagulation, metabolic acidosis may complicate
  - • Hemodynamic measurements depend upon underlying cause

- ■ Differential Diagnosis
  - • Numerous causes of the syndrome, as noted above
  - • Adrenal insufficiency

- ■ Treatment
  - • Correct cause of shock (ie, control hemorrhage, treat infection, correct metabolic disease)
  - • Empiric broad-spectrum antibiotics (gram-positive and gram-negative coverage) if cause not apparent
  - • Restore hemodynamics with fluids; vasopressor medications may be required; early hemodynamic correction associated with improved outcome
  - • Maintain urine output
  - • Treat contributing disease (eg, diabetes mellitus)

- ■ Pearl

A hypertensive patient who manifests the clinical appearance of shock raises the question of aortic dissection.

Reference

Wagner F, Baumgart K, Simkova V, Georgieff M, Radermacher P, Calzia E. Year in review 2007: Critical Care—shock. Crit Care 2008;12:227. [PMID: 18983707]

11

Genitourinary and Renal Disorders

GENITOURINARY DISORDERS

Bacterial Prostatitis

- **Essentials of Diagnosis**
  - Acute bacterial prostatitis: Fever, dysuria, urgency, frequency, perineal or suprapubic pain; tender prostate; leukocytosis, pyuria, bacteriuria, hematuria; caused by *Escherichia coli* most commonly, also *Neisseria gonorrhoeae, Chlamydia trachomatis, Proteus, Pseudomonas, Enterococcus*
  - Digital rectal exam essential; avoid vigorous prostatic massage
  - Chronic prostatitis: Usually in older men, may be asymptomatic; in some, urgency and frequency, dysuria, perineal or suprapubic pain; prostate boggy, not tender
  - Expressed prostatic secretions demonstrate increased numbers of leukocytes; culture often sterile

- **Differential Diagnosis**
  - Urethritis; cystitis; prostatodynia
  - Epididymitis; perirectal abscess; nonbacterial prostatitis

- **Treatment**
  - Urinary Gram stain can guide initial therapy; if no Gram stain available then treat as outlined below, but urine culture results should modify initial treatment
  - For acute bacterial prostatitis in men under 35 years of age, treat for *N. gonorrhoeae* and *C. trachomatis* infection
  - For acute bacterial prostatitis in men over age 35 years or homosexual men, treat for Enterobacteriaceae with systemic antibiotics
  - For chronic bacterial prostatitis, treat for Enterobacteriaceae with oral antibiotics
  - Treat symptoms with hot sitz baths, NSAIDs, stool softeners

- **Pearl**

Trimethoprim achieves one of the highest intraprostatic levels of all antibiotics; combined with sulfamethoxazole, it is the drug of choice.

Reference

Langer JE, Cornud F. Inflammatory disorders of the prostate and the distal genital tract. Radiol Clin North Am 2006;44:665. [PMID: 17030219]

Benign Prostatic Hyperplasia

- **Essentials of Diagnosis**
  - Urinary hesitancy, intermittent stream, straining to initiate micturition, reduced force and caliber of the urinary stream, nocturia, frequency, urgency
  - Palpably enlarged prostate
  - Urinalysis and serum creatinine should be obtained
  - High postvoid residual volume as determined by ultrasonography or excretory urography; not always prognostic of outcome
  - May be complicated by acute urinary retention or azotemia after prolonged obstruction

- **Differential Diagnosis**
  - Urethral stricture
  - Vesicular stone
  - Neurogenic bladder
  - Bladder neck contracture
  - Carcinoma of bladder of prostate
  - Urinary tract infection
  - Prostatitis

11

- **Treatment**
  - Treat associated infection if present; trimethoprim-sulfamethoxazole is usually best
  - Minimize evening fluid intake
  - Alpha$_1$-blockers for symptom relief; 5-α-reductase inhibitors (eg, finasteride) in patients with marked prostatic enlargement
  - Utilization of symptom scoring instruments to follow success of treatment
  - Transurethral resection for intolerable symptoms, refractory urinary retention, recurrent gross hematuria, and progressive renal insufficiency with demonstrated obstruction

- **Pearl**

In acute urinary retention in older men, ask about recent upper respiratory infections; over-the-counter remedies with anticholinergic properties may cause this, and stopping them may ward off a transurethral resection of the prostate.

Reference

Edwards JL. Diagnosis and management of benign prostatic hyperplasia. Am Fam Physician 2008;77:1403. [PMID: 18533373]

Infectious Epididymitis

- **Essentials of Diagnosis**
  - Acute to subacute unilateral testicular pain and palpable swelling of epididymis, with fever, dysuria, urinary urgency, and frequency of less than 6 weeks' duration
  - Subacute much more common than acute presentations
  - Marked epididymal, testicular, or spermatic cord tenderness with symptomatic relief upon elevation of scrotum (Prehn's sign); less pronounced in subacute presentations
  - Leukocytosis, pyuria, bacteriuria
  - Usually caused by *Neisseria gonorrhoeae* or *Chlamydia trachomatis* in heterosexual men under age 40 and by Enterobacteriaceae or *Pseudomonas* species in homosexual men of all ages and heterosexual men over age 40
  - Doppler ultrasonography differentiates from testicular torsion

- **Differential Diagnosis**
  - Testicular torsion
  - Testicular tumor
  - Orchitis
  - Prostatitis
  - Testicular trauma

11

- **Treatment**
  - Empiric antibiotics after culture of urine obtained
  - In men under age 40, treat for *N. gonorrhoeae* and *C. trachomatis* infection for 10–21 days
  - Consider examination and treatment of sexual partners
  - In men over age 40, treat for Enterobacteriaceae for 21–28 days
  - Analgesics, ice, and bed rest with elevation and support of scrotum

- **Pearl**

Consider a rapid plasma reagin and an HIV test for all patients with this disorder.

Reference

Luzzi GA, O'Brien TS. Acute epididymitis. BJU Int 2001;87:747. [PMID: 11350430]

Testicular Torsion

■ Essentials of Diagnosis

- Usually occurs in males under 25 years of age; may present as an acute abdomen
- Sudden onset of severe, unilateral scrotal or inguinal pain
- Exquisitely tender and swollen testicle and spermatic cord; pain worsened with elevation
- Asymmetric high-riding testis on affected side is classic
- Absence of cremasteric reflex
- Leukocytosis and pyuria
- Doppler ultrasonography is diagnostic test of choice

■ Differential Diagnosis

- Epididymitis
- Orchitis
- Testicular trauma
- Testicular tumor
- Torsion of the appendix testis

■ Treatment

- Inability to rule out testicular torsion requires surgical consult
- Diagnostic confirmation requires immediate surgery
- Irreversible damage after 12 hours of ischemia

■ Pearl

Probably the diagnosis most easily remembered by the affected patient in all of medicine.

Reference

Mansbach JM, Forbes P, Peters C. Testicular torsion and risk factors for orchiectomy. Arch Pediatr Adolesc Med 2005;159:1167. [PMID: 16330742]

Tuberculosis of the Genitourinary Tract

■ Essentials of Diagnosis

- Fever, malaise, night sweats, weight loss; evidence of pulmonary tuberculosis in 50%
- Symptoms or signs of urinary tract infection may be present
- Nodular, indurated epididymis, testes, or prostate
- Sterile pyuria or hematuria without bacteriuria; white blood cell casts can be seen with renal parenchymal involvement
- Positive culture of morning urine on one of three consecutive samples
- Proteinuria may indicate development of secondary amyloidosis
- Plain radiographs may show renal and lower tract calcifications
- Excretory urogram reveals "moth-eaten" calices, papillary necrosis, and beading of ureters
- Occasionally, ulcers or granulomas of bladder wall at cystoscopy

■ Differential Diagnosis

- Other causes of chronic urinary tract infections
- Interstitial nephritis, especially drug-induced
- Nonspecific urethritis
- Urinary calculi
- Epididymitis
- Bladder cancer

■ Treatment

- Standard combination antituberculosis therapy
- Surgical procedures for obstruction and severe hemorrhage
- Nephrectomy for extensive destruction of the kidney

■ Pearl

The common teaching about sterile pyuria and hematuria in this condition is only partially true; anatomic abnormalities in the collecting system often give rise to coinfection with more common bacteria.

Reference

Wise GJ. Urinary tuberculosis: modern issues. Curr Urol Rep 2009;10:313. [PMID: 19570494]

Urinary Calculi

- **Essentials of Diagnosis**

  - Most common in the stone belt, extending from central Ohio through mid-Florida
  - Sudden, severe colicky pain localized to the flank, commonly associated with nausea, vomiting, and fever; marked urinary urgency and frequency if stone lodged at ureterovesical junction
  - Occasionally asymptomatic
  - Hematuria in 90%, pyuria with concurrent infection; presence of crystals in urine may be diagnostically helpful
  - Plain films of the abdomen (stone seen in 90%), spiral CT, or sonography may be used to visualize location of stone
  - Depending on the metabolic abnormality (ie, hypercalcemia, hypercalciuria, hyperuricosuria, hypocitraturia, hyperoxaluria), stones can be composed of calcium oxalate or phosphate (> 80%), struvite, uric acid, or cystine; more than 50% of patients develop recurrent stones

- **Differential Diagnosis**

  - Acute pyelonephritis
  - Chronic prostatism
  - Tumor of genitourinary system
  - Renal tuberculosis
  - Renal infarction
  - Ectopic pregnancy

- **Treatment**

  - Stones usually pass spontaneously with analgesia and hydration
  - Antibiotics if concurrent infection present
  - Patient should filter urine and save stone for analysis
  - Hydration to produce at least 2 L/day of urine output is a mainstay to prevent recurrence; also dietary change, thiazides, allopurinol, citrate, or a combination of these may be used to prevent recurrence, depending on composition of the stone
  - Urinary stone risk profile (via 24-hour urine collection) should be sent if patients are at moderate to high risk for recurrence
  - Refer to specialist for recurrent stones
  - Lithotripsy or surgical lithotomy may be necessary in refractory cases

- **Pearl**

Instruct patients to retrieve passed stones when possible, and analyze them; it is a noninvasive metabolic biopsy of the disease process.

Reference

Moe OW. Kidney stones: pathophysiology and medical management. Lancet 2006;367:333. [PMID: 16443041]

RENAL DISORDERS

Acute and Chronic Tubulointerstitial Nephritis

- ■ Essentials of Diagnosis
  - Responsible for 10–15% of cases of acute kidney injury
  - Most drug-related (acutely, beta-lactam antibiotics or NSAIDs; chronically, lead or lithium), but may be associated with lupus, sarcoidosis, or certain infections (eg, *Staphylococcus*, *Streptococcus*, legionellosis, leptospirosis, various viruses)
  - Acute interstitial nephritis with sudden renal decline can present with fever, maculopapular rash, eosinophilia, flank pain
  - Hematuria, pyuria, proteinuria, white blood cell casts, and occasionally eosinophils in urine (seen with Hansel's or Wright's stain)
  - Chronic tubulointerstitial nephritis characterized by polyuria and nocturia, salt wasting, small kidneys, isosthenuria; mild proteinuria and hyperchloremic metabolic acidosis may also be present
  - Chronic form may result from prolonged obstruction, analgesic abuse, sickle cell trait, chronic hypercalcemia, uric acid nephropathy, or exposure to heavy metals
  - Signs of tubulointerstitial injury include Fanconi's syndrome and renal tubular acidosis
  - Clinical diagnosis that can only be confirmed by renal biopsy

- ■ Differential Diagnosis
  - Acute or chronic glomerulonephritis
  - Prerenal azotemia
  - Primary obstructive uropathy

- ■ Treatment
  - Discontinue all possible offending drugs or treat associated infection in patients with acute tubulointerstitial nephritis
  - Corticosteroids of questionable benefit but recommended for drug-induced acute interstitial nephritis without significant chronic component that does not improve after drug discontinuation; NSAID-induced nephritis much less likely to respond to steroids.
  - Temporary dialysis may be necessary in up to one-third of patients with drug-induced acute interstitial nephritis

- ■ Pearl

In ill-defined pain syndromes (headache, low back pain) with chronic kidney disease, over-the-counter analgesics used to great excess by the patient may be the cause.

Reference

John R, Herzenberg AM. Renal toxicity of therapeutic drugs. J Clin Pathol 2009;62:505. [PMID: 19474353]

Acute Cystitis and Pyelonephritis

■ Essentials of Diagnosis

- Dysuria with urinary frequency and urgency, hematuria, abdominal or flank pain
- Fever, flank or suprapubic tenderness, and vomiting with pyelonephritis
- Pyuria, bacteriuria, hematuria, positive urine culture, white cell casts on urinalysis (latter in pyelonephritis)
- Usually caused by gram-negative bacteria (eg, *E. coli, Proteus, Klebsiella,* Enterobacteriaceae) but may be due to gram-positive organisms (eg, *Enterococcus faecalis, Staphylococcus saprophyticus*)

■ Differential Diagnosis

- Urethritis
- Nephrolithiasis
- Prostatitis
- Pelvic inflammatory disease or vaginosis
- Lower lobe pneumonia
- Surgical abdomen due to any cause (eg, appendicitis)

■ Treatment

- Urine culture in complicated infections (pregnancy, male, elderly, hospital-acquired, recent antibiotics, immunocompromised, obstruction or instrumentation)
- Empiric oral antibiotics (eg, trimethoprim-sulfamethoxazole, ciprofloxacin) for 3 days for uncomplicated cystitis
- Oral or intravenous antibiotics (eg, fluoroquinolone or cephalosporin) for 7–14 days for pyelonephritis
- Intravenous antibiotics and fluids if dehydration or vomiting present
- Pyridium for early symptomatic relief
- Consider hospitalization for patients with single kidney, immunosuppression, or elderly
- Pursue evaluation for anatomic abnormalities in men who develop cystitis or pyelonephritis
- Recurrent episodes of cystitis (more than two per year) often treated with low-dose prophylactic antibiotics

■ Pearl

Pyelonephritis is one of the reasons no one should have an exploratory laparotomy without a urinalysis—white cell casts signify pyelonephritis, a non-surgical cause of acute abdomen.

Reference

Drekonja DM, Johnson JR. Urinary tract infections. Prim Care 2008;35:345. [PMID: 18486719]

Acute Glomerulonephritis

■ Essentials of Diagnosis

- History of preceding streptococcal or other infection, evidence of systemic vasculitis, or presence of occult malignancy
- Malaise, headache, fever, dark urine, hypertension, edema
- Acute decline in glomerular filtration rate (GFR), oligo/anuria with azotemia in severe cases
- Urine reveals: Hematuria (with or without dysmorphic red cells and red cell casts), proteinuria (usually mild)
- Depending on clinical situation, further tests include complement levels, antistreptolysin O (ASO) titer, antideoxyribonuclease B (anti-DNA B) titer, antinuclear antibody (ANA) titers, antiglomerular basement membrane (GBM) antibody levels, antineutrophil cytoplasmic antibodies (ANCA), hepatitis B and C antibodies, cryoglobulins, blood cultures; renal biopsy establishes the cause

■ Differential Diagnosis

- IgA nephropathy and Henoch-Schönlein purpura
- Systemic lupus erythematosus (SLE)
- Goodpasture syndrome (anti-GBM antibody syndrome)
- ANCA-associated vasculitides (eg, Wegener's granulomatosis, microscopic polyangiitis, Churg-Strauss syndrome)
- Membranoproliferative glomerulonephritis
- Hepatitis B– or C–associated glomerulonephritis, other postinfectious glomerulonephritides
- Infective endocarditis; tubulointerstitial disease

■ Treatment

- Start with therapy for underlying cause if possible; supportive therapy with fluid and sodium restriction, diuretics as needed; lower blood pressure slowly to prevent sudden decrease in renal perfusion
- Steroids and cytotoxic agents are used for rapidly progressive glomerulonephritis, more effective at higher GFRs
- Plasmapheresis occasionally of value in anti-GBM and ANCA-related disease

■ Pearl

Remember that a red cell cast in the urine is the equivalent of a biopsy showing glomerulonephritis; the first urine specimen after an oral water load with the patient in enforced lordosis may increase the yield of finding one, and most patients would prefer a urinalysis to a renal biopsy.

Reference

Beck LH Jr, Salant DJ. Glomerular and tubulointerstitial diseases. Prim Care 2008;35:265. [PMID: 18486716]

Acute Kidney Injury

■ Essentials of Diagnosis

- Most commonly caused by acute tubular necrosis (ATN)
- Nausea, vomiting, mental status changes, edema, hypertension
- History can include exposure to nephrotoxic agents, sepsis, trauma, surgery, shock, or hemorrhage
- Oliguria is a poor prognostic sign
- Pericardial friction rub, asterixis may be present with uremia
- Hyperkalemia, hyperphosphatemia, decreased serum bicarbonate
- Kidneys of normal size or enlarged on imaging studies; small kidneys or renal osteodystrophy suggests chronic renal failure
- Urinalysis with manual microscopy can guide diagnostic approach; ATN with pigmented granular casts; acute glomerulonephritis and interstitial nephritis as previously described

■ Differential Diagnosis

- Prerenal azotemia (eg, hypovolemia, heart failure, cirrhosis)
- Intrinsic causes (eg, tubulointerstitial, glomerular, vascular)
- Postrenal azotemia (eg, obstructive uropathy)

■ Treatment

- Volume resuscitation with isotonic fluid for hypovolemia
- Ultrasonography to rule out obstructive process
- Renal biopsy (when glomerulonephritis suspected or etiology unknown)
- Supportive care for uncomplicated cases: Minimize fluid intake, follow potassium, phosphorus, and bicarbonate levels
- Oliguric kidney injury with worse prognosis than a nonoliguric process; role of diuretics to convert to latter process unproven
- Dialysis for fluid overload, hyperkalemia, pericarditis, uremia
- Adjust dosage of renally metabolized medications
- Avoid contrast exposure; volume repletion and N-acetylcysteine prophylaxis in high-risk patients before unavoidable contrast studies

■ Pearl

The FENa can be inappropriately low in specific states of ATN (postischemic and radiocontrast nephropathy) and can be inappropriately high in prerenal disease (concurrent diuretic use).

Reference

Endre ZH. Acute kidney injury: definitions and new paradigms. Adv Chronic Kidney Dis 2008;15:213. [PMID: 18565473]

Anti–Glomerular Basement Membrane Nephritis (Goodpasture's Syndrome)

- ■ Essentials of Diagnosis
  - Triad of pulmonary hemorrhage with hemoptysis, circulating anti-GBM antibody, and glomerulonephritis due to anti-GBM
  - Most common in young (18–30) and middle-aged (50–60s) white men; smokers also have a predilection
  - Extrarenal manifestations may be absent
  - On immunofluorescence, renal biopsy reveals linear deposition of IgG with or without C3 deposition along the GBM
  - Serum anti-GBM antibody is pathognomonic

- ■ Differential Diagnosis
  - Wegener's granulomatosis
  - Polyarteritis nodosa
  - SLE
  - Endocarditis
  - Postinfectious glomerulonephritis
  - Primary pulmonary hemorrhage

- ■ Treatment
  - Plasmapheresis to remove circulating anti-GBM antibody
  - Prednisone and cyclophosphamide for at least 3 months
  - Recovery of renal function more likely if treatment is begun before serum creatinine reaches 6–7 mg/dL; hemodialysis as necessary
  - Renal transplant delayed for 12 months after disappearance of antibody from the serum

- ■ Pearl

One of the few causes in medicine of a dramatically elevated diffusion capacity of carbon monoxide, due to the increased amount of blood in the lungs.

Reference

Ooi JD, Holdsworth SR, Kitching AR. Advances in the pathogenesis of Goodpasture's disease: from epitopes to autoantibodies to effector T cells. J Autoimmun 2008;31:295. [PMID: 18502098]

Asymptomatic Bacteriuria

- ■ Essentials of Diagnosis
  - • History of recurring urinary tract infections may be present
  - • Bacteriuria with absence of symptoms or signs referable to the urinary tract
  - • May be associated with obstruction, anatomic or neurologic abnormalities, pregnancy, indwelling catheter, urologic procedures, diverted urinary stream (eg, ileal loop conduit), diabetes mellitus, or old age
  - • Usually caused by Enterobacteriaceae, *Pseudomonas,* or enterococci

- ■ Differential Diagnosis
  - • Drug-induced nephropathy, especially analgesics
  - • Contaminated urine specimen

- ■ Treatment
  - • Indications for treatment include pregnancy, persistent bacteriuria in certain patients and before urologic procedures
  - • Urine culture to guide antimicrobial therapy if treatment warranted
  - • Surgical relief of obstruction if present
  - • In selected cases, chronic antibiotic suppression

- ■ Pearl

Be certain that fresh urine is cultured before making this diagnosis; bacteria may grow with specimens not cultured promptly.

Reference

Lin K, Fajardo K; U.S. Preventive Services Task Force. Screening for asymptomatic bacteriuria in adults: evidence for the U.S. Preventive Services Task Force reaffirmation recommendation statement. Ann Intern Med 2008;149:W20. [PMID: 18591632]

Chronic Kidney Disease (CKD)

- ■ Essentials of Diagnosis
  - • Numerous causes, especially diabetes, hypertension; asymptomatic early
  - • National Kidney Foundation classification is useful:
    Stage I: GFR > 90 mL/min/1.73 m^2 plus kidney damage
    Stage II: GFR 60–89 mL/min/1.73 m^2 plus kidney damage
    Stage III: GFR 30–59 mL/min/1.73 m^2
    Stage IV: GFR 15–29 mL/min/1.73 m^2
    Stage V: GFR < 15 mL/min/1.73 m^2
  - • Advanced dysfunction with volume overload, hypertension, metabolic acidosis, hyperkalemia, hyperphosphatemia, hypocalcemia, anemia, CKD-related mineral and bone disorder
  - • Uremia: anorexia, nausea, hiccups, confusion, pericarditis
  - • Benign urinary sediment; bilateral shrunken kidneys in most

- ■ Differential Diagnosis
  - • Obstructive uropathy, prerenal azotemia, acute kidney injury

- ■ Treatment
  - • Slow progression by controlling underlying disease and hypertension, preferably with angiotensin-converting enzyme (ACE); regular estimation of GFR and proteinuria
  - • Attention to comorbid factors, especially cardiovascular disease, as well as hyperlipidemia, anemia, and bone disease
  - • Low-protein diet, salt and water restriction for patients with hypertension and edema
  - • Potassium, phosphorus, and magnesium restriction once GFR is below 30–60 mL/min; phosphorus binders for associated hyperphosphatemia with avoidance of chronic aluminum hydroxide if possible; calcium and vitamin D supplements to prevent osteodystrophy
  - • Erythropoietin after iron repletion and excluding other causes of anemia; bicarbonate therapy for chronic metabolic acidosis
  - • In progressive disease, referral for dialysis or renal transplantation

- ■ Pearl

Given its causes, patients with chronic kidney disease are more likely to die of cardiovascular disease than of the metabolic consequences of the renal problem.

Reference

Anothaisintawee T, et al. Prevalence of chronic kidney disease: a systematic review and meta-analysis. Clin Nephrol 2009;71:244. [PMID: 19281734]

Diabetic Nephropathy

■ Essentials of Diagnosis

- 20–30% of diabetics have microalbuminuria approximately 15 years after diabetes mellitus first diagnosed
- Diabetic retinopathy often present
- GFR increases initially, returns to normal as further renal damage occurs, then continues to fall
- Proteinuria > 1 g/d, often nephrotic range
- Normal to enlarged kidneys on ultrasound
- Biopsy can show mesangial matrix expansion, diffuse glomerulosclerosis, and nodular intercapillary glomerulosclerosis, the latter pathognomonic

■ Differential Diagnosis

- Nephrotic syndrome due to other cause, especially amyloidosis
- Glomerulonephritis with nephrotic features such as that seen in systemic lupus erythematosus, membranous glomerulonephritis, or IgA nephropathy

■ Treatment

- ACE inhibition or angiotensin II receptor blockade reduce hyperfiltration, proteinuria, and progression
- Strict glycemic and blood pressure control
- Supportive care for progression of chronic kidney disease—includes treatment of anemia, acidosis, and elevated phosphorus
- Transplantation an alternative to dialysis at end stage, but comorbid vasculopathy can be daunting; may have significant survival benefit with preemptive (before end-stage renal disease) transplantation

■ Pearl

One of medicine's few causes of massive albuminuria even at severe reduction of glomerular filtration rate.

Reference

Keane WF, Lyle PA. Recent advances in management of type 2 diabetes and nephropathy: lessons from the RENAAL study. Am J Kidney Dis 2003;41(suppl 1):S22. [PMID: 12612946]

Focal Segmental Glomerulosclerosis

- **Essentials of Diagnosis**
  - May be primary (idiopathic) or secondary (physiologic response to hyperfiltration or glomerular hypertrophy as in disorders with decreased renal mass such as unilateral renal agenesis, after nephrectomy, massive obesity, reflux nephropathy; or nonspecific healing from prior inflammatory injury)
  - Other causes include familial forms, toxin related (heroin), infections (HIV)
  - Along with membranous nephropathy, most common cause of nephrotic syndrome in nondiabetic adults
  - Primary form often presents with acute nephrotic syndrome: Proteinuria, hypoalbuminemia, edema, hyperlipidemia
  - Secondary forms often asymptomatic, presenting with non-nephrotic proteinuria and slowly progressive kidney disease
  - Depending on the history, further tests may include serologies (HIV), renal ultrasound, and renal biopsy

- **Differential Diagnosis**
  - Membranous nephropathy; diabetic nephropathy
  - Minimal change disease; amyloid; IgA nephropathy
  - Postinfectious glomerulonephritis (later stages)
  - Membranoproliferative glomerulonephritis

- **Treatment**
  - General measures similar to those for nephrotic syndrome, especially use of ACE inhibitor or angiotensin receptor blocker for proteinuria and lipid-lowering agents for hyperlipidemia
  - Steroid treatment initially for symptomatic idiopathic focal segmental glomerulosclerosis; favorable prognosis for complete or partial responders
  - Steroid resistance associated with poor renal prognosis; additional therapy with cyclosporine, tacrolimus, mycophenolate mofetil, cytotoxic agents (cyclophosphamide, chlorambucil), or plasmapheresis

- **Pearl**

Patients undergoing kidney transplant for this disorder have a higher incidence of rejection compared with most other nephropathies.

Reference

Braun N, Schmutzler F, Lange C, Perna A, Remuzzi G, Risler T, Willis NS. Immunosuppressive treatment for focal segmental glomerulosclerosis in adults. Cochrane Database Syst Rev 2008:CD003233. [PMID: 18646090]

Hypertensive Nephrosclerosis

- **Essentials of Diagnosis**
  - Poorly controlled hypertension for more than 15 years; alternatively, severe, aggressive hypertension, especially in young blacks
  - With extreme blood pressure elevation, papilledema and encephalopathy may occur
  - Ultrasound reveals bilateral small, echogenic kidneys in advanced disease
  - Proteinuria is usual
  - Biopsy can show thickened vessels and sclerotic glomeruli; malignant nephrosclerosis reveals characteristic onion-skinning

- **Differential Diagnosis**
  - Atheroembolic or atherosclerotic renal disease
  - Renal artery stenosis, especially bilateral
  - End-stage renal disease due to any other cause

- **Treatment**
  - Strict sodium restriction
  - Aggressive control of hypertension, including ACE inhibitor or angiotensin receptor blocker if possible
  - If patient presents with hypertensive urgency or emergency, decrease blood pressure slowly over several days to prevent decreased renal perfusion
  - May take up to 6 months of adequate blood pressure control to achieve improved baseline of renal function

- **Pearl**

In benign nephrosclerosis, the rule is for serum creatinine to rise slightly after beginning antihypertensive therapy; stay the course with blood pressure control and improved renal function will follow.

Reference

Hill GS. Hypertensive nephrosclerosis. Curr Opin Nephrol Hypertens 2008;17:266. [PMID: 18408477]

IgA Nephropathy (Berger's Disease)

- **Essentials of Diagnosis**
  - Most common form of acute and chronic glomerulonephritis in Caucasians and Asians
  - Focal proliferative glomerulonephritis of unknown cause
  - Secondary causes include hepatic cirrhosis, celiac disease, inflammatory bowel disease, dermatitis herpetiformis, psoriasis, minimal change disease
  - First episode: Macroscopic hematuria, often associated with a viral infection, with or without upper respiratory ("synpharyngitic") and gastrointestinal symptoms
  - Malaise, fatigue, myalgias, hypertension, edema may be present
  - Recurrent hematuria and mild proteinuria over decades, with same precipitants
  - Often detected incidentally with microscopic hematuria
  - Serum IgA increased in 30–50%; renal biopsy reveals inflammation and deposition of IgA with or without C3 and IgM in the mesangium of all glomeruli
  - Usually indolent; 20–30% of patients progress to end-stage renal disease over 2–3 decades

- **Differential Diagnosis**
  - Hereditary nephritis (Alport's syndrome)
  - Thin basement membrane disease; Henoch-Schönlein purpura
  - Poststreptococcal acute glomerulonephritis
  - Infective endocarditis; Goodpasture's syndrome
  - Other vasculitides (eg, polyarteritis nodosa, Wegener's)

- **Treatment**
  - Supportive therapy for patients with < 1 g/d of proteinuria with yearly monitoring of renal function
  - In patients with proteinuria > 1 g/d or hypertension, treat with ACE inhibitors
  - Fish oil of questionable benefit but not harmful
  - Steroids, cytotoxic agents, and immunosuppressants in selected cases with preserved GFR

- **Pearl**

IgA nephropathy commonly flares with upper respiratory infections— one patient may instruct many students in the appearance of red cell casts over decades of such events.

Reference

Glassock RJ. IgA nephropathy: challenges and opportunities. Cleve Clin J Med 2008;75:569. [PMID: 18756838]

Lupus Nephritis

- ■ Essentials of Diagnosis
  - • Can be the initial presentation of systemic lupus erythematosus
  - • WHO classification of renal biopsy: Normal renal biopsy (class I); mesangial proliferation (class II); focal proliferation (class III); diffuse proliferation (class IV); membranous (class V)
  - • Proteinuria or hematuria of glomerular origin; hypocomplementemia common
  - • Glomerular filtration rate need not be depressed
  - • Chronic tubulointerstitial changes on biopsy portend a worse prognosis

- ■ Differential Diagnosis
  - • Glomerulonephritis due to other diseases, including anti-GBM disease, microscopic polyangiitis, Wegener's granulomatosis, membranous nephropathy, IgA nephropathy, thrombotic thrombocytopenic purpura
  - • Nephrotic syndrome due to other causes
  - • Vascular thrombi secondary to antiphospholipid antibodies

- ■ Treatment
  - • Follow serial measures of renal function and urinalysis
  - • Strict control of hypertension
  - • ACE inhibitor to reduce proteinuria
  - • Steroids and cytotoxic agents for severe class III or any class IV; treatment for class V is still debatable
  - • Early treatment of renal relapses may prevent severe flare
  - • Repeat biopsy for flare of renal disease; lupus nephritis can change forms
  - • Upon reaching end-stage renal disease, renal transplantation is an excellent alternative to dialysis

- ■ Pearl

If kidney disease is encountered in drug-induced lupus, consider another cause; drug-induced SLE typically spares the kidney and brain.

Reference

Bagavant H, Fu SM. Pathogenesis of kidney disease in systemic lupus erythematosus. Curr Opin Rheumatol 2009;21:489. [PMID: 19584729]

Membranous Nephropathy

- ■ Essentials of Diagnosis
  - • Common; may be primary (idiopathic) or secondary (malignancy, usually solid organ; autoimmune diseases such as lupus or rheumatoid arthritis; systemic infections such as hepatitis B or C)
  - • Anorexia, dyspnea, foamy urine; anasarca
  - • Proteinuria, hypoalbuminemia, hyperlipidemia
  - • Hypercoagulability due to anticoagulant urinary loss; hematuria in half
  - • Renal ultrasound; renal biopsy to establish diagnosis
  - • Limit malignancy evaluation to age-appropriate screening or evaluation of abnormalities from history and physical

- ■ Differential Diagnosis
  - • Focal segmental glomerulosclerosis
  - • Diabetic nephropathy
  - • Minimal change disease
  - • Amyloidosis
  - • Membranoproliferative glomerulonephritis

- ■ Treatment
  - • General measures similar to those for nephrotic syndrome, further therapies reserved for idiopathic cases only
  - • Spontaneous or partial (≤ 2 g/d proteinuria) remission in 70%; thus if nonnephrotic proteinuria and asymptomatic, or symptoms of edema easily controlled, observe without treatment
  - • Risk factors for progressive disease: Men > age 50 years, proteinuria > 6 g/d, abnormal renal function at presentation, and tubulointerstitial disease on biopsy; active therapy with steroids and cytotoxic agent (cyclophosphamide or chlorambucil)
  - • Alternative agents in selected cases: Cyclosporine, mycophenolate mofetil, azathioprine, intravenous immunoglobulin
  - • Good long-term prognosis after spontaneous or drug-induced remission, although relapses may occur in one-quarter of cases

11

- ■ Pearl

At one time a paraneoplastic manifestation of this condition was thought its most common cause; though likely not still true, clinicians should be vigilant for tumor if no other explanation is present.

Reference

Waldman M, Austin HA 3rd. Controversies in the treatment of idiopathic membranous nephropathy. Nat Rev Nephrol 2009;5:469. [PMID: 19581908]

Myeloma Kidney

■ Essentials of Diagnosis

- May be initial presentation of multiple myeloma
- The systemic disease with the most renal and metabolic complications
- Classic definition: Light chain of immunoglobulins (Bence Jones proteins) directly toxic to tubules, or causing intratubular obstruction by precipitation
- Myeloma may also be associated with glomerular amyloidosis, hypercalcemia, nephrocalcinosis, nephrolithiasis, plasma cell infiltration of the renal parenchyma, hyperviscosity syndrome compromising renal blood flow, proximal (Fanconi-like syndrome) or distal renal tubular acidosis, type IV renal tubular acidosis, and progressive renal insufficiency
- Serum anion gap is low in the majority due to positively charged paraprotein
- Serum and urinary electrophoresis reveals monoclonal spike in more than 90% of patients; some cases are nonsecretory and are very aggressive clinically

■ Differential Diagnosis

- Interstitial nephritis
- Prerenal azotemia
- Obstructive nephropathy
- Nephrotic syndrome of other cause
- Drug-induced nephropathy

■ Treatment

- Therapy for myeloma; prognosis for renal survival is better if serum creatinine is < 2 mg/dL before treatment
- Treat hypertension and hypercalcemia if present
- Avoid contrast agents and other nephrotoxins
- Avoid dehydration and maintain adequate intravascular volume; remember that hypercalcemia causes nephrogenic diabetes insipidus, and this worsens dehydration

■ Pearl

Suspect if a dipstick test is negative in the face of an abnormal protein:creatinine ratio.

Reference

Dimopoulos MA, Kastritis E, Rosinol L, Bladé J, Ludwig H. Pathogenesis and treatment of renal failure in multiple myeloma. Leukemia 2008;22:1485. [PMID: 18528426]

11

Nephrotic Syndrome

- **Essentials of Diagnosis**

  - May be primary or secondary to systemic infections (eg, secondary syphilis, endocarditis), diabetes, multiple myeloma with or without amyloidosis, heavy metals, and autoimmune diseases
  - Anorexia, dyspnea, anasarca, foamy urine
  - Proteinuria (> 3 g/d), hypoalbuminemia (< 3 g/dL), edema, hyperlipidemia in ~50% upon presentation
  - Hypercoagulability with peripheral renal vein thrombosis, particularly in membranous nephropathy
  - Lipiduria with oval fat bodies, Maltese crosses, and fatty and waxy casts in urinary sediment
  - Further tests may include complement levels (CH50, C3, C4), serum and urine electrophoresis, antinuclear antibody (ANA), serologies (hepatitis B and C, syphilis), renal ultrasound, and renal biopsy if treatment implications present

- **Differential Diagnosis/Causes**

  - Congestive heart failure; cirrhosis; constrictive pericarditis
  - Minimal change disease; amyloidosis
  - Focal segmental glomerulosclerosis
  - Diabetic nephropathy; membranous nephropathy
  - Membranoproliferative glomerulonephritis

- **Treatment**

  - Supportive therapy with fluid and sodium restriction, diuretics to control edema, control of hypertension (with ACE inhibitor when possible), lipid-lowering agents, chronic anticoagulation for severe hypoalbuminemia or thrombotic events
  - Maintenance of adequate nutrition
  - Corticosteroids for minimal change disease; idiopathic membranous nephropathy may be treated with corticosteroids and cytotoxic agents

- **Pearl**

Given the therapeutic implications, renal biopsy should be seriously entertained in all patients with new onset of nephrotic syndrome.

Reference

Kodner C. Nephrotic syndrome in adults: diagnosis and management. Am Fam Physician 2009;80:1129. [PMID: 19904897]

Obstructive Nephropathy

■ Essentials of Diagnosis

- Most cases are postvesical and usually of prostatic origin
- A few cases result from bilateral ureteral obstruction, usually from stones, which can present with sudden pain
- Obstruction may be acute or chronic, partial or complete
- Postvesical obstruction presents with nocturia, incontinence, malaise, nausea, with normal 24-hour urine output, but in swings
- Palpable bladder, suprapubic pain
- Renal insufficiency, hypertension may be present
- Renal ultrasound localizes site of obstruction with proximal tract dilation and hydronephrosis
- Spectrum of causes includes anatomic abnormalities, stricture, retroperitoneal or pelvic tumor, prostatic hypertrophy, bilateral renal stones, drug effect (eg, anticholinergics, opioids), and neuromuscular disorders

■ Differential Diagnosis

- Prerenal azotemia
- Interstitial nephritis
- Acute or chronic kidney disease due to any cause

■ Treatment

- Urinary catheter or ultrasonography to rule out obstruction secondary to enlarged prostate
- Nephrostomy tubes if significant bilateral hydronephrosis present with bilateral ureteral obstruction
- Treatment of concurrent infection if present
- Observe for postobstructive diuresis; can be brisk

■ Pearl

Many clinicians believe obstructive uropathy is associated with anuria; such is the case only with bilateral ureteral obstruction, as postvesicular obstruction results in urinary overflow and often normal 24-hour urine volume.

Reference

Chevalier RL. Pathogenesis of renal injury in obstructive uropathy. Curr Opin Pediatr 2006;18:153. [PMID: 16601495]

Polycystic Kidney Disease

- ■ Essentials of Diagnosis
  - Autosomal-dominant inheritance and nearly complete penetrance, thus strikingly positive family history (autosomal-recessive form rare, usually discovered in childhood)
  - Abdominal or flank pain associated with hematuria, frequent urinary tract infections, nephrolithiasis
  - Hypertension, large palpable kidneys, positive family history
  - Renal insufficiency in 50% of patients by age 70 years; unlikely to develop renal disease if no cystic renal lesions by age 30 years
  - Normal or elevated hematocrit common: Interstitial cells near cysts may elaborate erythropoietin
  - Diagnosis confirmed by multiple renal cysts on ultrasonography or CT scan
  - Increased incidence of cerebral aneurysms (10% of affected patients), aortic aneurysms, and abnormalities of the mitral valve; 40–50% have concomitant hepatic cysts; colonic diverticula; abdominal wall hernias

- ■ Differential Diagnosis
  - Renal cell carcinoma
  - Simple renal cysts
  - Other causes of chronic kidney disease

- ■ Treatment
  - Treat hypertension and nephrolithiasis
  - Observe for urinary tract infection; if present, may require prolonged treatment
  - Avoid high-protein diet
  - Patients with family history of cerebral aneurysm should have screening cerebral CT or MR angiography
  - Occasional nephrectomy required for repeated episodes of pain and infection or before transplant for very large kidneys
  - Excellent outcome with transplant

- ■ Pearl

Hypertension, an abdominal mass, and azotemia should be considered to be polycystic disease until proven otherwise.

Reference

Patel V, Chowdhury R, Igarashi P. Advances in the pathogenesis and treatment of polycystic kidney disease. Curr Opin Nephrol Hypertens 2009;18:99. [PMID: 19430332]

11

Renal Tubular Acidosis

- **Essentials of Diagnosis**
  - Unexplained metabolic acidosis with a normal anion gap
  - Type I (distal): Impaired urinary acidification, plasma bicarbonate may be < 10–15 mEq/L, hypokalemia, abnormal (positive) urinary anion gap; may be familial or secondary to autoimmune disease, obstructive uropathy, drugs (eg, amphotericin B), hyperglobulinemia, hypercalciuria, renal transplantation, or sickle cell anemia
  - Type II (proximal): Bicarbonaturia with serum bicarbonate usually 12–20 mEq/L, hypokalemia, often with Fanconi's syndrome (glycosuria, aminoaciduria, phosphaturia, uricosuria, and tubular proteinuria); may be secondary to myeloma, drugs, or renal transplant
  - Type IV: Low renin and aldosterone; impaired ammoniagenesis with serum bicarbonate usually > 17 mEq/L; hyperkalemia, abnormal (positive) urinary anion gap; typical of renal insufficiency; others due to diabetes mellitus, drugs (eg, ACE inhibitors, NSAIDs, cyclosporine), tubulointerstitial disease, or nephrosclerosis

- **Differential Diagnosis**
  - Diarrhea
  - Ileal loop constriction after surgery for bladder cancer
  - Hypokalemia or hyperkalemia from other causes

- **Treatment**
  - Discontinue offending drug or treat underlying disease if present
  - Bicarbonate or citrate and potassium replacement for types I and II
  - Vitamin D and phosphate supplementation for type I to prevent osteomalacia, not type II because of possible hypercalcemia and further damage to the distal tubule
  - Thiazides may increase bicarbonate reabsorption for type II
  - Fludrocortisone for type IV only if volume repletion is difficult

- **Pearl**

Multiple myeloma may cause all three types of RTA in adults.

Reference

Laing CM, Unwin RJ. Renal tubular acidosis. J Nephrol 2006;19(suppl 9):S46. [PMID: 16736441]

Uric Acid and Kidney Disease

■ Essentials of Diagnosis

- Three distinct syndromes, as described below; terminology confusing
- Uric acid nephrolithiasis: Radiolucent urate stones in 3% of patients with gout
- Gouty kidney (chronic urate nephropathy): Interstitial sodium urate crystals of uncertain significance in patients with gout and interstitial nephropathy; no clear correlation with degree of elevation of serum uric acid
- Uric acid nephropathy: Uric acid sludge within nephron due to cellular necrosis, typically after chemotherapy or radiation has induced rapid cell lysis

■ Differential Diagnosis

- Kidney disease due to other cause
- Hypertensive nephrosclerosis
- Nephrolithiasis due to other cause
- Myeloma kidney

■ Treatment

- Depends on syndrome
- Intravenous hydration and alkalinization of urine for uric acid stones
- Pretreatment with allopurinol and intravenous hydration for selected patients at risk for tumor lysis syndrome; maintain urine pH > 6.5 and urine output > 2 L/d
- In patients with gout, allopurinol and colchicine adjusted for renal function; NSAID use minimized in patients with renal dysfunction
- Uricase prophylaxis in high-risk patients or treatment of acute uric acid nephropathy

■ Pearl

Hyperuricemia is not synonymous with gout; there is only fair correlation between the height of the serum uric acid and the occurrence of that condition.

Reference

Gaffo AL, Saag KG. Management of hyperuricemia and gout in CKD. Am J Kidney Dis 2008;52:994. [PMID: 18971014]

12

Neurologic Diseases

Arteriovenous Malformations

- **Essentials of Diagnosis**
  - Congenital vascular malformations that consist of arteriovenous communications without intervening capillaries
  - Patients typically under age 30 years and normotensive
  - Unruptured arteriovenous malformations (AVMs) present incidentally or with headache or seizure; ruptured AVMs present with acute headache, seizure, hemiparesis, or coma
  - May also present as transverse myelopathy (spinal cord arteriovenous malformation)
  - Non-contrast CT of the brain will show blood in cases of rupture; CT or MRI with contrast will show tangle of blood vessels; angiography characteristically diagnostic

- **Differential Diagnosis**
  - Dural arteriovenous fistulas
  - Cavernous malformation
  - Hypertensive intracerebral hemorrhage
  - Ruptured intracranial aneurysm
  - Intracranial tumor
  - Brain abscess

- **Treatment**
  - Ruptured AVMs have a high risk of re-rupture and are usually excised; treatment of patients with unruptured AVMs depends on symptoms and neurologic risk of surgery
  - Endovascular embolization in selected malformations
  - Radiosurgery for small malformations
  - Ongoing clinical trial is comparing surgery with watchful waiting for unruptured AVMs (study name is "ARUBA")

- **Pearl**

The most common cause of intracranial hemorrhage between ages 15 and 30 years.

Reference

Choi JH, Mohr JP. Brain arteriovenous malformations in adults. Lancet Neurol 2005;4:299. [PMID: 15847843]

Bell's Palsy (Idiopathic Facial Paresis)

- ▪ Essentials of Diagnosis
  - An idiopathic facial paresis
  - Abrupt onset of hemifacial weakness including the forehead, difficulty closing eye; ipsilateral ear pain may precede or accompany weakness
  - Examination shows unilateral peripheral seventh nerve palsy; taste lost on the anterior two-thirds of the tongue, eye irritation due to decreased lacrimation and hyperacusis may occur; absence of other neurologic signs

- ▪ Differential Diagnosis
  - Carotid distribution stroke
  - Intracranial mass lesion
  - Basilar meningitis, especially that associated with sarcoidosis
  - Lyme disease
  - First of multiple cranial neuropathies
  - Guillain-Barré syndrome

- ▪ Treatment
  - Treatment with corticosteroids is beneficial when initiated early (48–72 hours)
  - Antiviral agents (eg, acyclovir, valacyclovir) probably not helpful
  - Supportive measures with frequent eye lubrication and nocturnal eye patching
  - Only 10% of patients are dissatisfied with the final outcome of their disability or disfigurement

- ▪ Pearl

The Bell phenomenon: the eye on the affected side moves superiorly and laterally when the patient attempts to close his eyes.

Reference

Hernández RA, Sullivan F, Donnan P, Swan I, Vale L; BELLS Trial Group. Economic evaluation of early administration of prednisolone and/or acyclovir for the treatment of Bell's palsy. Fam Pract 2009;26:137. [PMID: 19244470]

Brain Abscess

- **■ Essentials of Diagnosis**
  - History of sinusitis, otitis, endocarditis, chronic pulmonary infection, or congenital heart defect common
  - Headache, focal neurologic symptoms, seizures may occur
  - Examination may show hemiparesis, sensory loss, visual field cut, aphasia, ataxia depending on location of lesion
  - The most common organisms are streptococci, staphylococci, and anaerobes; *Toxoplasma* in AIDS patients; commonly polymicrobial
  - Tuberculosis can also cause an isolated ring-enhancing lesion
  - Ring-enhancing lesion on CT scan or MRI; lumbar puncture potentially dangerous because of mass effect and not usually helpful diagnostically

- **■ Differential Diagnosis**
  - Primary or metastatic tumor
  - Cerebral infarction
  - Contusion
  - Resolving hematoma
  - Demyelination (eg, multiple sclerosis)

- **■ Treatment**
  - Intravenous broad-spectrum antibiotics (with coverage to include anaerobic organisms) may be curative if abscess smaller than 2 cm in diameter
  - Surgical aspiration through burr hole if no response to antibiotic drugs, either clinically or by CT scan

- **■ Pearl**

Brain abscess may mimic glioblastoma on MRI; take a careful history for predisposing conditions to this curable condition.

Reference

Carpenter J, Stapleton S, Holliman R. Retrospective analysis of 49 cases of brain abscess and review of the literature. Eur J Clin Microbiol Infect Dis 2007;26:1. [PMID: 17180609]

Combined System Disease (Posterolateral Sclerosis)

■ Essentials of Diagnosis

- Numbness (pins and needles), tenderness, weakness; feeling of heaviness in toes, feet, fingers, and hands
- Stocking and glove distribution of sensory loss in some patients
- Extensor plantar response and hyperreflexia typical, as is loss of position and vibratory senses
- May develop myelopathy in severe cases
- Serum vitamin B_{12} level low; methylmalonic acid and homocysteine levels high
- Megaloblastic anemia may be present but does not parallel neurologic dysfunction

■ Differential Diagnosis

- Cervical spondylosis
- Epidural tumor or abscess
- Multiple sclerosis
- Transverse myelitis of viral or other origin
- Polyneuropathy due to toxin or metabolic abnormality
- Tabes dorsalis
- Nitrous oxide abuse

■ Treatment

- Vitamin B_{12} replacement, usually intramuscular

■ Pearl

Pernicious anemia is not identical to vitamin B_{12} deficiency; the former is an autoimmune disorder and is only one of many causes of deficiency of this vitamin.

Reference

Vasconcelos OM, Poehm EH, McCarter RJ, Campbell WW, Quezado ZM. Potential outcome factors in subacute combined degeneration: review of observational studies. J Gen Intern Med 2006;21:1063. [PMID: 16970556]

Guillain-Barré Syndrome (Acute Inflammatory Polyneuropathy)

- **Essentials of Diagnosis**
  - Approximately two-thirds of cases are preceded by a respiratory tract or gastrointestinal infection, often *Campylobacter jejuni* enteritis
  - Pathophysiology thought to be molecular mimicry with antibodies raised against an infectious organism cross reacting with nerve tissue
  - Progressive, usually ascending, symmetric weakness with areflexia and variable paresthesia or dysesthesia; autonomic involvement (eg, cardiac irregularities, hypertension, or hypotension) may be prominent
  - Spinal imaging (both of cervical and lumbar spine) is often necessary to rule out myelopathy or cauda equina syndrome, especially if there is bowel or bladder involvement
  - Electromyography consistent with demyelinating injury; also a less common axonal form with worse prognosis for full recovery
  - Lumbar puncture shows high protein, normal cell count

- **Differential Diagnosis**
  - Myelopathy or cauda equina syndrome of any cause
  - Bickerstaff's brainstem encephalitis or Miller Fisher syndrome
  - Diphtheria, poliomyelitis, West Nile virus (where endemic)
  - HIV
  - Porphyria
  - Heavy metal poisoning
  - Botulism
  - Periodic paralysis
  - Tick paralysis

- **Treatment**
  - Plasmapheresis or intravenous immunoglobulin
  - Pulmonary function is closely monitored, with intubation for impending respiratory failure
  - Respiratory toilet with physical therapy
  - Up to 20% of patients are left with persistent disability

- **Pearl**

In what appears to be rapid-onset Guillain-Barré in an Asian man, be sure the serum potassium is normal before starting expensive therapy: the patient may have thyrotoxic periodic paralysis.

Reference

Gupta D, Nair M, Baheti NN, Sarma PS, Kuruvilla A. Electrodiagnostic and clinical aspects of Guillain-Barré syndrome: an analysis of 142 cases. J Clin Neuromuscul Dis 2008;10:42. [PMID: 19169089]

Hemorrhagic Stroke

- ■ Essentials of Diagnosis
  - • Risk factors: Hypertension, excessive alcohol use, cocaine and methamphetamine abuse, antiplatelet or anticoagulation therapy
  - • Sudden onset of neurologic deficit, variably including focal weakness, sensory abnormalities, visual field cut, aphasia, or altered mentation; often with headache
  - • CT of the head will show intracranial hemorrhage immediately; MRI, MR angiogram, or catheter angiogram is often necessary to exclude an arteriovenous malformation, aneurysm, or underlying tumor
  - • Check prothrombin time and platelet count immediately

- ■ Differential Diagnosis
  - • Head trauma
  - • Hypertensive hemorrhage
  - • Iatrogenic (therapeutic anticoagulation) or toxic (cocaine, methamphetamine)
  - • Arteriovenous malformation
  - • Cerebral amyloid angiopathy (in the elderly and those with Down's syndrome)
  - • Hemorrhagic conversion of ischemic infarct
  - • Primary or metastatic tumor
  - • Septic emboli
  - • Aneurysm
  - • Dural venous sinus thrombosis
  - • Vasculitis

12

- ■ Treatment
  - • If present, reversal of coagulopathy should be considered with factor IX complex or fresh-frozen plasma and vitamin K; platelets can be transfused if thrombocytopenic
  - • Neurosurgical decompression often indicated for cerebellar hemorrhage
  - • An external ventricular drain may be necessary for hydrocephalus or intracranial pressure monitoring
  - • Blood pressure is usually lowered acutely

- ■ Pearl

The most common locations for hypertensive hemorrhage are in the internal capsule, basal ganglia, thalamus, pons, and cerebellum.

Reference

Burns JD, Manno EM. Primary intracerebral hemorrhage: update on epidemiology, pathophysiology, and treatment strategies. Compr Ther 2008;34:183. [PMID: 19137762]

Huntington's Disease

- ■ Essentials of Diagnosis
  - Family history usually present (autosomal dominant with anticipation)
  - Onset at age 30–50 years, with gradual progressive chorea and dementia; death usually occurs within 20 years after onset
  - Caused by a CAG trinucleotide-repeat expansion in a gene located on the short arm of chromosome 4 that encodes the protein huntingtin
  - The earliest mental changes are often behavioral, including depression, emotional lability, delusions and hypersexuality
  - CT/MRI scan shows cerebral atrophy, particularly in the caudate

- ■ Differential Diagnosis
  - Sydenham's chorea
  - Tardive dyskinesia
  - Lacunar infarcts of subthalamic nuclei
  - Wilson's disease
  - Thyrotoxicosis
  - Central nervous system lupus
  - Antiphospholipid antibody syndrome
  - Polycythemia vera
  - Neuroacanthocytosis
  - Other causes of dementia

- ■ Treatment
  - Primarily supportive
  - Antidopaminergic agents (eg, haloperidol, olanzapine) or monoamine-depleting agents (eg, reserpine, tetrabenazine) may reduce severity of movement abnormality
  - Genetic counseling for offspring

- ■ Pearl

On rare occasions, a Huntington's Münchhausen has been noted in a patient who is educated about the disease.

Reference

Squitieri F, Ciarmiello A, Di Donato S, Frati L. The search for cerebral biomarkers of Huntington's disease: a review of genetic models of age at onset prediction. Eur J Neurol 2006;13:408. [PMID: 16643321]

Idiopathic Epilepsy

- ■ Essentials of Diagnosis
  - • Epilepsy is the tendency toward recurrent seizures
  - • Seizures are paroxysmal, transitory alterations of central nervous system function; may be generalized or focal with or without alteration of consciousness
  - • Metabolic panel to rule out sodium, glucose, or calcium disorders; urine toxicology screen; antiepileptic drug levels may be helpful
  - • CT or MRI important to rule out structural lesion; lumbar puncture important to rule out meningitis or encephalitis
  - • Characteristic electroencephalography during seizures; often abnormal during interictal periods

- ■ Differential Diagnosis
  - • Syncope; migraine; narcolepsy; hypoglycemia
  - • Stroke (when patient first seen postictally) or transient ischemic attack (TIA); psychiatric abnormalities (pseudoseizures, panic attack)

- ■ Treatment
  - • For newly diagnosed epilepsy, multiple options (eg, carbamazepine, phenytoin, lamotrigine, for initial monotherapy)
  - • Other newer-generation anticonvulsants and phenobarbital may be helpful in patients unresponsive to other medications
  - • Valproic acid should be avoided in women considering pregnancy
  - • Status epilepticus is treated as a medical emergency with intravenous diazepam or lorazepam and fosphenytoin

- ■ Pearl

Remember that a generalized seizure produces temporary lactic acidosis; an undetectable post-ictal bicarbonate may completely normalize within an hour.

Reference

Ben-Menachem E, Schmitz B, Tomson T, Vajda F. Role of valproate across the ages. Treatment of epilepsy in adults. Acta Neurol Scand Suppl 2006;184:14. [PMID: 16776493]

Intracranial Aneurysms and Subarachnoid Hemorrhage

- ■ Essentials of Diagnosis
  - • Synonymous with berry aneurysm
  - • Asymptomatic until expansion or rupture; sometimes preceded by abrupt onset of headaches that resolve (sentinel leaks)
  - • Rupture characterized by sudden, severe headache ("the worst headache of my life"), confusion, photophobia, and vomiting
  - • Focal neurologic signs unusual except for third nerve palsy with posterior communicating artery aneurysm
  - • CT scan is 95% sensitive for subarachnoid blood in the first 24 hours, less sensitive thereafter; a lumbar puncture looking for blood is the definitive test; cerebral catheter angiography indicates size, location, and number of aneurysms

- ■ Differential Diagnosis
  - • Traumatic subarachnoid hemorrhage
  - • Ruptured arteriovenous malformation
  - • Ruptured mycotic aneurysm; brain tumor
  - • Vasculitis; migraine headache; meningitis

- ■ Treatment
  - • Definitive therapy with surgical clipping or endovascular coil embolization of aneurysm to prevent re-rupture; re-rupture associated with high mortality
  - • Nimodipine (calcium channel blocker) may improve outcome
  - • Aggressive fluid resuscitation, induced hypertension, and intracranial angioplasty may be useful for treating vasospasm after subarachnoid hemorrhage
  - • An external ventricular drain is often necessary to treat hydrocephalus
  - • Monitor sodium closely for cerebral salt wasting; fluid restriction is contraindicated in subarachnoid hemorrhage so hyponatremia is treated with hypertonic saline or sodium tablets
  - • Small unruptured aneurysms may not require treatment

- ■ Pearl

When a patient complains of "the worst headache of my life," it is a ruptured berry aneurysm . . . less than 50% of the time.

Reference

Salary M, Quigley MR, Wilberger JE Jr. Relation among aneurysm size, amount of subarachnoid blood, and clinical outcome. J Neurosurg 2007;107:13. [PMID: 17639867]

Ischemic Stroke and Transient Ischemic Attack

- ■ Essentials of Diagnosis
  - • Risk factors: Tobacco, hypertension, diabetes, hypercholes-terolemia, carotid atherosclerosis, valvular heart disease, atrial fibrillation
  - • Sudden onset of neurologic deficit, may include focal weakness, sensory defects, visual field cut, aphasia, confusion
  - • If stroke-like symptoms resolve in < 24 hours, defined as a transient ischemic attack (TIA)
  - • CT of the head is necessary to rule out hemorrhage; may not show ischemia in the first 24 hours but hemorrhage visible immediately; MRI a superior imaging modality, especially in posterior fossa
  - • Etiology may be cardioembolic, artery-to-artery embolus, or thrombotic
  - • ECG or telemetry to rule out atrial fibrillation; carotid imaging to rule out stenosis; echo to rule out patent foramen ovale

- ■ Differential Diagnosis
  - • Hemorrhagic stroke; subarachnoid hemorrhage
  - • Seizure (and postictal state); migraine; vasculitis
  - • Subdural or epidural hematoma
  - • Primary or metastatic brain tumor
  - • Multiple sclerosis; neurosyphilis
  - • Any metabolic abnormality, especially hypoglycemia

12

- ■ Treatment
  - • Tissue plasminogen activator for selected patients with ischemic stroke who can be treated within 4.5 hours after onset
  - • Secondary prevention with aspirin, clopidogrel, or the combination of dipyridamole and aspirin for all ischemic stroke or TIA without an indication for anticoagulation
  - • Anticoagulation for stroke or TIA due to atrial fibrillation, metal heart valve
  - • Control of risk factors, especially hypertension, hypercholes-terolemia, and tobacco use
  - • Carotid endarterectomy for patients with carotid stenosis

- ■ Pearl

A stroke is never a stroke until it's had 50 of D50.

Reference

Biller J. Antiplatelet therapy in ischemic stroke. J Neurol Sci 2009;284:1. [PMID: 19380153]

Migraine Headache

- **Essentials of Diagnosis**
  - Onset usually in adolescence or early adulthood
  - May be triggered by stress, foods (chocolate, red wine), smells (eg, perfume, car exhaust), dehydration, lack of sleep, menses
  - Common migraine: Lasts 4–72 hours, unilateral, throbbing, moderate to severe intensity, aggravated by routine physical activity, associated with nausea, vomiting, photophobia, phonophobia
  - Classic migraine (only approximately 20% of cases): Same symptoms as common migraine with a prodrome (aura) that includes a homonymous visual disturbance, unilateral numbness, paresthesias, or weakness
  - Basilar variant: Brainstem and cerebellar findings followed by occipital headache
  - Ophthalmic variant: Painless loss of vision, scotomas, usually unilateral

- **Differential Diagnosis**
  - Cluster headache or other trigeminal autonomic cephalgia
  - Giant cell arteritis
  - Subarachnoid hemorrhage
  - Mass lesion (eg, tumor or abscess)
  - Meningitis
  - Increased intracranial pressure of other cause

- **Treatment**
  - Avoidance of triggers
  - Acute treatment: Triptans, ergotamine with caffeine, NSAIDs (preferably at onset of prodrome)
  - Prophylaxis should be considered for more than three migraines per month and includes propranolol, amitriptyline, verapamil, valproic acid, and many others

- **Pearl**

Interesting etymology: Hemi (mi) cranium (graine), a linguistic corruption here indicating the unilaterality of the process.

Reference

Bigal ME, Lipton RB. The epidemiology, burden, and comorbidities of migraine. Neurol Clin 2009;27:321. [PMID: 19289218]

Multiple Sclerosis

- ■ Essentials of Diagnosis
  - • Patient usually under 50 years of age at onset
  - • Episodic symptoms that may include sensory abnormalities, blurred vision due to optic neuritis, urinary sphincter disturbances, and upper motor neuron weakness; 15% are steadily progressive from onset (primary progressive)
  - • Diagnosis can be made if there are two clinical deficits separated by time and space with supportive imaging data; multiple foci in white matter best demonstrated radiographically by MRI
  - • Finding of oligoclonal bands or elevated IgG index on lumbar puncture is a nonspecific marker of inflammation

- ■ Differential Diagnosis
  - • Vasculitis or systemic lupus erythematosus
  - • Small vessel ischemic disease; B_{12} deficiency
  - • Neurosyphilis, Lyme disease, HIV-related illness, human T-lymphotropic virus (HTLV)
  - • Primary or metastatic central nervous system neoplasm
  - • Optic neuritis due to other causes
  - • Cord compression, radiculopathy due to mechanical compression

- ■ Treatment
  - • Beta-interferon and glatiramer acetate reduce exacerbation rate
  - • Natalizumab also reduces exacerbation rate but carries risk of progressive multifocal leukoencephalopathy
  - • Other immunosuppressants, including mitoxantrone, may be effective
  - • Steroids may hasten recovery from relapses, but do not change long-term disability
  - • Symptomatic treatment of spasticity and bladder dysfunction

12

- ■ Pearl

If you first diagnose multiple sclerosis in a patient whose symptoms began over age 50 years, diagnose something else.

Reference

Langer-Gould A, et al. Clinical and demographic predictors of long-term disability in patients with relapsing-remitting multiple sclerosis: a systematic review. Arch Neurol 2006;63:1686. [PMID: 17172607]

Myasthenia Gravis

- ■ Essentials of Diagnosis
  - • Due to autoimmune destruction of acetylcholine receptors at the neuromuscular junction; often associated with other autoimmune conditions such as Graves' disease
  - • Fatigable weakness of most-commonly used muscles: Diplopia, dysphagia, ptosis, facial weakness with chewing and speaking; sensation and reflexes are preserved
  - • Electromyography and nerve conduction studies demonstrate decremental muscle response with repetitive stimulation at 3 Hz
  - • Elevated acetylcholine receptor antibody assay confirmatory but not completely sensitive; some have antibodies to MuSK
  - • Chest CT is necessary to rule out thymoma
  - • Any infection and some medications can exacerbate myasthenia and precipitate myasthenic crisis, characterized by neuromuscular respiratory failure

- ■ Differential Diagnosis
  - • Botulism; Lambert-Eaton syndrome
  - • Drug-induced myasthenia (penicillamine)
  - • Motor neuropathy due to other causes
  - • Amyotrophic lateral sclerosis
  - • Primary myopathy (eg, polymyositis)
  - • Bulbar poliomyelitis; thyrotoxicosis

- ■ Treatment
  - • Avoid medications that are known to worsen myasthenia (eg, aminoglycosides)
  - • Anticholinesterase drugs (eg, pyridostigmine) provide symptomatic benefit
  - • Consider thymectomy in an otherwise healthy patient under age 60 years if weakness not restricted to extraocular muscles
  - • Corticosteroids and immunosuppressants if response to above measures not ideal
  - • Plasmapheresis or intravenous immunoglobulin therapy provides short-term benefit in some; especially useful in myasthenic crisis

- ■ Pearl

All skeletal muscles are involved in this disorder; only the ones used most frequently cause the symptoms.

Reference

Díaz-Manera J, Rojas-García R, Illa I. Treatment strategies for myasthenia gravis. Expert Opin Pharmacother 2009;10:1329. [PMID: 19445561]

Normal Pressure Hydrocephalus

■ Essentials of Diagnosis

- Subacute loss of higher cognitive function
- Urinary incontinence
- Gait apraxia
- In some, history of head trauma or meningitis
- Normal opening pressure on lumbar puncture
- Enlarged ventricles without atrophy by CT or MRI

■ Differential Diagnosis

- High pressure hydrocephalus
- Alzheimer's or other dementia
- Parkinson's disease
- Alcoholic cerebellar degeneration
- Wernicke-Korsakoff syndrome
- Chronic meningitis

■ Treatment

- Lumbar puncture provides temporary amelioration of symptoms
- Ventriculoperitoneal shunting, most effective when precipitating event is identified and recent; gait is most likely symptom to improve

■ Pearl

The sole cause of a magnetic gait; the patient walks as though the floor were a magnet, and his shoes made of metal, this being gait apraxia.

Reference

Shprecher D, Schwalb J, Kurlan R. Normal pressure hydrocephalus: diagnosis and treatment. Curr Neurol Neurosci Rep 2008;8:371. [PMID: 18713572]

12

Parkinson's Disease

- **Essentials of Diagnosis**
  - Insidious onset in older patient of pill-rolling tremor (3–5 Hz), rigidity, bradykinesia, and progressive postural instability; tremor is the least disabling feature
  - Masklike facies, cogwheeling of extremities on passive motion; cutaneous seborrhea characteristic
  - Absence of tremor—not uncommon—may delay diagnosis
  - Mild intellectual deterioration often noted, but concurrent Alzheimer's disease may account for this in many

- **Differential Diagnosis**
  - Essential tremor; hypothyroidism; depression
  - Phenothiazine, metoclopramide toxicity; also carbon monoxide, manganese poisoning
  - Multiple system atrophy, progressive supranuclear palsy
  - Dementia with Lewy bodies; small-vessel ischemic disease
  - Repeated head trauma; normal pressure hydrocephalus

- **Treatment**
  - Carbidopa-levodopa, dopamine agonists (pramipexole, ropinirole), or MAO-B inhibitors (selegiline, rasagiline) are all reasonable as first-line therapy
  - No treatment necessary in early disease if symptoms not bothersome or disabling
  - Carbidopa-levodopa is most effective treatment for disabling symptoms; dopamine agonists and MAO-B inhibitors may permit reduction of carbidopa-levodopa dose; anticholinergics and amantadine also useful adjuncts
  - Catechol O-methyl transferase inhibitors (entacapone) are useful to extend the duration of carbidopa-levodopa effect
  - Selected patients with good cognitive function who have a good response to levodopa but have dose-limiting side effects are candidates for deep brain stimulators (usually in the subthalamic nucleus)

- **Pearl**

An important reason for testing the first cranial nerve: Anosmia may be the first symptom of Parkinson's disease, appearing years before the tremor and rigidity.

Reference

Rodriguez-Oroz MC, et al. Initial clinical manifestations of Parkinson's disease: features and pathophysiological mechanisms. Lancet Neurol 2009;8:1128. [PMID: 19909911]

12

Periodic Paralysis Syndromes

- ■ Essentials of Diagnosis
  - • Episodes of flaccid weakness or paralysis with strength normal between attacks
  - • Hypokalemic variety: Infrequent, prolonged, severe attacks; usually upon awakening, during rest after exercise, or after carbohydrate meals; typically autosomal dominant but can be associated with hyperthyroidism, especially in Asian men
  - • Hyperkalemic or normokalemic variety: Frequent, short-duration, less severe attacks often with rest after exercise or during fasting; autosomal dominant

- ■ Differential Diagnosis
  - • Myasthenia gravis
  - • Polyneuropathies due to other causes, especially Guillain-Barré syndrome
  - • Seizure
  - • Myopathy, especially metabolic myopathies

- ■ Treatment
  - • Hypokalemic variant: Potassium replacement for acute episode; low-carbohydrate, low-salt diet chronically, acetazolamide prophylactically; treatment of hyperthyroidism, when associated, reduces attacks, as does therapy with propranolol
  - • Hyperkalemic-normokalemic variant: Intravenous calcium, intravenous diuretics useful for acute therapy; prophylactic acetazolamide beneficial

- ■ Pearl

The only cause of hypokalemia this marked in the absence of vomiting or diarrhea.

Reference

Jurkat-Rott K, Weber MA, Fauler M, et al. K+-dependent paradoxical membrane depolarization and Na+ overload, major and reversible contributors to weakness by ion channel leaks. Proc Natl Acad Sci U S A 2009;106:4036. [PMID: 19225109]

Peripheral Neuropathy

- **Essentials of Diagnosis**
  - Exam shows sensory loss, lower motor neuron weakness, atrophy, and normal to decreased tone; diminished reflexes dependant on the nerves involved
  - Polyneuropathies: Distal, symmetric (often subacute, slowly progressive) abnormalities of sensation, strength, or both usually secondary to metabolic, toxic, or inherited disorders
  - Mononeuropathies: Dysfunction of a single nerve (eg, carpal tunnel syndrome) usually secondary to focal nerve compression or stretch
  - Mononeuritis multiplex: Multiple individual nerves affected asymmetrically either at the same time or stepwise, usually secondary to inflammatory disorders; requires workup for vasculitis
  - Electromyography and nerve conduction studies can be helpful extension of neurologic exam

- **Causes**
  - Diabetes mellitus; alcohol; thyroid disease; HIV
  - Alcohol
  - B_{12} deficiency; liver disease; syphilis
  - Dysimmune (usually monoclonal gammopathy of unknown significance, but also multiple myeloma, amyloid, Waldenström's)
  - Chronic inflammatory demyelinating polyneuropathy
  - Medication (especially chemotherapy)
  - Liver or renal disease
  - Autoimmune disease (SLE, Sjögren's, vasculitis)
  - Inherited (Charcot-Marie-Tooth)
  - Heavy metals and other toxins

- **Treatment**
  - Treat underlying cause if known (eg, stop alcohol or replace vitamin B_{12})
  - Treat pain with tricyclic antidepressants, gabapentin, duloxetine
  - Other anticonvulsants, topical capsaicin, or lidocaine also may be tried
  - Bracing/padding and surgery for mononeuropathies (eg, carpal tunnel syndrome)

Pearl

The metabolic neuropathies affect the longest nerves first; feet, then hands, then sternum become symptomatic in that order.

Reference

Haanpää ML, Backonja MM, Bennett MI, et al. Assessment of neuropathic pain in primary care. Am J Med 2009;122(suppl):S13. [PMID: 19801048]

12

Pseudotumor Cerebri (Benign Intracranial Hypertension)

- ■ Essentials of Diagnosis
  - • Headache, diplopia, nausea, blurry vision or transient visual obscuration
  - • Papilledema, sixth nerve palsy, enlarged blind spot, and/or reduced peripheral vision
  - • Brain MRI brain and MR venogram normal except for small ventricles
  - • Lumbar puncture with elevated pressure but normal cerebrospinal fluid
  - • Associations include endocrinopathy (hypoparathyroidism, Addison's disease), hypervitaminosis A, drugs (tetracyclines, oral contraceptives, corticosteroids), chronic pulmonary disease, obesity; often idiopathic
  - • Untreated pseudotumor cerebri may lead to secondary optic atrophy and permanent visual loss

- ■ Differential Diagnosis
  - • Venous sinus thrombosis
  - • Chronic meningitis (eg, coccidioidomycosis, cryptococcosis)
  - • Brain abscess or basilar meningitis
  - • Primary or metastatic tumor
  - • Optic neuritis or other causes of papillitis
  - • Migraine headache (would not cause papilledema)

- ■ Treatment
  - • Treat underlying cause if present
  - • Acetazolamide or furosemide to reduce cerebrospinal fluid formation
  - • Repeat lumbar puncture with removal of cerebrospinal fluid
  - • Weight loss in obese patients
  - • Monitor visual fields and visual acuity closely
  - • Surgical therapy with placement of ventriculoperitoneal shunt or optic nerve sheath fenestration in refractory cases

- ■ Pearl

Be meticulous in the history before making this diagnosis; be sure to inquire about surgically resected moles or breast lumps in the past.

Reference

Ball AK, Clarke CE. Idiopathic intracranial hypertension. Lancet Neurol 2006;5:433. [PMID: 16632314]

Spinal Cord Compression

- **Essentials of Diagnosis**
  - Weakness in legs or both arms and legs, sensory level, hyper-reflexia
  - Often early bowel/bladder dysfunction
  - Common causes: Trauma, vertebra or disc fragment, primary or metastatic tumor, epidural abscess, epidural hematoma
  - Risk factors for cord compression in patient presenting with back pain: Pain worse at rest, history of malignancy or trauma, presence of chronic infection, age > 50 years, pain for more than 1 month, current corticosteroid use, history of intravenous drug use, unexplained fever/weight loss, rapidly progressive neurologic deficit
  - Emergent MRI of spine diagnostic
  - Delayed diagnosis results in more severe neurologic impairment

- **Differential Diagnosis**
  - Cord contusion
  - Spinal cord infarction
  - Transverse myelitis
  - Infectious: HIV, HTLV-1 or -2, Lyme disease
  - Vitamin B_{12} deficiency
  - Vascular malformation
  - Intracranial midline anterior mass
  - Polyradiculopathy

- **Treatment**
  - Acute surgical decompression in cases of rapid neurologic deterioration
  - High-dose intravenous corticosteroids for metastatic cord compression or traumatic cases
  - Chemotherapy/radiation if tumor-associated
  - Bowel and bladder regimen

- **Pearl**

When caused by a tumor, if a patient walks into the hospital, they may walk out; if paralysis is already present, it is unlikely to be reversed, unless the tumor is benign.

Reference

George R, Jeba J, Ramkumar G, Chacko AG, Leng M, Tharyan P. Interventions for the treatment of metastatic extradural spinal cord compression in adults. Cochrane Database Syst Rev 2008:CD006716. [PMID: 18843728]

12

Syringomyelia

- **Essentials of Diagnosis**
  - Expansion of the central canal of the spinal cord results in destruction or degeneration of the adjacent gray and white matter
  - Initial loss of pain and temperature sense with preservation of other sensory function, often in a cape-like distribution over the shoulders and lateral arms and hands; unrecognized burning or injury of hands a characteristic presentation
  - Weakness, hyporeflexia or areflexia, atrophy of muscles at level of spinal cord involvement (usually upper limbs and hands); hyperreflexia and spasticity below the level of the lesion
  - Thoracic kyphoscoliosis common; associated with Arnold-Chiari malformation
  - Secondary to trauma in some cases, especially neck hyperextension/hyperflexion injuries
  - MRI of cervical cord confirms diagnosis

- **Differential Diagnosis**
  - Spinal cord tumor or arteriovenous malformation
  - Transverse myelitis
  - Multiple sclerosis
  - Neurosyphilis
  - Degenerative arthritis of the cervical spine
  - Polyradiculopathy

- **Treatment**
  - Surgical decompression of the foramen magnum
  - Syringotomy in selected cases

- **Pearl**

Test the contralateral eye for blink in corneal abrasion; the cause may be syring bulbar omyelia involving the brainstem causing anesthesia in the distribution of the trigeminal nerve.

Reference

Kunert P, Janowski M, Zakrzewska A, Marchel A. Syringoperitoneal shunt in the treatment of syringomyelia. Neurol Neurochir Pol 2009;43:258. [PMID: 19618309]

Tourette's Syndrome

- ■ Essentials of Diagnosis
  - Motor and vocal tics; onset in childhood or adolescence and persistence for more than 1 year
  - Compulsive utterances are typical
  - Hyperactivity, nonspecific electroencephalographic abnormalities in 50%
  - Obsessive-compulsive disorder common

- ■ Differential Diagnosis
  - Simple tic disorder
  - Wilson's disease
  - Focal seizures

- ■ Treatment
  - Tics usually do not require treatment
  - Neuroleptics (eg, risperidone) and tetrabenazine are beneficial
  - Alpha-2-adrenergic agonists (eg, clonidine, guanfacine) and clonazepam may also be tried
  - Selective serotonin reuptake inhibitors for obsessive-compulsive symptoms

12

- ■ Pearl

When a child has no neurologic signs other than tics, and Wilson's disease has been excluded, think Tourette's syndrome.

Reference

Porta M, Sassi M, Cavallazzi M, Fornari M, Brambilla A, Servello D. Tourette's syndrome and role of tetrabenazine: review and personal experience. Clin Drug Investig 2008;28:443. [PMID: 18544005]

Trigeminal Neuralgia (Tic Douloureux)

- ■ Essentials of Diagnosis
  - Characterized by momentary episodes of lancinating facial pain in the distribution of the trigeminal nerve, usually the second or third division
  - Commonly affects women more than men in middle and later life
  - Triggered by touch, movement, and eating
  - Occasionally caused by multiple sclerosis or a brainstem tumor; thus MRI is often obtained

- ■ Differential Diagnosis
  - SUNCT (short-lasting, unilateral, neuralgiform headache attacks with conjunctival injection and tearing) or SUNA (short-lasting unilateral neuralgiform) headache
  - Cluster-tic headache
  - Glossopharyngeal neuralgia
  - Postherpetic neuralgia
  - Giant cell arteritis
  - Multiple sclerosis or cerebellopontine angle tumor

- ■ Treatment
  - Carbamazepine is the drug of choice; if this is ineffective or poorly tolerated, oxcarbazepine, phenytoin, lamotrigine, or baclofen can be tried
  - Surgical microvascular decompression of the trigeminal nerve successful in selected patients; radiosurgery may also be effective

- ■ Pearl

Virtually the only cause of unilaterally unshaven face in men: even the pressure of the razor may trigger an attack.

Reference

Dhople AA, Adams JR, Maggio WW, Naqvi SA, Regine WF, Kwok Y. Long-term outcomes of Gamma Knife radiosurgery for classic trigeminal neuralgia: implications of treatment and critical review of the literature. J Neurosurg 2009;111:351. [PMID: 19326987]

13

Geriatrics

Constipation

- **Essentials of Diagnosis**
  - Infrequent stools (less than three times a week) and causing discomfort
  - Straining with defecation more than 25% of the time

- **Differential Diagnosis**
  - Normal bowel function that does not match patient expectations of bowel function
  - Anorectal dysfunction
  - Slow bowel transit
  - Dietary factors, including low-calorie diet
  - Obstructing cancer
  - Metabolic disorder, such as hypercalcemia
  - Medications (calcium, calcium channel blockers, diuretics, opioids, iron, others)

- **Treatment**
  - In absence of pathology, increase fiber and liquid intake
  - In presence of slow transit constipation, use osmotic agents such as sorbitol and lactulose
  - Docusate stool softeners may help some but generally are limited in efficacy
  - In refractory cases or with opioid use, stimulant laxatives (eg, senna) may be necessary
  - In presence of anorectal dysfunction, suppositories often necessary

- **Pearl**

One patient's constipation is another's diarrhea, and vice versa.

Reference

Gallagher P, O'Mahony D. Constipation in old age. Best Pract Res Clin Gastroenterol 2009;23:875. [PMID: 19942165]

Delirium

- ■ Essentials of Diagnosis
  - Acute-onset confusional state, usually lasting less than 1 week
  - Fluctuating mental status with marked deficit of short-term memory
  - Inability to concentrate, maintain attention, or sustain purposeful behavior
  - Increased anxiety and irritability or withdrawal
  - Risk factors include dementia, organic brain lesion, alcohol dependence, medications, and various medical problems
  - Mild to moderate delirium at night ("sundowning") is often precipitated by hospitalization, drugs, or sensory deprivation

- ■ Differential Diagnosis
  - Depression or other psychiatric disorder
  - Alcohol or benzodiazepine withdrawal
  - Medication side effect
  - Subclinical status epilepticus
  - Pain

- ■ Treatment
  - Identify and treat underlying cause
  - Manage pain; undertreatment or overtreatment of pain may contribute to delirium
  - Promote restful sleep; keep patient up and interactive during day
  - Frequent reorientation by staff, family, clocks, calendars
  - When medication needed, low-dose haloperidol or atypical antipsychotic; avoid benzodiazepines except in alcohol and benzodiazepine withdrawal
  - Avoid potentially offending medications, particularly anticholinergic and psychoactive medications
  - Avoid restraints, lines, and tubes

- ■ Pearl

Although hyperactive delirium (agitation and delusions) is most often recognized, hypoactive delirium (sleepiness and being subdued) is the most common subtype.

Reference

Miller MO. Evaluation and management of delirium in hospitalized older patients. Am Fam Physician 2008;78:1265. [PMID: 19069020]

Dementia

- ■ Essentials of Diagnosis
  - • Persistent and progressive impairment in intellectual function, including loss of short-term memory, word-finding difficulties, apraxia (inability to perform previously learned tasks), agnosia (inability to recognize objects), and visuospatial problems (becoming lost in familiar surroundings)
  - • Impaired function in activities of daily living
  - • Behavioral disturbances or psychiatric symptoms can be common
  - • Alzheimer's disease accounts for more than half of cases; vascular dementia second most common; other causes include Lewy body and frontotemporal dementia

- ■ Differential Diagnosis
  - • Normal age-related cognitive changes or drug effects
  - • Depression or other psychiatric disorder
  - • Delirium
  - • Metabolic disorder (eg, hypercalcemia, hyper- and hypothyroidism, or vitamin B_{12} deficiency)
  - • Sensory impairment
  - • Parkinson's disease
  - • Rare CNS process such as chronic subdural hematoma, meningioma, metastasis; or neurologic process such as temporal lobe epilepsy

- ■ Treatment
  - • Correct sensory deficits, treat underlying disease, remove offending medications, and treat depression, when present
  - • Caregiver education, referral to Alzheimer's Association, advanced care planning early
  - • Consider anticholinesterase inhibitors (eg, donepezil) in Alzheimer's type dementia, vascular dementia, or dementia with Lewy bodies
  - • Consider memantine in more advanced Alzheimer's type dementia
  - • Treat behavioral problems (eg, agitation) with environmental and behavioral interventions; use medications for targeted symptoms that are disturbing to the patient or endanger the patient or others
  - • Advanced dementia can benefit from a palliative approach

- ■ Pearl

In the demented patient, assess for reversible cases and start long-term care planning early.

Reference

Kester MI, Scheltens P. Dementia: the bare essentials. Pract Neurol 2009;9:241. [PMID: 19608778]

Falls

- **Essentials of Diagnosis**
    - Frequently not mentioned to physicians
    - Evidence of trauma or fractures, but this may be subtle, especially in the hip
    - Decreased activity, social isolation
    - Fear of falling
    - Functional decline

- **Differential Diagnosis**
    - Visual impairment
    - Gait impairment due to muscular weakness, podiatric disorder, or neurologic dysfunction
    - Environmental hazards such as poor lighting, stairways, rugs, warped floors
    - Polypharmacy (especially with use of sedative-hypnotics)
    - Postural hypotension, particularly postprandial hypotension
    - Presyncope, vertigo, disequilibrium, and syncope

- **Treatment**
    - Prescribe an exercise program and appropriate assistive devices and refer as needed for physical therapy
    - Evaluate for and treat osteoporosis
    - Evaluate vision
    - Review medications
    - Assess home and environmental safety and prescribe modifications as indicated

- **Pearl**

Regularly ask older adults and caregivers about falls; and consider falls with occult injury in the older adult who suddenly "takes to bed" or has altered cognition.

Reference

Ganz DA, Bao Y, Shekelle PG, Rubenstein LZ. Will my patient fall? JAMA 2007;297:77-86 [PMID: 17200478]

Hearing Impairment

- ■ Essentials of Diagnosis
  - • Difficulty understanding speech, difficulty listening to television or talking on the telephone, tinnitus, hearing loss limiting personal or social life
  - • "Whisper test": Patient is unable to repeat numbers whispered with one ear occluded
  - • Refer patient for formal audiologic evaluation; hearing loss of > 40 dB will cause difficulty understanding normal speech
  - • Hearing handicap reflects the impact of hearing loss on performing activities of daily living

- ■ Differential Diagnosis
  - • Sensorineural hearing loss (presbycusis, ototoxicity due to medications, tumors or infections of cranial nerve VIII, injury by vascular events)
  - • Conductive hearing loss (cerumen impaction, otosclerosis, chronic otitis media, Ménière's disease, trauma, tumors)

- ■ Treatment
  - • Cerumen removal if impaction present (carbamide peroxide drops, gentle irrigation with warm water)
  - • Consider assistive listening devices (amplifiers, amplified telephone, low-frequency doorbells, closed-captioned television decoders) and hearing aids
  - • Refer patients with sudden or asymmetric hearing loss to a specialist for further evaluation
  - • Educate family to speak slowly and to face the patient directly when speaking

- ■ Pearl

Loss of hearing and vision in the older patient contracts the environment and may lead to the misdiagnosis of dementia.

Reference

Bagai A, Thavendiranathan P, Detsky AS. Does this patient have hearing impairment? JAMA 2006;295:416. [PMID: 16434632]

Inappropriate Prescribing and Polypharmacy

- ■ Essentials of Diagnosis
  - • Risk factors: Older age, cognitive impairment, taking five or more medications, multiple prescribing physicians, and recent discharge from a hospital
  - • A medical regimen that includes unnecessary or inappropriate medications, such that the likelihood of adverse effects (from the number or type of medications) exceeds the likelihood of benefit
  - • Medications used to prevent illness without improving symptoms have increasingly marginal risk-benefit profiles in patients with limited life expectancies
  - • Over-the-counter drugs and supplements often added on by a patient without physician's awareness

- ■ Differential Diagnosis
  - • Appropriate use of multiple medications to treat older adults for multiple comorbid conditions
  - • Underuse of potentially useful medications is also common among older patients

- ■ Treatment
  - • Regularly review all medications, instructions, and indications (including prescriptions from other providers)
  - • Involve pharmacists in medication review, especially for medication reconciliation during transitions of care
  - • Keep dosing regimens as simple as possible
  - • Avoid managing an adverse drug reaction with another drug
  - • Select medications that can treat more than one problem
  - • Consider if benefits of adding a medication justifies the increase in complexity of the regimen and risk of side effects

13

- ■ Pearl

For any new symptom or lab abnormality in an older patient, a medication side effect or drug-drug interaction is the simplest—and most overlooked—cause.

Reference

Kaur S, Mitchell G, Vitetta L, Roberts MS. Interventions that can reduce inappropriate prescribing in the elderly. Drugs Aging 2009;26:1013. [PMID: 19929029]

Insomnia

- ■ Essentials of Diagnosis
  - Difficulty in initiating or maintaining sleep or nonrestorative sleep lasting at least 1 month and causing impairment of social or occupational functioning
  - For acute insomnia (< 3 weeks), presence of recent life stress, new symptoms (such as cough, pain, acid reflux), or new medications
  - Related to psychiatric disorder, such as major depression or posttraumatic stress disorder

- ■ Differential Diagnosis
  - Primary sleep disorders (sleep apnea, restless legs)
  - Psychiatric illness (depression, anxiety, mania, psychoses, stress, panic attacks, posttraumatic stress disorder)
  - Comorbid disease causing chronic pain, dyspnea, urinary frequency, reflux esophagitis, or delirium
  - Drug effect (beta-blockers, bronchodilators, caffeine, corticosteroids, theophylline, selective serotonin reuptake inhibitors, diuretics, others); withdrawal from sedative-hypnotic medications or alcohol
  - Noisy environment, excessive daytime napping
  - Disordered circadian rhythms (jet lag, shift work, dementia)

- ■ Treatment
  - Treat underlying cause of insomnia by removing or modifying mitigating factors
  - Maintain good sleep hygiene (avoid stimulants, minimize noise, keep regular sleep schedule, avoid daytime naps, exercise regularly)
  - Refer for cognitive behavioral therapy for insomnia
  - Refer for polysomnography if a primary sleep disorder, such as sleep apnea, is suspected
  - Consider short-term (< 4 weeks) intermittent use of ramelteon (melatonin receptor agonist), zolpidem, or eszopiclone (nonbenzodiazepine)
  - Avoid diphenhydramine because of anticholinergic effects

- ■ Pearl

The necessary hours of sleep for an individual often diminish with age; it is more useful to ask someone if they have adequate wakefulness to function during the day than the number of hours they slept.

Reference

Bloom HG, Ahmed I, Alessi CA, et al. Evidence-based recommendations for the assessment and management of sleep disorders in older persons. J Am Geriatr Soc 2009;57:761. [PMID: 19484833]

Pressure Ulcers

- ■ Essentials of Diagnosis
  - Ulcers over bony or cartilaginous prominences (sacrum, hips, heels)
  - Stage I (nonblanchable erythema of intact skin); stage II (partial-thickness skin loss involving the epidermis or dermis); stage III (full-thickness skin loss extending to the deep fascia); stage IV (full-thickness skin loss involving muscle or bone)
  - Risk factors: Immobility, incontinence, malnutrition, cognitive impairment, older age, impaired sensory perception

- ■ Differential Diagnosis
  - Herpes simplex virus ulcers
  - Venous insufficiency ulcers
  - Underlying osteomyelitis
  - Ulcerated skin cancer
  - Pyoderma gangrenosum

- ■ Treatment
  - Reduce pressure (reposition patient every 2 hours, use special support mattress)
  - Treat underlying conditions that may prevent wound healing (infection, malnutrition, poor functional status, incontinence, comorbid illnesses)
  - Control pain
  - Select dressing to keep the wound moist and the surrounding tissue intact (hydrocolloids, silver sulfadiazine, or, if heavy exudate, calcium alginate or foams)
  - Debridement if necrotic tissue present (sharp debridement with scalpel, enzymatic debridement with collagenase, bio-debridement with maggot therapy, or autolytic debridement with occlusive dressings)
  - Surgical procedures may be necessary to treat extensive pressure ulcers

13

- ■ Pearl

There is no "early" decubitus; pathogenesis begins from within, and skin breakdown is the last part of the process.

Reference

Reddy M, Gill SS, Kalkar SR, et al. Treatment of pressure ulcers: a systematic review. JAMA 2008;300:2647. [PMID: 19066385.]

Weight Loss (Involuntary)

- ■ Essentials of Diagnosis
  - • Weight loss exceeding 5% in 1 month or 10% in 6 months
  - • Weight should be measured regularly
  - • The cause of weight loss is usually diagnosed by history and physical examination
  - • Most useful tests for further evaluation: Chest x-ray, complete blood count, comprehensive metabolic panel (including glucose and calcium), thyroid-stimulating hormone, urinalysis, and fecal occult blood testing

- ■ Differential Diagnosis
  - • Physiologic changes of aging (reduced smell, taste, and chewing efficiency; slower gastric emptying; reduced ability to recover from acute undernutrition)
  - • Medical disorders (congestive heart failure, chronic lung disease, chronic renal failure, peptic ulcers, dementia, dysphagia, malignancy, diabetes mellitus, hyperthyroidism, malabsorption, systemic infections, hospitalization)
  - • Social problems (poverty, isolation, inability to obtain food, alcoholism, abuse and neglect, dietary restrictions)
  - • Psychiatric disorders (depression, schizophrenia, bereavement, anorexia nervosa, bulimia)
  - • Drug effects (selective serotonin reuptake inhibitors, NSAIDs, digoxin, antibiotics, acetylcholinesterase inhibitors)

13

- ■ Treatment
  - • Direct at underlying etiology—usually multifactorial
  - • Frequent meals, protein-calorie supplements, multivitamins, enhancement of food flavor
  - • Family-style dining (rather than eating alone), hand-feeding, and occupational and swallow therapy to modify utensils and teach swallow techniques
  - • Referral to senior centers and meal programs as indicated
  - • Exercise prescription to help restore or preserve muscle
  - • "Watchful waiting" when cause is unknown after basic evaluation (25% of cases)
  - • Consider enteral tube feedings if treatment would improve quality of life and is in line with goals of care

- ■ Pearl

The gradual weight loss due to diminished muscle mass is typical of aging; too detailed evaluations may be unnecessary and even harmful.

Reference

Visvanathan R, McPhee Chapman I. Undernutrition and anorexia in the older person. Gastroenterol Clin N Am 2009;38:393. [PMID: 19699404]

14

Psychiatric Disorders

Alcohol Dependence

- **Essentials of Diagnosis**
  - Intoxication: Mood lability, impaired judgment, somnolence, slurred speech, ataxia, attention or memory deficits, coma
  - Symptoms of withdrawal when intake is interrupted
  - Tolerance to the effects of alcohol
  - Presence of alcohol-associated medical illnesses (eg, liver disease, neuropathy, cerebellar ataxia, pancreatitis)
  - Recurrent use resulting in multiple legal problems, hazardous situations, or failure to fulfill role obligations
  - Continued drinking despite strong medical and social contraindications and life disruptions
  - High comorbidity with depression

- **Differential Diagnosis**
  - Alcohol use secondary to psychiatric illness
  - Other sedative-hypnotic dependence or intoxication
  - Withdrawal from other substances (eg, cocaine, amphetamine)
  - Pathophysiologic disturbance such as hypoxia, hypoglycemia, stroke, central nervous system infection or neoplasm, or subdural hematoma

- **Treatment**
  - Total abstinence is the safest course
  - Substance abuse counseling and groups (eg, Alcoholics Anonymous)
  - Naltrexone if patient is not taking opioids; disulfiram in selected patients
  - Treat underlying depression if present

- **Pearl**

Healed rib fractures on a chest x-ray without a history of trauma suggests forgotten injury due to intoxication.

Reference

Coder B, Freyer-Adam J, Rumpf HJ, John U, Hapke U. At-risk and heavy episodic drinking, motivation to change, and the development of alcohol dependence among men. J Stud Alcohol Drugs 2009;70:937. [PMID: 19895771]

Alcohol Withdrawal

- **Essentials of Diagnosis**
  - Symptoms when patient with dependence abruptly stops drinking
  - Tremor, wakefulness, psychomotor agitation, anxiety, seizures, hallucinations or delusions
  - Severe withdrawal: Disorientation, frightening visual hallucinations, marked autonomic hyperactivity (delirium tremens)

- **Differential Diagnosis**
  - Delirium secondary to other medical illness (eg, infection, hypoglycemia, hepatic disease)
  - Withdrawal from other sedative-hypnotics (eg, benzodiazepines) or opioids
  - Substance intoxication (eg, cocaine, amphetamine)
  - Anxiety disorders
  - Manic episode
  - Psychotic disorders
  - Seizure disorder

- **Treatment**
  - Benzodiazepines, with target of keeping vital signs normal
  - Haloperidol if hallucinations or delusions are present
  - Folic acid, multivitamins, and parenteral thiamin
  - Encourage hydration

- **Pearl**

The longer the period between the discontinuation and the appearance of symptoms, the more marked they are, especially delirium tremens.

14

Reference

Walker L, Brown P, Beeching NJ, Beadsworth MB. Managing alcohol withdrawal syndromes: the place of guidelines. Br J Hosp Med (Lond) 2009;70:444. [PMID: 19684533]

Attention-Deficit/Hyperactivity Disorder

- ■ Essentials of Diagnosis
  - Inattention with school, home, or work obligations
  - Difficulty organizing tasks and activities
  - Easily distracted or forgetful in daily activities
  - Hyperactivity: Fidgeting, inappropriate running about, excessive talking, subjective feelings of restlessness
  - Impulsivity, interrupting others
  - Onset of symptoms before age 7 years
  - Impairment present in two or more settings (eg, school, home, work)

- ■ Differential Diagnosis
  - Major depressive disorder
  - Anxiety disorder
  - Bipolar disorder
  - Other childhood mental disorders (eg, autistic, learning, conduct, oppositional-defiant disorders)
  - Dementia in adults
  - Medical illness (eg, hyperthyroidism, seizure, central nervous system neoplasm, stroke)

- ■ Treatment
  - Stimulants (eg, methylphenidate, dextroamphetamine)
  - Atomoxetine and guanfacine have no abuse potential
  - Bupropion or tricyclic antidepressants may provide additional benefit
  - Cognitive-behavioral therapy

14

- ■ Pearl

Attention-deficit/hyperactivity disorder may be diagnosed in adults, but onset of symptoms dates to childhood with careful history-taking.

Reference

Goodman DW, Thase ME. Recognizing ADHD in adults with comorbid mood disorders: implications for identification and management. Postgrad Med 2009;121:20. [PMID: 19820271]

Bipolar Disorder

- **Essentials of Diagnosis**
    - History of manic episode: Grandiosity, decreased need for sleep, pressured speech, racing thoughts, distractibility, increased activity, excessive spending, or hypersexuality
    - A single manic episode establishes the diagnosis
    - Depressive episodes may alternate with periods of mania
    - Manic episode may have psychotic component

- **Differential Diagnosis**
    - Substance intoxication and/or withdrawal (eg, cocaine, amphetamine, alcohol)
    - Medication use (eg, steroids, thyroxine, methylphenidate)
    - Infectious disease (eg, neurosyphilis, complications of HIV infection)
    - Endocrinopathies (eg, hyperthyroidism, Cushing's syndrome)
    - Central nervous system neoplasm
    - Complex partial seizures
    - Personality disorders (eg, borderline, narcissistic)

- **Treatment**
    - Mood stabilizer: Lithium, valproic acid, carbamazepine
    - Antipsychotic medication (eg, olanzapine, quetiapine) for acute mania or psychotic component
    - Lamotrigine useful for bipolar depression
    - Psychotherapy may be helpful once acute mania is controlled

- **Pearl**

    14

    Consider this in a patient superficially similar to marked hyperthyroidism but normal TSH and T4.

Reference

Hirschfeld RM. Screening for bipolar disorder. Am J Manag Care 2007; 13(suppl):S164. [PMID: 18041877]

Eating Disorders

- ◼ Essentials of Diagnosis
  - • Severe abnormalities in eating behavior
  - • Includes anorexia nervosa and bulimia nervosa
  - • Disturbance in perception of body shape or weight
  - • Anorexia: Refusal to maintain a minimally normal body weight
  - • Bulimia: Repeated binge eating, followed by compensatory behavior to prevent weight gain (eg, vomiting, use of laxatives, excessive exercise, fasting)
  - • Medical sequelae include gastrointestinal disturbances, electrolyte imbalance, cardiovascular abnormalities, amenorrhea or oligomenorrhea, caries or periodontitis

- ◼ Differential Diagnosis
  - • Major depressive disorder
  - • Body dysmorphic disorder: Excessive preoccupation with an imagined defect in appearance
  - • Obsessive-compulsive disorder
  - • Weight loss secondary to medical illness (eg, neoplasm, gastrointestinal disease, hyperthyroidism, diabetes)

- ◼ Treatment
  - • Psychotherapy (eg, cognitive-behavioral, interpersonal)
  - • Family therapy, particularly for adolescent patients
  - • Selective serotonin reuptake inhibitors (eg, fluoxetine) may be of benefit, particularly for bulimic patients
  - • Medical management of associated physical sequelae
  - • Consider inpatient or partial hospitalization for severe cases

- ◼ Pearl

In younger patients with discolored teeth and perioral dermatitis, consider bulimia.

Reference

Waxman SE. A systematic review of impulsivity in eating disorders. Eur Eat Disord Rev 2009;17:408. [PMID: 19548249]

Factitious Disorder

- ### Essentials of Diagnosis
  - Also known as Munchausen's syndrome
  - Intentional production or feigning of symptoms
  - Motivation for symptoms is unconscious, to assume the sick role
  - External incentives for symptom production are absent
  - Patient may produce symptoms in another person in order to indirectly assume the sick role (Munchausen's by proxy)
  - High correlation with personality disorders

- ### Differential Diagnosis
  - Somatoform disorders
  - Malingering
  - Organic disease producing symptoms

- ### Treatment
  - Gentle confrontation regarding diagnosis
  - Emphasis on patient's strengths
  - Empathy with patient's long history of suffering
  - Attention to building therapeutic relationship between patient and a single primary provider
  - Psychotherapy; seldom decisive
  - Many with less severe forms eventually stop or decrease self-destructive behaviors upon confrontation

- ### Pearl

When a symptom complex eludes diagnosis in a patient with recent training in an allied health field, a factitious cause tops the list of possibilities.

14

Reference

Velazquez MD, Bolton J. Factitious disorder. Br J Hosp Med (Lond) 2006;67:548. [PMID: 17069136]

Generalized Anxiety Disorder

- **Essentials of Diagnosis**
  - Excessive, persistent worry about numerous things
  - Worry is difficult to control
  - Physiologic symptoms of restlessness, fatigue, irritability, muscle tension, sleep disturbance

- **Differential Diagnosis**
  - Endocrinopathies (eg, hyperthyroidism)
  - Pheochromocytoma
  - Medication or substance use (eg, caffeine, nicotine, amphetamine, pseudoephedrine)
  - Medication or substance withdrawal (eg, alcohol, benzodiazepines)
  - Major depressive disorder
  - Adjustment disorder
  - Other anxiety disorders (eg, obsessive-compulsive disorder)
  - Somatoform disorders
  - Personality disorders (eg, avoidant, dependent, obsessive-compulsive)

- **Treatment**
  - Psychotherapy, especially cognitive-behavioral
  - Relaxation techniques (eg, biofeedback)
  - Buspirone, paroxetine, extended-release venlafaxine, duloxetine, benzodiazepines

- **Pearl**

In patients with both anxiety and depression, treating the anxiety first may markedly exaggerate the depression; treat the latter first.

14

Reference

Weisberg RB. Overview of generalized anxiety disorder: epidemiology, presentation, and course. J Clin Psychiatry 2009;70(suppl 2):4. [PMID: 19371500]

Major Depressive Disorder

- ■ Essentials of Diagnosis
  - Depressed mood or anhedonia (loss of interest or pleasure in usual activities), with hopelessness, intense feelings of sadness
  - Poor concentration, thoughts of suicide, worthlessness, guilt
  - Sleep or appetite disturbance (increased or decreased), malaise, psychomotor retardation or agitation
  - Increased isolation and social withdrawal, decreased libido
  - May have psychotic component (eg, self-deprecatory auditory hallucinations), or multiple somatic complaints
  - Symptoms last longer than 2 weeks and impair functioning

- ■ Differential Diagnosis
  - Bipolar disorder
  - Adjustment disorder, bereavement, or dysthymic disorder
  - Substance abuse or withdrawal
  - Medication use (eg, steroids, interferon)
  - Medical illness (eg, hypothyroidism, stroke, Parkinson's disease, neoplasm, polymyalgia rheumatica)
  - Delirium or dementia
  - Anxiety, psychotic, or personality disorders

- ■ Treatment
  - Assess suicidal risk; specific plans indicate higher probability
  - Antidepressant medications: Selective serotonin reuptake inhibitors, tricyclic antidepressants, venlafaxine, nefazodone, bupropion, mirtazapine, duloxetine, monoamine oxidase inhibitors
  - Psychotherapy (eg, cognitive-behavioral, interpersonal)
  - Interventions to help with resocialization (eg, supportive groups, day treatment programs)
  - Education of patient and family about depression
  - Electroconvulsive therapy for refractory cases
  - Antipsychotic medication if psychotic component present

- ■ Pearl

The manic patient may appear very productive and personally engaging; it may erroneously be ascribed to the patient's baseline personality.

Reference

Fournier JC, DeRubeis RJ, Hollon SD, Dimidjian S, Amsterdam JD, Shelton RC, Fawcett J. Antidepressant drug effects and depression severity: a patient-level meta-analysis. JAMA 2010;303:47. [PMID: 20051569]

14

Nicotine Dependence and Withdrawal

- ■ Essentials of Diagnosis
  - Symptoms of withdrawal when intake is interrupted
  - Tolerance to the effects of nicotine
  - Persistent desire or unsuccessful efforts to decrease use
  - Continued use despite nicotine-associated medical illnesses (eg, pulmonary, cardiovascular)
  - Withdrawal: Dysphoric mood, anxiety, insomnia, irritability, difficulty concentrating, slowed heart rate, increased appetite

- ■ Differential Diagnosis
  - Other substance dependence, intoxication, or withdrawal
  - For withdrawal: Anxiety or mood disorder

- ■ Treatment
  - Cognitive-behavioral therapy, groups, brief clinician counseling
  - Nicotine replacement (eg, patch, lozenge, gum, inhaler, nasal spray)
  - Sustained-release bupropion or varenicline

- ■ Pearl

Choosing a quit date and engaging social supports in efforts to cease tobacco use may help the patient succeed.

Reference

Zhou X, Nonnemaker J, Sherrill B, Gilsenan AW, Coste F, West R. Attempts to quit smoking and relapse: factors associated with success or failure from the ATTEMPT cohort study. Addict Behav 2009;34:365. [PMID: 19097706]

14

Obsessive-Compulsive Disorder

- ■ Essentials of Diagnosis
  - • Obsessions: Recurrent, distressing, intrusive thoughts
  - • Compulsions: Repetitive behaviors (eg, hand washing, checking) that patient cannot resist performing
  - • Patient recognizes obsessions and compulsions as excessive
  - • Obsessions and compulsions cause distress and interfere with functioning

- ■ Differential Diagnosis
  - • Psychotic disorders
  - • Other anxiety disorders (eg, generalized anxiety disorder, phobia)
  - • Major depressive disorder
  - • Somatoform disorders
  - • Obsessive-compulsive personality disorder: Lifelong pattern of preoccupation with orderliness and perfectionism but without presence of true obsessions or compulsions
  - • Substance intoxication
  - • Tic disorder (eg, Tourette's syndrome)

- ■ Treatment
  - • Behavioral therapy (eg, exposure, response prevention)
  - • Selective serotonin reuptake inhibitors or clomipramine

- ■ Pearl

Presence of insight is typical; its absence makes psychotic disorders more likely.

14

Reference

Storch EA, Mariaskin A, Murphy TK. Psychotherapy for obsessive-compulsive disorder. Curr Psychiatry Rep 2009;11:296. [PMID: 19635238]

Opioid Dependence and Withdrawal

- ■ Essentials of Diagnosis
  - • Intoxication: Mood lability, impaired judgment, psychomotor disturbance, attention or memory deficits, somnolence, slurred speech, miotic pupils, hallucinations, respiratory depression, coma
  - • Physical dependence with tolerance
  - • Continued use despite disruptions in social and occupational functioning
  - • Withdrawal: Nausea, vomiting, abdominal cramps, diarrhea, lacrimation, rhinorrhea, dilated pupils, dysphoria, irritability, diaphoresis, insomnia, tachycardia, fever
  - • Withdrawal uncomfortable but not life-threatening

- ■ Differential Diagnosis
  - • Alcohol or other sedative-hypnotic intoxication, dependence, or withdrawal
  - • Intoxication by or withdrawal from other substances or medications
  - • For intoxication: medical abnormalities (eg, hypoxia, hypoglycemia, stroke, central nervous system infection, or hemorrhage); for withdrawal: gastrointestinal or infectious disease

- ■ Treatment
  - • Naloxone for suspected overdose with close medical observation
  - • Methadone maintenance after withdrawal for selected patients
  - • Buprenorphine may also be used for maintenance treatment
  - • Clonidine may be helpful in alleviating the autonomic symptoms of withdrawal
  - • NSAIDs, antidiarrheals, antiemetics, and sleeping medication with low abuse potential may alleviate other symptoms of withdrawal
  - • Methadone may be used to treat acute withdrawal, but only under specific federal guidelines
  - • Substance abuse counseling and groups (eg, Narcotics Anonymous)

- ■ Pearl

Many opioids are prescribed in fixed-drug combinations with acetaminophen; a blood level of the latter should be obtained in any overdose because treatment is effective only before liver chemistries become abnormal.

Reference

Madlung-Kratzer E, Spitzer B, Brosch R, Dunkel D, Haring C. A double-blind, randomized, parallel group study to compare the efficacy, safety and tolerability of slow-release oral morphine versus methadone in opioid-dependent in-patients willing to undergo detoxification. Addiction 2009;104:1549. [PMID: 19686525]

Panic Disorder

- ■ Essentials of Diagnosis
    - Sudden, recurrent, unexpected panic attacks
    - Characterized by palpitations, tachycardia, sensation of dyspnea or choking, chest pain or discomfort, nausea, dizziness, diaphoresis, numbness, depersonalization
    - Sense of doom; fear of losing control or of dying
    - Persistent worry about future attacks
    - Change in behavior due to anxiety about being in places where an attack might occur (agoraphobia)

- ■ Differential Diagnosis
    - Endocrinopathies (eg, hyperthyroidism)
    - Supraventricular tachycardia
    - Asthma, chronic obstructive pulmonary disease exacerbation
    - Pheochromocytoma
    - Medication or substance use or withdrawal
    - Other anxiety disorders (eg, generalized anxiety disorder, post-traumatic stress disorder)
    - Major bipolar or depressive disorder
    - Somatoform disorders

- ■ Treatment
    - Cognitive-behavioral therapy
    - Antidepressant medication (selective serotonin reuptake inhibitors, tricyclic antidepressants, monoamine oxidase inhibitors)
    - Benzodiazepines as adjunctive treatment
    - May have only a single attack; reassurance, education thus important early

- ■ Pearl

In younger patients with many clinic visits with negative evaluations, for non-specific symptoms panic attack ranks high on the list.

Reference

Katon WJ. Clinical practice. Panic disorder. N Engl J Med 2006;354:2360. [PMID: 16738272]

Personality Disorders

- **Three Types**
    1. Odd, eccentric ("weird"): Paranoid, schizoid, schizotypal
    2. Dramatic ("wild"): Borderline, histrionic, narcissistic, antisocial
    3. Anxious, fearful ("worried"): Avoidant, dependent, obsessive-compulsive

- **Essentials of Diagnosis**
    - History dating from childhood or adolescence of recurrent maladaptive behavior
    - Minimal introspective ability
    - Major recurrent difficulties with interpersonal relationships
    - Enduring pattern of behavior stable over time, deviating markedly from cultural expectations
    - Increased risk of substance abuse

- **Differential Diagnosis**
    - Anxiety, major depressive, bipolar, or psychotic disorders
    - Dissociative disorders
    - Substance use or withdrawal
    - Personality change due to medical illness (eg, central nervous system neoplasm, stroke)

- **Treatment**
    - Maintenance of a highly structured environment and clear, consistent interactions with the patient
    - Individual or group therapy (eg, cognitive-behavioral, interpersonal)
    - Antipsychotic medications may be required transiently in times of stress or decompensation
    - Serotonergic medications if depression or anxiety is prominent
    - Serotonergic medications or mood stabilizers if emotional lability is prominent

14

- **Pearl**

Just as no pearl captures the essence of this problem, no treatment is consistently valuable or effective.

Reference

Tackett JL, Balsis S, Oltmanns TF, Krueger RF. A unifying perspective on personality pathology across the life span: developmental considerations for the fifth edition of the Diagnostic and Statistical Manual of Mental Disorders. Dev Psychopathol 2009;21:687. [PMID: 19583880]

Phobic Disorders

- ■ Essentials of Diagnosis
    - • Includes specific and social phobias
    - • Persistent, irrational fear due to the presence or anticipation of an object or situation
    - • Exposure to the phobic object or situation results in excessive anxiety
    - • Avoidance of phobic object or situation
    - • Social phobia (social anxiety disorder): Fear of humiliation or embarrassment in a performance or social situation (eg, speaking or eating in public)

- ■ Differential Diagnosis
    - • Other anxiety disorders (eg, generalized anxiety disorder, panic disorder, posttraumatic stress disorder)
    - • Psychotic disorders
    - • Personality disorders (eg, avoidant)

- ■ Treatment
    - • Behavioral therapy (eg, exposure)
    - • Hypnosis
    - • Benzodiazepines as necessary for anticipated situations that cannot be avoided (eg, flying)
    - • Beta-blockers for anticipated, circumscribed social phobia (performance anxiety)
    - • Paroxetine, sertraline, extended-release venlafaxine for social phobia

14

- ■ Pearl

The most common phobia in clinical medicine is the fear of public speaking; it is even the content of dreams in some affected patients.

Reference

Choy Y, Fyer AJ, Lipsitz JD. Treatment of specific phobia in adults. Clin Psychol Rev 2007;27:266. [PMID: 17112646]

Psychotic Disorders

- ■ Essentials of Diagnosis
  - Includes schizophrenia, schizoaffective and schizophreniform disorders, delusional disorder, brief psychotic disorder, and shared psychotic disorder
  - Loss of ego boundaries, gross impairment in reality testing
  - Prominent delusions or hallucinations
  - May have flat or inappropriate affect and disorganized speech, thought processes, or behavior
  - Brief psychotic disorder: Symptoms last less than 1 month, then resolve completely

- ■ Differential Diagnosis
  - Major depressive or manic episode with psychotic features
  - Medication or substance use (eg, steroids, levodopa, cocaine, amphetamines)
  - Medication or substance withdrawal (eg, alcohol)
  - Heavy metal toxicity
  - Psychotic symptoms associated with dementia
  - Delirium
  - Complex partial seizures or central nervous system neoplasm
  - Multiple sclerosis
  - Systemic lupus erythematosus
  - Endocrinopathies (eg, hypercalcemia, Cushing's syndrome)
  - Infectious disease (eg, neurosyphilis)
  - Acute intermittent porphyria
  - Personality disorders (eg, paranoid, schizoid, schizotypal)

- ■ Treatment
  - Antipsychotic medications: Newer agents (risperidone, olanzapine, quetiapine, clozapine, ziprasidone, aripiprazole) less likely to cause extrapyramidal symptoms
  - Attempt to provide structured environment
  - Behavioral therapy (eg, skills training)

- ■ Pearl
  - *Hallucinations or delusions diagnose psychosis generically specific; its organic or functional cause is then determined.*

Reference

Thomas P, Alptekin K, Gheorghe M, Mauri M, Olivares JM, Riedel M. Management of patients presenting with acute psychotic episodes of schizophrenia. CNS Drugs 2009;23:193. [PMID: 19320529]

14

Sexual Dysfunction

■ Essentials of Diagnosis

- Includes hypoactive sexual desire disorder, sexual aversion disorder, female sexual arousal disorder, male erectile disorder, orgasmic disorder, premature ejaculation
- Persistent disturbance in the phases of the sexual response cycle (eg, absence of desire, arousal, or orgasm)
- Causes significant distress or interpersonal difficulty
- Conditioning may cause or exacerbate dysfunction

■ Differential Diagnosis

- Underlying medical condition (eg, chronic illness, various hormone deficiencies, diabetes mellitus, hypertension, peripheral vascular disease, pelvic pathology)
- Medication (eg, selective serotonin reuptake inhibitors, numerous antihypertensives) or substance use (eg, alcohol)
- Depression

■ Treatment

- Encourage increased communication with sexual partner
- Decrease performance anxiety via sensate focus, relaxation exercises
- Sex or couples therapy, especially if life or relationship stressors are present
- Hormone replacement if levels are low
- Erectile dysfunction in men: Consider oral medication (eg, sildenafil, vardenafil, tadalafil), alprostadil pellet or injection, vacuum device, penile implant
- Premature ejaculation: Selective serotonin reuptake inhibitors may help

■ Pearl

As this is commonly under-diagnosed in women, gentle inquiries should be made in the presence of ill-characterized somatic symptoms.

Reference

DeLamater J, Karraker A. Sexual functioning in older adults. Curr Psychiatry Rep 2009;11:6. [PMID: 19187702]

14

Somatoform Disorders (Psychosomatic Disorders)

- ■ Essentials of Diagnosis
  - • Includes conversion, somatization, pain disorder with psychologic factors, hypochondriasis, and body dysmorphic disorder
  - • Symptoms may involve one or more organ systems and are unintentional
  - • Subjective complaints exceed objective findings
  - • Symptom development may correlate with psychosocial stress, and symptoms are real to the patient

- ■ Differential Diagnosis
  - • Major depressive disorder
  - • Anxiety disorders (eg, generalized anxiety disorder)
  - • Psychotic disorders
  - • Factitious disorder or malingering (See Table 14-1)
  - • Organic disease producing symptoms

- ■ Treatment
  - • Attention to building therapeutic relationship between patient and a single primary provider
  - • Acknowledgment that patient's distress is real
  - • Avoidance of confrontation regarding reality of the symptoms
  - • Follow-up visits at regular intervals
  - • Focus on patient's level of functioning
  - • Empathy regarding patient's psychosocial difficulties
  - • Continued vigilance about organic disease
  - • Psychotherapy, especially group cognitive-behavioral
  - • Biofeedback; hypnosis

- ■ Pearl

Vigilance about anatomic disease is essential; this disorder commonly results in a psychiatric label and therefore missed organic disease.

Table 14-1. Somatoform disorders

		Symptom Production	
		Unconscious	**Conscious**
Motivation	**Unconscious**	Somatoform disorders	Factitious disorders
	Conscious	Not applicable	Malingering

Reference

Lieb R, Meinlschmidt G, Araya R. Epidemiology of the association between somatoform disorders and anxiety and depressive disorders: an update. Psychosom Med 2007;69:860. [PMID: 18040095]

14

Stress Disorders

- ■ Essentials of Diagnosis
  - Includes acute stress disorder and posttraumatic stress disorder
  - Exposure to a traumatic event
  - Intrusive thoughts, nightmares, flashbacks
  - Mental distress or physiologic symptoms or signs (eg, tachycardia, diaphoresis) when exposed to stimuli that cue the trauma
  - Avoidance of thoughts, feelings, or situations associated with the trauma
  - Isolation, detachment from others, emotional numbness
  - Sleep disturbance, irritability, hypervigilance, startle response, poor concentration
  - Comorbid depression and substance abuse common

- ■ Differential Diagnosis
  - Other anxiety disorders (eg, panic disorder, generalized anxiety disorder)
  - Major depressive disorder
  - Adjustment disorder
  - Psychotic disorders
  - Substance use or withdrawal
  - Dissociative disorders
  - Neurologic syndrome secondary to head trauma

- ■ Treatment
  - Individual and group psychotherapy
  - Cognitive-behavioral therapy
  - Antidepressant medication (selective serotonin reuptake inhibitors, tricyclic antidepressants, phenelzine)
  - Use of prazosin may be associated with fewer nightmares and less sleep disturbance

- ■ Pearl

Although posttraumatic stress disorder has been only recently recognized as a consequence of war, it has clearly been present in all armed conflicts in history, if under different names.

Reference

Smid GE, Mooren TT, van der Mast RC, Gersons BP, Kleber RJ. Delayed posttraumatic stress disorder: systematic review, meta-analysis, and meta-regression analysis of prospective studies. J Clin Psychiatry 2009;70:1572. [PMID: 19607763]

Dermatologic Disorders

Acanthosis Nigricans

- **Essentials of Diagnosis**
  - Symmetric velvety hyperpigmented plaques on axillae, groin, and neck; the face, umbilicus, inner thighs, anus, flexor surfaces of elbows and knees, and mucosal surfaces may also be affected
  - Usually a cutaneous marker of insulin-resistant state (obesity, type 2 diabetes, polycystic ovarian syndrome, metabolic syndrome)
  - Also associated with several less common insulin resistance syndromes, such as type A (hyperandrogenism) and type B (autoimmune disease), and with fibroblast growth factor receptor mutations
  - Associated with some drugs (testosterone, nicotinic acid, oral contraceptives, corticosteroids, protease inhibitors)
  - Widespread lesions, palmar involvement, or disease occurring in a nonobese patient arouse suspicion of malignant acanthosis nigricans associated with adenocarcinomas of the stomach, lung, and breast
  - Basic work-up may include fasting glucose and insulin, blood pressure, lipid profile, and androgen levels depending on presentation

- **Differential Diagnosis**
  - Confluent and reticulated papillomatosis (Gougerot-Carteaud syndrome)
  - Epidermal nevus
  - Dowling-Degos disease

- **Treatment**
  - Weight loss for obese patients
  - Malignant form often responds to treatment of the causal tumor
  - Metformin, retinoids, and laser treatments are sometimes helpful

- **Pearl**

A harbinger of impending diabetes before fasting glucose levels are elevated, but occasionally, a paraneoplastic manifestation of a number of tumors.

Reference

Higgins SP, Freemark M, Prose NS. Acanthosis nigricans: a practical approach to evaluation and management. Dermatol Online J 2008;14:2. [PMID: 19061584]

Acne Vulgaris

- **Essentials of Diagnosis**
  - Often occurs at puberty, though onset may be delayed until the third or fourth decade
  - Open and closed comedones the hallmarks
  - Severity varies from comedone to papular or pustular inflammatory acne to cysts or nodules
  - Face, neck, upper chest, and back may be affected
  - Pigmentary changes and severe scarring can occur

- **Differential Diagnosis**
  - Acne rosacea, perioral dermatitis, gram-negative folliculitis, tinea faciei, and pseudofolliculitis
  - Trunk lesions may be confused with staphylococcal folliculitis, miliaria, or eosinophilic folliculitis
  - May be induced by topical, inhaled, or systemic steroids, oily topical products, and anabolic steroids
  - Foods neither cause nor exacerbate acne (except possibly cow's milk)
  - In women with resistant acne, hyperandrogenism should be considered; may be accompanied by hirsutism and irregular menses

- **Treatment**
  - Improvement usually requires 4–6 weeks
  - Topical treatment options include benzoyl peroxide, retinoids, dapsone, and antibiotics (primarily clindamycin)
  - Oral antibiotics (tetracycline, doxycycline, minocycline) for moderate inflammatory acne; erythromycin is an alternative when tetracyclines are contraindicated
  - Low-dose oral contraceptives containing a nonandrogenic progestin can be effective in women. Oral spironolactone may be added.
  - Diluted intralesional corticosteroids effective in reducing highly inflammatory papules and cysts
  - Oral isotretinoin useful in some who fail antibiotic therapy; pregnancy prevention and monitoring essential
  - Surgical and laser techniques available to treat scarring

- **Pearl**

Don't waste time continuing failing therapies in scarring acne—treat aggressively to prevent further scars.

Reference

Haider A, Shaw JC. Treatment of acne vulgaris. JAMA 2004;292:726. [PMID: 15304471]

Actinic Keratosis (Solar Keratosis)

- ■ Essentials of Diagnosis
  - Most common in older, fair-skinned individuals; also increased in organ transplant recipients and other immunocompromised patients
  - Discrete keratotic, scaly papules; red, pigmented, or skin-colored
  - Found primarily on the face, ears, scalp, dorsal hands, and forearms
  - Induced by chronic sun exposure
  - Lesions may become hypertrophic or develop a cutaneous horn
  - Lower lip actinic keratosis (actinic cheilitis) presents as diffuse, slight scaling of the entire lip
  - Actinic keratoses are precancerous, as some develop into squamous cell carcinoma or basal cell carcinoma

- ■ Differential Diagnosis
  - Squamous cell carcinoma
  - Bowen's disease (squamous cell carcinoma in-situ)
  - Seborrheic keratosis
  - Discoid lupus erythematosus
  - Pemphigus foliaceus

- ■ Treatment
  - Cryotherapy when limited number of lesions present
  - Topical fluorouracil or imiquimod effective for extensive disease; usually causes a severe inflammatory reaction; photodynamic therapy emerging as an additional treatment option
  - Laser therapy for severe actinic cheilitis
  - Keep a low threshold for biopsy of atypical lesions or those that do not respond to therapy
  - Sun protection, sunscreen use

15

- ■ Pearl

Although topical fluorouracil or imiquimod can be very effective for patients with extensive disease, patient education and selection are critical—certain individuals are more willing than others to endure a few weeks of extensive inflammation induced by these agents.

Reference

Criscione VD, Weinstock MA, Naylor MF, Luque C, Eide MJ, Bingham SF. Actinic keratoses: natural history and risk of malignant transformation in the Veterans Affairs Topical Tretinoin Chemoprevention Trial. Cancer 2009;115:2523. [PMID: 19382202]

Allergic Contact Dermatitis

- ■ Essentials of Diagnosis
  - • Erythema, edema, and vesicles in an area of contact with suspected agent
  - • Weeping, crusting, or secondary infection may follow
  - • Intense pruritus
  - • Pattern of eruption may be diagnostic (eg, linear streaked vesicles in poison oak or ivy)
  - • History of previous reaction to suspected contactant, though patients may be exposed to allergens for years before developing hypersensitivity
  - • Consider patch testing for chronic or recurrent disease
  - • Common allergens include nickel, plants, neomycin, bacitracin, topical anesthetics, fragrances, preservatives, hair dyes, textile dyes, nail care products, adhesives, gold, cobalt, chrome, and constituents of rubber and latex products

- ■ Differential Diagnosis
  - • Nonallergic (irritant) contact dermatitis
  - • Scabies
  - • Impetigo
  - • Dermatophytid reaction
  - • Atopic dermatitis
  - • Seborrheic dermatitis

- ■ Treatment
  - • Identify and avoid contactant
  - • Topical corticosteroids for localized involvement
  - • Wet compresses with aluminum acetate solutions for weeping lesions
  - • Systemic corticosteroids for acute, severe cases; tapering may require 2–3 weeks to avoid rebound
  - • Antihistaminic ointments should be avoided because of their sensitization potential

- ■ Pearl

If the agent can be aerosolized, as with Rhus (poison oak and ivy vines in a campfire), noncardiogenic pulmonary edema may result.

Reference

Zug KA, Warshaw EM, Fowler JF Jr, et al. Patch-test results of the North American Contact Dermatitis Group 2005-2006. Dermatitis 2009;20:149. [PMID: 19470301]

15

Alopecia Areata

- **Essentials of Diagnosis**
  - Usually occurs without associated disease, but patients with alopecia areata have an increased incidence of atopic dermatitis, Down's syndrome, lichen planus, vitiligo, autoimmune thyroiditis, and systemic lupus erythematosus
  - Rapid and complete hair loss in one or several round or oval patches
  - Occurs on the scalp or in the beard, eyebrows, or eyelashes; other hair-bearing areas less frequently affected
  - Short broken hairs on patch periphery
  - During active disease, telogen hairs near the patches easily pulled
  - The patches show preservation of follicles and normal scalp
  - Some patients have nail pitting
  - Some progress to total loss of scalp hair (alopecia totalis); a few lose all body hair (alopecia universalis)
  - Biopsy with horizontal sectioning if diagnosis unclear

- **Differential Diagnosis**
  - Tinea capitis
  - Discoid lupus erythematosus, early lesions
  - Lichen planopilaris, early lesions
  - Secondary syphilis
  - Trichotillomania
  - Metastatic or cutaneous malignancy
  - Loose anagen syndrome
  - Androgenic alopecia

- **Treatment**
  - Course is variable: Some patches regrow spontaneously, others resist therapy
  - Intralesional steroid injections (monthly) are primary treatment
  - Topical anthralin, corticosteroids, or minoxidil, contact sensitization with squaric acid, and psoralen plus UVA
  - Psychologic stress can be devastating; emotional support and patient education essential

15

- **Pearl**

Because the disease affects dark hairs and frequently spares white hairs, some patients with salt-and-pepper hair will present complaining of "sudden whitening" of their hair.

Reference

Norris D. Alopecia areata: current state of knowledge. J Am Acad Dermatol 2004;51(suppl):S16. [PMID: 15243493]

Androgenetic Alopecia (Common Pattern Baldness)

- ■ Essentials of Diagnosis
  - Genetic predisposition plus probable excessive response of androgen receptor
  - Men in third and fourth decades: Gradual loss of hair, chiefly from vertex and frontotemporal regions; rate variable
  - Women: Diffuse hair loss throughout the mid scalp, sparing frontal hairline
  - Appropriate laboratory work-up for women with signs of hyperandrogenism (hirsutism, acne, abnormal menses)
  - Hair pull test may show a normal or increased number of telogen hairs; hair shafts narrow but not fragile

- ■ Differential Diagnosis
  - Telogen effluvium
  - Alopecia induced by hypothyroidism
  - Alopecia induced by iron deficiency
  - Secondary syphilis
  - Trichotillomania
  - Tinea capitis
  - Alopecia areata in evolution
  - Anagen effluvium due to chemotherapy or other drugs

- ■ Treatment
  - Early topical minoxidil effective in most with limited disease
  - Oral finasteride prevents further loss and increases hair counts (except on the temples); contraindicated in women of childbearing potential; lacks efficacy in postmenopausal women
  - Wigs or interwoven hair for cosmetic purposes
  - Hair transplantation with minigrafts
  - Women with hyperandrogenism may respond to antiandrogen therapies

- ■ Pearl

Anxious patients with this condition support an enormous market for uninvestigated—and ineffective—products.

Reference

Rogers NE, Avram MR. Medical treatments for male and female pattern hair loss. J Am Acad Dermatol 2008;59:547. [PMID: 18793935]

15

Atopic Dermatitis (Atopic Eczema)

- ■ Essentials of Diagnosis
  - Pruritic, exudative, or lichenified eruption on face, neck, upper trunk, wrists, hands, antecubital and popliteal folds
  - Involves face and extensor surfaces more typically in infants
  - Personal or family history of allergies or asthma
  - Recurring; remission possible in adolescence
  - Peripheral eosinophilia, increased serum IgE—not needed for diagnosis

- ■ Differential Diagnosis
  - Seborrheic dermatitis
  - Contact dermatitis
  - Scabies
  - Impetigo
  - Eczema herpeticum may be superimposed on atopic dermatitis
  - Eczematous dermatitis may be presenting feature of immunodeficiency syndromes in infants

- ■ Treatment
  - Avoidance of anything that dries or irritates skin
  - Frequent emollients
  - Topical corticosteroids are first-line therapy
  - Topical tacrolimus and pimecrolimus are effective but expensive alternatives to steroids
  - Phototherapy sometimes helpful
  - Sedative antihistamines relieve pruritus, especially when sleep is disturbed
  - Atopic patients frequently colonized with staphylococci; systemic antibiotics and bleach baths helpful in flares
  - Systemic steroids, cyclosporine, or other immunosuppressives in highly selected cases
  - Dietary restrictions may be of benefit in few limited cases when specific food allergies are implicated

- ■ Pearl

A small subset of pediatric atopic dermatitis may be associated with food allergy, but dietary restrictions are difficult to effect.

Reference

Krakowski AC, Eichenfield LF, Dohil MA. Management of atopic dermatitis in the pediatric population. Pediatrics 2008;122:812. [PMID: 18829806]

15

Basal Cell Carcinoma

- **Essentials of Diagnosis**
  - Dome-shaped semitranslucent or pink papule with overlying telangiectases, or a plaque of such nodules with a rolled border around a central depression; may crust or ulcerate
  - Most occur on head and neck, but the trunk and extremities also affected
  - Most common in older, light-skinned individuals, but occurs in people of all ages and ethnicities
  - Several variants (nodular, superficial, micronodular, infiltrative, sclerosing, pigmented, etc.)
  - Immunosuppressive medications increase frequency and aggressiveness; patients with albinism or xeroderma pigmentosum or exposed to radiation therapy or arsenic also at increased risk
  - Chronic, local spread typical; metastasis rare
  - Biopsy critical for diagnosis

- **Differential Diagnosis**
  - Squamous cell carcinoma
  - Actinic keratosis
  - Seborrheic keratosis
  - Paget's disease
  - Melanoma
  - Nevus
  - Psoriasis
  - Nevoid basal cell carcinoma syndrome

- **Treatment**
  - Excisional surgery with histologic examination of margins
  - Curettage with electrodesiccation in superficial lesions of trunk or small nodular tumors in select locations
  - Mohs micrographic surgery for lesions with aggressive histology, recurrences, or in areas where tissue conservation is important
  - Imiquimod cream in selected superficial lesions with close follow-up
  - Ionizing radiation is an alternative
  - Sun protection, regular sunscreen use, regular skin screening

- **Pearl**

An extremely common malignancy, with millions of cases annually worldwide.

Reference

Rubin AI, Chen EH, Ratner D. Basal cell carcinoma. N Engl J Med 2005;353:2262. [PMID: 16306523]

15

Bullous Drug Reactions (Erythema Multiforme Major, Stevens-Johnson Syndrome, and Toxic Epidermal Necrolysis)

- **Essentials of Diagnosis**
  - Flulike symptoms frequently precede eruption
  - Initial lesions macular and erythematous or dusky; may become targetoid, form bullae, or desquamate
  - Two or more mucosal surfaces (oral, conjunctival, anogenital) usually affected; in severe cases, pneumonitis, arthritis, hepatitis, nephritis, or GI bleeding may occur
  - Skin biopsies confirm diagnosis
  - Stevens-Johnson syndrome: < 10% of body surface involvement; toxic epidermal necrolysis: > 30% of body surface involvement
  - Sulfonamides, phenytoin, carbamazepine, phenobarbital, penicillins, allopurinol, NSAIDs, bupropion, terbinafine, tetracyclines, and nevirapine are frequent offenders

- **Differential Diagnosis**
  - Staphylococcal scalded skin syndrome
  - Infection-induced erythema multiforme major (most frequently associated with *Mycoplasma pneumoniae* infection)
  - Early disease may be confused with morbilliform drug eruptions or erythema multiforme minor
  - Bullous pemphigoid and pemphigus vulgaris
  - Graft-versus-host disease

- **Treatment**
  - Discontinuation of provocative agent
  - Extensive involvement may require transfer to a burn unit for fluid, electrolyte, and nutritional management
  - Systemic corticosteroids are controversial
  - Wet dressings, oral and ophthalmologic care, pain relief
  - Intravenous immunoglobulin should be given early in severe cases

15

- **Pearl**

Beware of rechallenge with phenytoin, carbamazepine, or phenobarbital in any patient with anticonvulsant hypersensitivity given cross-reactivity; valproic acid is sometimes a safer alternative.

Reference

Borchers AT, Lee JL, Naguwa SM, Cheema GS, Gershwin ME. Stevens-Johnson syndrome and toxic epidermal necrolysis. Autoimmun Rev 2008;7:598. [PMID: 18603022]

Bullous Pemphigoid

- **Essentials of Diagnosis**
  - Age at onset seventh or eighth decade, though also occurs in young children
  - Caused by autoantibodies to two specific components of the hemidesmosome
  - Occasionally drug-induced (penicillamine, furosemide, captopril, enalapril, penicillin, sulfasalazine, nalidixic acid)
  - Large, tense blisters that rupture, leaving denuded areas that heal without scarring
  - Erythematous patches and urticarial plaques can be precursors or occur without bullae
  - Predilection for groin, axillae, flexor forearms, thighs, and shins; may occur anywhere; some have oral involvement
  - Frequently pruritic
  - Diagnosis by lesional biopsy, perilesional direct immunofluorescence, and indirect immunofluorescence

- **Differential Diagnosis**
  - Epidermolysis bullosa acquisita
  - Cicatricial pemphigoid
  - Herpes gestationis
  - Linear IgA dermatosis
  - Dermatitis herpetiformis
  - Early disease may mimic drug reactions, urticaria, contact dermatitis, or scabies

- **Treatment**
  - Prednisone initially
  - Nicotinamide plus tetracycline are steroid sparing
  - Some patients require other immunosuppressives to permit steroid tapering (azathioprine, low-dose methotrexate, or mycophenolate mofetil); monitor patients for side effects and infections
  - Topical steroids for localized mild disease that breaks through medical treatment
  - Pemphigoid usually self-limited, lasting months to years

- **Pearl**

Many patients present in the early stages with only intractable pruritus; vesicles or bullae come later.

Reference

Olasz EB, Yancey KB. Bullous pemphigoid and related subepidermal autoimmune blistering diseases. Curr Dir Autoimmun 2008;10:141. [PMID: 18460884]

15

Common Warts (Verrucae Vulgaris)

- ■ Essentials of Diagnosis
  - Scaly, rough, spiny papules or plaques
  - Most frequently seen on hands, may occur anywhere on skin
  - Caused by human papillomavirus

- ■ Differential Diagnosis
  - Actinic keratosis
  - Squamous cell carcinoma
  - Seborrheic keratosis
  - Acrochordon (skin tag)
  - Nevus
  - Molluscum contagiosum
  - Amelanotic melanoma
  - Verrucous zoster in HIV-infected patients
  - Extensive warts may suggest epidermodysplasia verruciformis, HIV infection, or lymphoproliferative disorders

- ■ Treatment
  - Cryotherapy
  - Patient-applied salicylic acid products
  - Office-applied cantharidin
  - Curettage and electrodesiccation
  - Pulsed dye laser therapy
  - Sensitization with topical squaric acid or intralesional Candida in resistant cases
  - Intralesional bleomycin
  - Oral cimetidine has low efficacy but may be a useful adjunct
  - Topical imiquimod much less effective in common warts than genital warts

- ■ Pearl

Avoid aggressive destructive treatment in young children when possible—spontaneous resolution is common, and the parents are often more bothered by the warts than the patient.

Reference

Gibbs S, Harvey I, Sterling J, Stark R. Local treatments for cutaneous warts: systematic review. BMJ 2002;325:461. [PMID: 12202325]

Cutaneous Candidiasis

- **Essentials of Diagnosis**
    - Candidal intertrigo causes superficial, denuded, pink to beefy-red patches that may be surrounded by tiny satellite pustules in genitocrural, subaxillary, gluteal, interdigital, and submammary areas
    - Oral candidiasis shows grayish white plaques that scrape off to reveal a raw, erythematous base
    - Oral candidiasis more common in elderly, debilitated, malnourished, diabetic, or HIV-infected patients, as well as those taking antibiotics, systemic steroids, or chemotherapy
    - Angular cheilitis (perlèche) sometimes due to *Candida*
    - Perianal candidiasis may cause pruritus ani
    - Candidal paronychia causes thickening and erythema of the nail fold and occasional discharge of thin pus

- **Differential Diagnosis**
    - Candidal intertrigo: Dermatophytosis, bacterial skin infections, seborrheic dermatitis, contact dermatitis, deep fungal infection, inverse psoriasis, erythrasma, eczema
    - Oral candidiasis: Lichen planus, leukoplakia, geographic tongue, herpes simplex infection, erythema multiforme, pemphigus
    - Candidal paronychia: Acute bacterial paronychia, paronychia associated with hypoparathyroidism, celiac disease, acrodermatitis enteropathica, or reactive arthritis
    - Chronic mucocutaneous candidiasis

- **Treatment**
    - Control exacerbating factors (eg, hyperglycemia in diabetics, chronic antibiotic use, estrogen-dominant oral contraceptives, systemic steroids, ill-fitting dentures, malnutrition)
    - Treat localized skin disease with topical azoles or polyenes
    - Soaks with aluminum acetate solutions for raw, denuded lesions
    - Fluconazole or itraconazole for systemic therapy
    - Nystatin suspension or clotrimazole troches for oral disease
    - Treat chronic paronychia with topical imidazoles or 4% thymol in chloroform
    - Avoid chronic water exposure

- **Pearl**

Look for adjacent pustules and the absence of much scale; it helps differentiate candidal intertrigo from tinea cruris.

Reference

Huang DB, Ostrosky-Zeichner L, Wu JJ, Pang KR, Tyring SK. Therapy of common superficial fungal infections. Dermatol Ther 2004;17:517. [PMID: 15571501]

15

Cutaneous Kaposi's Sarcoma

- **■** Essentials of Diagnosis
  - Vascular neoplasm presenting with one or several red to purple macules that progress to papules or nodules
  - Classic form occurs on legs of elderly men of Mediterranean, East European, or Jewish descent
  - African endemic form cutaneous and locally aggressive in young adults or lymphadenopathic and fatal in children
  - AIDS-associated form shows cutaneous lesions on head, neck, trunk, and mucous membranes; may progress to nodal, pulmonary, and gastrointestinal involvement
  - The form associated with iatrogenic immunosuppression can mimic either classic or AIDS-associated type
  - Human herpesvirus 8 the causative agent in all types
  - Skin biopsy for diagnosis

- **■** Differential Diagnosis
  - Dermatofibroma
  - Bacillary angiomatosis
  - Pyogenic granuloma
  - Prurigo nodularis
  - Blue nevus
  - Melanoma
  - Cutaneous lymphoma

- **■** Treatment
  - In AIDS-associated cases, combination antiretroviral therapy—increasing CD4 counts—is the treatment of choice
  - Intralesional vinblastine or interferon, radiation therapy, cryotherapy, alitretinoin gel, laser ablation, or excision
  - Systemic therapy with liposomal doxorubicin, vinblastine, vincristine, bleomycin, etoposide, or other cytotoxic drugs in certain cases with rapid progression or visceral involvement; several targeted agents are being investigated

15

- **■** Pearl

The first alert to the HIV epidemic was a New York dermatologist reporting two cases of atypical Kaposi's sarcoma to the Centers for Disease Control and Prevention; a single physician giving thought to a patient's problem can still make a difference.

Reference

Schwartz RA, Micali G, Nasca MR, Scuderi L. Kaposi sarcoma: a continuing conundrum. J Am Acad Dermatol 2008;59:179. [PMID: 18638627]

Cutaneous T-Cell Lymphoma (Mycosis Fungoides)

- ■ Essentials of Diagnosis
  - • Early stage: Erythematous 1- to 5-cm patches, sometimes pruritic, on lower abdomen, buttocks, upper thighs, and in women, breasts
  - • Middle stages: Infiltrated, erythematous, scaly plaques
  - • Advanced stages: Skin tumors, erythroderma, lymphadenopathy, or visceral involvement
  - • Skin biopsy with immunohistochemical studies critical; serial biopsies over months to years may be required to confirm diagnosis
  - • CD4:CD8 ratios, tests to detect clonal rearrangement of the T-cell receptor gene
  - • Mycosis fungoides is the classic and most common type, but there are several other forms of CTCL

- ■ Differential Diagnosis
  - • Psoriasis
  - • Drug eruption
  - • Eczematous dermatoses
  - • Leprosy
  - • Tinea corporis
  - • Other lymphoreticular malignancies

- ■ Treatment
  - • Treatment depends on stage of disease
  - • Early and aggressive therapy may control cutaneous lesions—not shown to prevent progression
  - • High-potency corticosteroids, mechlorethamine, or carmustine (BCNU) topically
  - • Phototherapy in early stages
  - • Options for advanced disease include total skin electron beam radiation, extracorporeal photophoresis, systemic chemotherapy, retinoids, alpha interferon, histone deacetylase inhibitors, and denileukin diftitox (diphtheria toxin fused to recombinant IL-2)

- ■ Pearl

  Be careful of psoriasis in adults that fails to respond to therapy or hypopigmented patches in young patients; this may be the diagnosis.

Reference

Girardi M, Heald PW, Wilson LD. The pathogenesis of mycosis fungoides. N Engl J Med 2004;350:1978. [PMID: 15128898]

Diffuse Pruritus

- ■ Essentials of Diagnosis
  - Excoriations are an objective sign of pruritus, but not always present
  - May be systemic (metabolic, endocrine, drug-induced, paraneoplastic, etc.), dermatologic (on diseased or inflamed skin), neuropathic (burning, stinging, dysesthetic), or psychogenic

- ■ Differential Diagnosis
  - Hepatic disease, especially cholestatic
  - Hepatitis C with or without liver dysfunction
  - Chronic renal insufficiency or failure
  - Hypothyroidism or hyperthyroidism
  - Intestinal parasites
  - Polycythemia rubra vera
  - Lymphomas, leukemias, myeloma, other malignancies
  - Neuropsychiatric diseases (anorexia nervosa, delusions of parasitosis)
  - Scabies or other infestations

- ■ Treatment
  - For itch associated with skin disease, treat the primary condition
  - Sedative antihistamines for symptomatic relief, especially at night
  - Topical menthol lotions, topical capsaicin
  - Opioid antagonists (naltrexone) may help cholestatic, uremic, or other itch
  - Antidepressants (selective serotonin reuptake inhibitors or mirtazapine)
  - Anticonvulsants (gabapentin, carbamazepine)
  - Optimization of dialysis, erythropoietin (epoetin alfa), emollients, cholestyramine, phosphate binders, and phototherapy helpful in some with uremic pruritus
  - Aspirin for pruritus of polycythemia vera

- ■ Pearl

Excoriations spare areas out of the patient's reach, such as the "butterfly zone" on the back, and show that the pruritus is primary.

Reference

Ikoma A, Steinhoff M, Ständer S, Yosipovitch G, Schmelz M. The neurobiology of itch. Nat Rev Neurosci 2006;7:535. [PMID: 16791143]

Discoid (Chronic Cutaneous) Lupus Erythematosus

- **Essentials of Diagnosis**
  - Dull red macules or papules developing into sharply demarcated hyperkeratotic plaques with follicular plugs
  - Lesions heal from the center with atrophy, dyspigmentation, and telangiectasias
  - Localized lesions most common on scalp, nose, cheeks, ears, lower lip, and neck
  - Scalp lesions cause scarring alopecia
  - Generalized disease involves trunk and upper extremities
  - Abnormal serologies, leukopenia, and albuminuria identify DLE patients likely to progress; children with DLE more likely to progress
  - Skin biopsy for diagnosis; direct immunofluorescence

- **Differential Diagnosis**
  - Seborrheic dermatitis
  - Rosacea
  - Lupus vulgaris (cutaneous tuberculosis)
  - Sarcoidosis
  - Bowen's disease (squamous cell carcinoma in-situ)
  - Polymorphous light eruption
  - Tertiary syphilis
  - Lichen planopilaris of the scalp

- **Treatment**
  - Screen for systemic disease with history, physical, and laboratory tests
  - Aggressive sun protection, including a high-SPF sunscreen
  - Potent topical corticosteroids or intralesional steroids for localized lesions
  - Systemic therapy with antimalarials is standard; monitor laboratory studies; ophthalmologic consultation every 6 months; smoking decreases efficacy
  - Immunosuppressives in resistant cases (methotrexate, azathioprine, or mycophenolate mofetil)
  - Thalidomide in severe cases; pregnancy prevention and monitoring for side effects critical

- **Pearl**

Fewer than 10% of patients with DLE progress to SLE—focus on reassurance and adequate treatment to limit disfiguring scars.

Reference

Walling HW, Sontheimer RD. Cutaneous lupus erythematosus: issues in diagnosis and treatment. Am J Clin Dermatol 2009;10:365. [PMID: 19824738]

Erysipelas and Cellulitis

- ■ Essentials of Diagnosis
  - Cellulitis: An acute infection of the subcutaneous tissue, most frequently caused by *Streptococcus pyogenes* or *Staphylococcus aureus*
  - Erythema, edema, tenderness are the hallmarks of cellulitis; vesicles, exudation, purpura, necrosis may follow
  - Lymphangitic streaking may be seen
  - Demarcation from uninvolved skin indistinct
  - Erysipelas: Involves superficial dermal lymphatics
  - Erysipelas characterized by a warm, red, tender, edematous plaque with a sharply demarcated, raised, indurated border; classically occurs on the face
  - Both erysipelas and cellulitis require a portal of entry
  - Recurrence seen in lymphatic damage or venous insufficiency
  - A prodrome of malaise, fever, and chills may accompany either
  - Atypical presentations or failure to respond to therapy require expansion of differential diagnosis and possibly laboratory tests (blood count, liver function, blood cultures, skin biopsies, tissue cultures, or imaging)

- ■ Differential Diagnosis
  - Early necrotizing fasciitis or clostridial gangrene
  - Underlying osteomyelitis
  - Deep fungal or mycobacterial infections, especially in the immunocompromised
  - Acute febrile neutrophilic dermatosis (Sweet's syndrome)
  - Erythema migrans
  - Erythema nodosum
  - Venous thrombosis
  - Chronic venous insufficiency and stasis dermatitis (many of these patients are misdiagnosed with leg cellulitis and unnecessarily treated with several rounds of antibiotics)
  - Contact dermatitis, evolving zoster, and connective tissue disease may mimic erysipelas

15

- ■ Treatment
  - Appropriate systemic antibiotics (*Staphylococcus aureus* isolates are increasingly methicillin-resistant)
  - Local wound care and elevation

- ■ Pearl

Look for tinea pedis as a portal of entry in patients with leg cellulitis.

Reference

Kroshinsky D, Grossman ME, Fox LP. Approach to the patient with presumed cellulitis. Semin Cutan Med Surg 2007;26:168. [PMID: 18070684]

Erythema Multiforme Minor

■ Essentials of Diagnosis

- Most often associated with herpes simplex infection (orolabial more than genital)
- Episodes follow orolabial herpes by 1–3 weeks and may recur with succeeding outbreaks
- Early sharply demarcated erythematous papules that become edematous
- Later "target" lesions with three zones: Central duskiness that may vesiculate; edematous, pale ring; and surrounding erythema
- Dorsal hands, dorsal feet, palms, soles, and extensor surfaces most frequently affected, with few to hundreds of lesions
- Mucosal involvement (usually oral) in 25%
- Biopsies often diagnostic, but usually not required

■ Differential Diagnosis

- Stevens-Johnson in evolution
- Pemphigus vulgaris
- Bullous pemphigoid
- Urticaria
- Acute febrile neutrophilic dermatosis (Sweet's syndrome)
- Subacute cutaneous lupus
- Granuloma annulare
- Fixed drug eruption

■ Treatment

- Chronic suppressive antiherpetic therapy prevents 90% of recurrences (episodic treatment begun after symptoms appear is ineffective)
- Facial and lip sunscreens may also decrease recurrences by limiting herpes outbreaks
- Episodes usually self-limited (resolving in 1–4 weeks) and do not require therapy
- Systemic corticosteroids discouraged

■ Pearl

Even when a history of clinical herpes cannot be elicited, empiric antivirals may prevent recurring target lesions.

Reference

Nikkels AF, Pierard GE. Treatment of mucocutaneous presentations of herpes simplex virus infections. Am J Clin Dermatol 2002;3:475. [PMID: 12180895]

Erythema Nodosum

- ■ Essentials of Diagnosis
  - A reactive inflammation of the subcutis associated with infections (streptococcal, *Mycoplasma*, tuberculous, *Yersinia,* coccidioidomycosis), drugs (oral contraceptives, sulfonamides, bromides), sarcoidosis, and inflammatory bowel disease
  - Symmetric, erythematous, tender plaques or nodules 1–10 cm in diameter on anterior shins
  - Lesions also occasionally seen on upper legs, neck, and arms
  - Onset may be accompanied by malaise, leg edema, and arthralgias
  - Lesions flatten over a few days, leaving a violaceous patch, then heal without atrophy or scarring
  - All lesions generally resolve within 6 weeks, but recurrences are common
  - Chronic form with prolonged course not associated with underlying diseases
  - Deep skin biopsy for diagnosis
  - Many cases are idiopathic

- ■ Differential Diagnosis
  - Erythema induratum or nodular vasculitis (secondary to tuberculosis)
  - Poststeroid panniculitis
  - Lupus panniculitis
  - Erythema multiforme
  - Syphilis
  - Behçet's disease
  - Subcutaneous fat necrosis associated with pancreatitis

- ■ Treatment
  - Treat underlying causes
  - Bed rest, gentle support hose; avoid vigorous exercise
  - NSAIDs
  - Potassium iodide
  - Intralesional steroids in persistent cases
  - Systemic steroids in severe cases; contraindicated when the underlying cause is infectious

- ■ Pearl

Persistent lesions should prompt consideration of a pulmonary cause, such as subclinical tuberculosis.

Reference

Requena L, Sánchez Yus E. Erythema nodosum. Semin Cutan Med Surg 2007;26:114. [PMID: 17544964]

Exfoliative Dermatitis (Erythroderma)

■ Essentials of Diagnosis

- Erythema and scaling over most of the body
- Itching is common
- Systemic manifestations may include malaise, fever, chills, lymphadenopathy, weight loss
- Preexisting dermatosis causes more than half of cases
- Skin biopsy to identify cause
- Leukocyte gene rearrangement studies if Sézary's syndrome suspected and biopsies nondiagnostic
- Not a single disease—erythroderma is the clinical presentation of one of the conditions below

■ Differential Diagnosis

- Erythrodermic psoriasis
- Pityriasis rubra pilaris
- Drug eruption (including DRESS [Drug Rash with Eosinophilia and Systemic Symptoms] syndrome)
- Atopic dermatitis
- Contact dermatitis
- Severe seborrheic dermatitis
- Sézary's syndrome of cutaneous T-cell lymphoma
- Hodgkin's disease

■ Treatment

- Soaks and emollients
- Mid-potency topical steroids, possibly under occlusive suit
- Hospitalization may be required for fluid, electrolyte, and nutritional management
- Specific systemic therapies depending on cause
- Discontinue offending agent in drug-induced cases
- Antibiotics for secondary bacterial infections

15

■ Pearl

Unexplained erythroderma in a middle-aged or elderly person raises the index of suspicion for a visceral malignancy.

Reference

Sehgal VN, Srivastava G, Sardana K. Erythroderma/exfoliative dermatitis: a synopsis. Int J Dermatol 2004;43:39. [PMID: 14693020]

Fixed Drug Eruption

- ■ Essentials of Diagnosis
  - • Lesions recur at the same site with each repeat exposure to the causative medication
  - • From one to six lesions
  - • Oral, genital, facial, and acral lesions most common
  - • Lesions begin as erythematous, edematous, round, sharply demarcated patches or plaques
  - • May evolve to become targetoid, bullous, or erosive
  - • Postinflammatory hyperpigmentation common
  - • Offending agents: NSAIDs, sulfonamides, barbiturates, tetracyclines, erythromycin, metronidazole, antifungals, pseudoephedrine, carbamazepine, and laxatives with phenolphthalein

- ■ Differential Diagnosis
  - • Bullous pemphigoid
  - • Erythema multiforme
  - • Sweet's syndrome (acute febrile neutrophilic dermatosis)
  - • Residual hyperpigmentation can appear similar to pigmentation left behind by numerous other inflammatory disorders
  - • The differential of genital lesions includes psoriasis, lichen planus, and syphilis

- ■ Treatment
  - • Avoidance of the causative agent
  - • Symptomatic care of lesions

- ■ Pearl

An often overlooked source of penile erosions.

15

Reference

Sehgal VN, Srivastava G. Fixed drug eruption (FDE): changing scenario of incriminating drugs. Int J Dermatol 2006;45:897. [PMID: 16911371]

Folliculitis, Furuncles, and Carbuncles

- ■ Essentials of Diagnosis
    - Folliculitis: Thin-walled pustules at follicular orifices, particularly extremities, scalp, face, and buttocks; develop in crops and heal in a few days
    - Furuncle: Acute, round, tender, circumscribed, perifollicular abscess; most undergo central necrosis and rupture with purulent discharge
    - Carbuncle: Two or more confluent furuncles
    - Classic folliculitis caused by *S. aureus*

- ■ Differential Diagnosis
    - Pseudofolliculitis barbae
    - Acne vulgaris and acneiform drug eruptions
    - Pustular miliaria (heat rash)
    - Fungal folliculitis
    - Herpes folliculitis
    - Hot tub folliculitis caused by *Pseudomonas*
    - Gram-negative folliculitis (in acne patients on long-term antibiotic therapy)
    - Eosinophilic folliculitis (HIV-infected patients)
    - Nonbacterial folliculitis (occlusion or oil-induced)
    - Hidradenitis suppurativa of axillae or groin
    - Dissecting cellulitis of scalp

- ■ Treatment
    - Thorough cleansing with antibacterial soaps
    - Mupirocin ointment in limited disease
    - Oral antibiotics (dicloxacillin or cephalexin) for more extensive involvement
    - Warm compresses and systemic antibiotics for furuncles and carbuncles
    - Culture for methicillin-resistant strains in unresponsive lesions
    - Selected larger, fluctuant lesions may require incision and drainage

- ■ Pearl

Culture anterior nares in recurrent cases to rule out S. aureus *carriage; if positive, consider applying mupirocin to nares and adding oral rifampin as a second systemic agent.*

Reference

Elston DM. Community-acquired methicillin-resistant Staphylococcus aureus. J Am Acad Dermatol 2007;56:1. [PMID: 17190619]

Genital Warts (Condylomata Acuminata)

- ■ Essentials of Diagnosis
    - Gray, yellow, or pink exophytic papules or broad-based confluent plaques
    - Occur on the penis, vulva, cervix, perineum, crural folds, or perianal area; also may be intraurethral or intra-anal
    - Caused by human papillomavirus; sexually transmitted
    - Increased risk of progression to cervical cancer, anal cancer, or bowenoid papulosis in certain HPV subtypes (primarily 16, 18, and 31)
    - Children with genital warts should be evaluated for sexual abuse, but childhood infection can also be acquired via perinatal vertical transmission or digital autoinoculation

- ■ Differential Diagnosis
    - Molluscum contagiosum
    - Bowenoid papulosis and squamous cell carcinoma
    - Seborrheic keratosis
    - Pearly penile papules (circumferential around base of glans)
    - Acrochordon (skin tag)
    - Secondary syphilis (condyloma latum)

- ■ Treatment
    - Treatment may remove lesions but has not been shown to reduce transmission or prevent progression to cancer
    - Cryotherapy, topical podophyllum resin, topical trichloroacetic acid, electrofulguration, and carbon dioxide laser; plume generated by lasers or electrofulguration is potentially infectious to health care personnel
    - Topical imiquimod; women have a higher response rate than men
    - Emphasis on pap smear for women with genital warts and female sexual partners of men with genital warts
    - Biopsy suspicious lesions; HIV-infected patients with genital warts are at increased risk of HPV-induced carcinomas

15

- ■ Pearl

Pearly penile papules are normal anatomic structures consisting of rows of small papules around the proximal edge of the glans—they are frequently mistaken for warts and treated unnecessarily.

Reference

Brodell LA, Mercurio MG, Brodell RT. The diagnosis and treatment of human papillomavirus-mediated genital lesions. Cutis 2007;79(suppl):5. [PMID: 17508490]

Granuloma Annulare

- **Essentials of Diagnosis**
  - Skin-colored or red flat-topped, asymptomatic papules that spread with central clearing to form annular plaques; cause unknown
  - May coalesce, then involute spontaneously
  - Predilection for dorsum of fingers, hands, or feet; elbows or ankles also favored sites
  - Most common in young women (under age 30)
  - Generalized form sometimes associated with diabetes; subcutaneous form most common in children
  - Atypical presentations have been associated with lymphomas and with HIV infection
  - Skin biopsy secures diagnosis

- **Differential Diagnosis**
  - Necrobiosis lipoidica
  - Tinea corporis
  - Erythema migrans (Lyme disease)
  - Sarcoidosis
  - Secondary syphilis
  - Erythema multiforme
  - Subacute cutaneous lupus erythematosus
  - Annular lichen planus
  - Leprosy (Hansen's disease)
  - Rheumatoid nodules (subcutaneous form)

- **Treatment**
  - None required in mild cases; 75% of patients with localized disease clear in 2 years (though recurrence is common)
  - Intralesional or potent topical corticosteroids effective for limited disease
  - Prednisone contraindicated due to relapse upon withdrawal
  - Anecdotal success with dapsone, nicotinamide, potassium iodide, systemic retinoids, antimalarials, and psoralen plus UVA (PUVA)

- **Pearl**

Many patients are misdiagnosed with tinea infections because the lesions of granuloma annulare can be strikingly annular.

Reference

Dahl MV. Granuloma annulare: long-term follow-up. Arch Dermatol 2007;143:946. [PMID: 17638746]

15

Herpes Simplex

■ Essentials of Diagnosis

- Orolabial herpes: Initial infection varies from asymptomatic to severe gingivostomatitis
- Recurrent grouped blisters on erythematous base (cold sore or fever blister); lips most frequently involved
- UV exposure a common trigger
- Genital herpes: Primary infection presents as systemic illness with grouped blisters and erosions on penis, rectum, or vagina
- Recurrences common; present with painful grouped vesicles
- Asymptomatic infection (and asymptomatic infectious shedding) common
- A prodrome of tingling, itching, or burning
- More severe and persistent in immunocompromised patients
- Eczema herpeticum is diffuse, superimposed upon a preexisting inflammatory dermatosis
- Herpetic whitlow; infection of fingers or hands
- Tzanck smears, fluorescent antibody tests, viral cultures, and skin biopsies diagnostic

■ Differential Diagnosis

- Impetigo
- Zoster
- Syphilis, chancroid, lymphogranuloma venereum, or granuloma inguinale
- Oral aphthosis, coxsackievirus infection (herpangina), erythema multiforme, pemphigus, or primary HIV infection

■ Treatment

- Sunblock to prevent orolabial recurrences
- Early acute intermittent therapy with oral acyclovir, famciclovir, or valacyclovir
- Prophylactic suppressive therapy for patients with frequent recurrences or immunosuppressed patients
- Short-term prophylaxis before intense sun exposure, dental procedures, and laser resurfacing for patients with recurrent orolabial disease
- IV foscarnet for resistance in severely immunosuppressed

15

■ Pearl

For uninfected sexual partners, chronic suppressive therapy has the potential to reduce the risk of transmission.

Reference

Fatahzadeh M, Schwartz RA. Human herpes simplex virus infections: epidemiology, pathogenesis, symptomatology, diagnosis, and management. J Am Acad Dermatol 2007;57:737. [PMID: 17939933]

Leg Ulcers from Venous Insufficiency

- ■ Essentials of Diagnosis
  - • Occurs in patients with signs of venous insufficiency
  - • Irregular ulcerations, often on medial aspect of lower legs; fibrinous eschar at the base
  - • Light rheography to assess venous insufficiency
  - • Measure ankle-brachial index to exclude arterial disease
  - • Biopsy atypical or persistent ulcers to rule out other causes

- ■ Differential Diagnosis
  - • Arterial insufficiency
  - • Pyoderma gangrenosum
  - • Diabetic neuropathy and microangiopathy
  - • Vasculitis or vasculopathy (hypercoagulable state)
  - • Cryofibrinogenemia
  - • Infection (mycobacteria, fungi)
  - • Hypercoagulable state
  - • Neoplasm (eg, basal cell, squamous cell, melanoma, lymphoma)

- ■ Treatment
  - • Occlusive semipermeable biosynthetic dressing (such as hydrocolloid) to create moist environment
  - • Elastic compression bandage or Unna boot essential
  - • Mechanical debridement only if eschar present
  - • Topical metronidazole reduces odor; topical steroids when inflammation is present; topical honey becoming popular but evidence in venous ulcers is unconvincing; topical becaplermin in refractory diabetics ulcers
  - • Oral pentoxifylline may be useful adjunct
  - • Uncomplicated ulcers do not benefit from oral antibiotics
  - • Cultured epidermal cell grafts or bilayered skin substitutes in highly refractory ulcers
  - • Compression stockings for life to prevent recurrence

- ■ Pearl

Superimposed allergic contact dermatitis (caused by neomycin, bacitracin, or lanolin) can impede wound healing.

Reference

O'Meara S, Cullum NA, Nelson EA. Compression for venous leg ulcers. Cochrane Database Syst Rev 2009:CD000265. [PMID: 19160178]

15

Lichen Planus

- ■ Essentials of Diagnosis
  - • Small pruritic, violaceous, polygonal, flat-topped papules; may show white streaks (Wickham's striae) on surface
  - • Common sites: Flexor wrists, dorsal hands, forearms, shins, ankles
  - • Oral mucosa affected with ulcers or reticulated white patches in half of patients
  - • Vulvovaginal and perianal lesions show leukoplakia or erosions
  - • Lesions on glans penis may be annular
  - • Scalp involvement (lichen planopilaris) causes scarring alopecia
  - • Nail changes infrequent (10%) but can include pterygium
  - • Trauma may induce additional lesions (Koebner's phenomenon)
  - • Linear, annular, actinic, atrophic, and hypertrophic variants
  - • Skin biopsy when diagnosis not clear

- ■ Differential Diagnosis
  - • Lichenoid drug eruption (due to beta-blockers, antimalarials, thiazides, furosemide, and others)
  - • Pityriasis rosea
  - • Psoriasis
  - • Secondary syphilis
  - • Mucosal lesions: Lichen sclerosus, candidiasis, erythema multiforme, leukoplakia, pemphigus vulgaris, bullous pemphigoid
  - • Discoid lupus erythematosus

- ■ Treatment
  - • Topical or intralesional steroids or topical calcineurin inhibitors for limited cutaneous or mucosal lesions
  - • Systemic corticosteroids, psoralen plus UVA, oral isotretinoin or acitretin, antimalarials for generalized disease
  - • Cyclosporine for severe cases
  - • Monitor for malignant transformation to squamous cell carcinoma in erosive mucosal disease
  - • Aggressive management to avoid debilitating scarring in vulvar lichen planus

15

- ■ Pearl

Hepatitis C infection appears to be associated with lichen planus—consider testing for it in patients with this disorder.

Reference

Shengyuan L, Songpo Y, Wen W, Wenjing T, Haitao Z, Binyou W. Hepatitis C virus and lichen planus: a reciprocal association determined by a meta-analysis. Arch Dermatol 2009;145:1040. [PMID: 19770446]

Lichen Simplex Chronicus and Prurigo Nodularis

■ Essentials of Diagnosis

- Chronic, severe, localized itching; lesions result from habitual scratching, rubbing, or picking
- Lichen simplex chronicus: Well-circumscribed, erythematous, and hyperpigmented plaques with accentuated skin markings, often on the extremities and posterior neck
- Prurigo nodularis: Multiple pea-sized firm, erythematous or brownish, dome-shaped, excoriated nodules, typically on the extremities

■ Differential Diagnosis

- Lichen simplex chronicus: Secondary phenomenon in atopic dermatitis, stasis dermatitis, insect bite reactions, contact dermatitis, or pruritus of other cause
- Lesions of psoriasis, cutaneous lymphoma, lichen planus, and tinea corporis may resemble lichen simplex chronicus
- Prurigo nodularis: Associated with HIV infection, hyperthyroidism, renal dysfunction, hepatic disease, atopic dermatitis, lymphoma, anemia, emotional stress, pregnancy, and gluten enteropathy
- Lesions of hypertrophic lichen planus, perforating disorders, keratoacanthomas, and scabietic nodules may resemble prurigo nodularis

■ Treatment

- Avoid scratching involved areas—occlusion with steroid tape, semipermeable dressings, or even Unna boots may be of value
- Intralesional steroids or topical superpotent steroids helpful in treating individual lesions
- Oral antihistamines of limited benefit
- Phototherapy, isotretinoin, topical calcipotriene, and oral cyclosporine are alternatives
- Thalidomide in recalcitrant, severe prurigo nodularis; pregnancy prevention and monitoring for side effects are critical

■ Pearl

These lesions are a response to chronic rubbing or picking; a specific cause is seldom suggested by the morphology alone.

Reference

Lee MR, Shumack S. Prurigo nodularis: a review. Australas J Dermatol 2005;46:211. [PMID: 16197418]

Malignant Melanoma

- **Essentials of Diagnosis**
  - Higher incidence in those with fair skin, blue eyes, blond or red hair, blistering sunburns, chronic sun exposure, family history, immunodeficiency, many nevi, dysplastic nevi, giant congenital nevus, and certain genetic diseases such as xeroderma pigmentosum
  - ABCD warning signs: Asymmetry, Border irregularity, Color variegation, and Diameter over 6 mm
  - Clinical characteristics vary depending on subtype and location
  - Early detection is critical; advanced-stage disease has high mortality
  - Epiluminescence microscopy can help identify high-risk lesions
  - Biopsies for diagnosis must be deep enough to permit measurement of thickness; partial biopsies should be avoided

- **Differential Diagnosis**
  - Seborrheic keratosis
  - Basal cell carcinoma, pigmented type
  - Benign or dysplastic (Clark's) nevi
  - Solar lentigo
  - Pyogenic granuloma
  - Kaposi's sarcoma
  - Dermatofibroma
  - Pregnancy-associated darkening of nevi

- **Treatment**
  - For localized disease, prognosis determined by histologic features (microstaging)
  - Appropriate staging work-up including history and physical; consider laboratory tests, radiologic studies, and sentinel lymph node biopsy to evaluate for metastatic spread (not indicated for stage 0 or IA)
  - Reexcision with appropriate margins determined by histologic characteristics of the tumor
  - Adjuvant therapy for high-risk lesions
  - Close follow-up
  - Consider genetic counseling and assessment in familial melanoma

15

- **Pearl**

When a mole is suspicious or changing, it belongs in formalin.

Reference

Balch CM, Gershenwald JE, Soong SJ, et al. Final version of 2009 AJCC Melanoma Staging and Classification. J Clin Oncol 2009;27:6199. [PMID: 19917835]

Melasma (Chloasma Faciei)

- ■ Essentials of Diagnosis
    - • Most frequently seen in women who are pregnant, taking oral contraceptives, or on hormone replacement therapy
    - • Well-demarcated symmetric brown patches with irregular borders
    - • Typically on cheeks and forehead, but may also involve nipples, genitals, or forearms
    - • Exacerbated by sun exposure
    - • More common in Asian and Hispanic patients

- ■ Differential Diagnosis
    - • Postinflammatory hyperpigmentation
    - • Contact photodermatitis from perfumes
    - • Exogenous ochronosis (from hydroquinones, phenol, or resorcinol)
    - • Drug-induced hyperpigmentation (minocycline, gold, Dilantin, etc.)

- ■ Treatment
    - • Sun protection, including broad-spectrum sunscreen with UVA coverage
    - • Bleaching creams with 4% hydroquinone moderately effective, sometimes combined with topical retinoids and mild topical steroid (contraindicated during pregnancy or lactation)

- ■ Pearl

Pregnancy-induced melasma clears within months; untreated medication-induced disease may persist for years, even after medication has been discontinued.

Reference

Balch CM Gupta AK, Gover MD, Nouri K, Taylor S. The treatment of melasma: a review of clinical trials. J Am Acad Dermatol 2006;55:1048. [PMID: 17097400]

15

Molluscum Contagiosum

- ■ Essentials of Diagnosis
  - • Smooth, firm, dome-shaped, pearly papules; characteristic central umbilication and white core
  - • Sexually transmitted in immunocompetent adults; usually with fewer than 20 lesions; on lower abdomen, upper thighs, and penile shaft
  - • Frequently generalized in young children
  - • Immunosuppressed patients, especially those with AIDS and a CD4 count of less than 100/µL, are at highest risk; large disfiguring lesions on face and genitalia
  - • Patients with malignancies, sarcoidosis, extensive atopic dermatitis, or history of diffuse topical steroid use are also predisposed

- ■ Differential Diagnosis
  - • Warts
  - • Varicella
  - • Bacterial infection
  - • Basal cell carcinoma
  - • Lichen planus

- ■ Treatment
  - • Avoid aggressive treatment in young children; possible therapies for children include topical tretinoin or cantharidin, or continuous application of occlusive tape
  - • Cryotherapy or curettage for adults with genital disease
  - • Antiretroviral therapies resulting in increasing CD4 counts are most effective for HIV-infected patients, though response may be delayed 6 months or more

- ■ Pearl

Disseminated cryptococcal infection may mimic molluscum lesions in patients with HIV/AIDS.

Reference

Hanna D, Hatami A, Powell J, et al. A prospective randomized trial comparing the efficacy and adverse effects of four recognized treatments of molluscum contagiosum in children. Pediatr Dermatol 2006;23:574. [PMID: 17156002]

15

Morbilliform (Exanthematous) Drug Eruption

- ■ Essentials of Diagnosis
  - • Begins with erythematous small macules or faint papules that later become confluent
  - • Eruption symmetric, beginning on trunk and then generalizing
  - • Often occurs within first 2 weeks of drug treatment; may appear later
  - • Pruritus usually prominent
  - • Ampicillin, amoxicillin, allopurinol, sulfonamides, cephalosporins most common causes
  - • Amoxicillin eruptions more frequent in patients with infectious mononucleosis; sulfonamide rashes common in HIV-infected patients

- ■ Differential Diagnosis
  - • Viral exanthems often indistinguishable
  - • Early stages of erythema multiforme major or drug hypersensitivity syndrome
  - • Scarlet fever
  - • Toxic shock syndrome
  - • Kawasaki's disease
  - • Acute graft-versus-host disease

- ■ Treatment
  - • Discontinue offending agent unless this represents a greater risk to the patient than the eruption
  - • Topical corticosteroids and oral antihistamines
  - • Avoid rechallenge in complex exanthems and with certain antiretroviral medications

15

- ■ Pearl

Fever, lymphadenopathy, and eosinophilia should prompt evaluation for hepatitis and pneumonitis, signs of the DRESS syndrome; mucosal involvement or painful dusky skin may be signs of Stevens-Johnson syndrome.

Reference

Cotliar J. Approach to the patient with a suspected drug eruption. Semin Cutan Med Surg 2007;26:147. [PMID: 18070681]

Nevi (Congenital Nevi, Acquired Nevi)

- **Essentials of Diagnosis**
  - Common acquired nevi have homogeneous surfaces and color patterns, smooth and sharp borders, and are round or oval in shape
  - Color may vary from flesh-colored to brown
  - Flat or raised depending on the subtype or stage of evolution
  - Excisional biopsy to rule out melanoma in changing nevi or those with suspicious features (see Malignant Melanoma)
  - Congenital nevi darkly pigmented, sometimes hairy papules or plaques that may be present at birth
  - Large congenital nevi (those whose longest diameter will be greater than 20 cm in adulthood) are at increased risk for melanoma; when found on head, neck, or posterior midline, associated with underlying leptomeningeal melanocytosis

- **Differential Diagnosis**
  - Dysplastic (Clark's) nevus
  - Melanoma
  - Lentigo simplex
  - Solar lentigo
  - Dermatofibroma
  - Basal cell carcinoma
  - Molluscum contagiosum
  - Blue nevus
  - Café au lait spot
  - Epidermal nevus
  - Becker's nevus

- **Treatment**
  - Excision of bothersome nevi and those at high risk of developing melanoma
  - Biopsy suspicious lesions
  - Head or spinal scans in children with large congenital nevi occurring on the head, neck, or posterior midline

15

- **Pearl**

Partial biopsies of suspicious lesions may make histologic diagnosis difficult; avoid them in favor of excisional biopsies.

Reference

Marghoob AA, Borrego JP, Halpern AC. Congenital melanocytic nevi: treatment modalities and management options. Semin Cutan Med Surg 2007;26:231. [PMID: 18395671]

Nummular Eczema

- **Essentials of Diagnosis**
  - Middle-aged and older men most frequently affected
  - Discrete coin-shaped, crusted, erythematous, 1- to 5-cm plaques that may contain vesicles
  - Usually begins on lower legs, dorsal hands, or extensor surfaces of arms, but may spread to involve all extremities and the trunk over several months
  - Pruritus often severe

- **Differential Diagnosis**
  - Tinea corporis
  - Psoriasis
  - Xerotic dermatitis
  - Impetigo
  - Contact dermatitis

- **Treatment**
  - Avoidance of agents capable of drying or irritating skin (hot or frequent baths, extensive soaping, etc.)
  - Frequent emollients
  - Topical corticosteroids (potency appropriate to location and severity) applied twice daily and tapered as tolerated; ointment formulations preferred
  - Topical tacrolimus and pimecrolimus are effective but expensive alternatives to steroids
  - Topical tar preparations
  - Phototherapy may be helpful in severe cases
  - Sedative antihistamines to relieve pruritus, given at bedtime
  - Antibiotics when signs of impetiginization are present (fissures, crusts, erosions, or pustules)
  - Systemic steroids only in highly selected, refractory cases

- **Pearl**

If it scales, scrape it; KOH (Potassum Hydroxide) preparation should always be examined to rule out tinea corporis.

Reference

Gutman AB, Kligman AM, Sciacca J, James WD. Nummular eczema: soak and smear: a standard technique revisited. Arch Dermatol 2005;141:1556. [PMID: 16365257]

Onychomycosis (Tinea Unguium)

- **Essentials of Diagnosis**
  - Yellowish discoloration, piling up of subungual keratin, friability, and separation of the nail plate
  - May show only overlying white scale if superficial
  - Nail shavings for immediate microscopic examination, culture, or histologic examination with periodic acid-Schiff stain to establish diagnosis; repeated sampling may be required

- **Differential Diagnosis**
  - Candidal onychomycosis or paronychia
  - Psoriasis
  - Lichen planus
  - Allergic contact dermatitis from nail polish
  - Contact urticaria from foods or other sensitizers
  - Nail changes associated with reactive arthritis (Reiter's), Darier's disease, crusted scabies

- **Treatment**
  - Confirm diagnosis before initiating therapy
  - Antifungal creams not effective; topical ciclopirox lacquer approved but has low efficacy
  - Oral terbinafine and itraconazole are effective, though re-infection is common
  - Weekly prophylactic topical antifungals to suppress tinea pedis may limit recurrences after oral treatment
  - Adequate informed consent critical; patients must decide if benefits of oral therapy outweigh risks (including liver failure)

- **Pearl**

Given the risks of systemic therapy and the number of diseases that mimic this disorder, accurate diagnosis is essential pretreatment.

15

Reference

Finch JJ, Warshaw EM. Toenail onychomycosis: current and future treatment options. Dermatol Ther 2007;20:31. [PMID: 17403258]

Pediculosis (Lice)

- **Essentials of Diagnosis**
  - Three types of lice (*Pediculus humanus*), each with a predilection for certain body parts
  - Dermatitis caused by inflammatory response to louse saliva
  - Pediculosis capitis (head lice): Intense scalp pruritus, presence of nits, possible secondary impetigo and cervical lymphadenopathy; most common in children, rare in blacks
  - Pediculosis corporis (body lice): Rarely found on skin, causes generalized pruritus, erythematous macules or urticarial wheals, excoriations, and lichenification; homeless persons and those living in crowded conditions most frequently affected
  - Pediculosis pubis (crabs): Usually sexually transmitted; generally limited to pubic area, axillae, and eyelashes; lice may be observed on skin and nits on hairs; maculae ceruleae (blue macules) may be seen
  - Body lice can transmit trench fever, relapsing fever, and epidemic typhus

- **Differential Diagnosis**
  - Head lice: Impetigo, hair casts, seborrheic dermatitis
  - Body lice: Scabies, urticaria, impetigo, dermatitis herpetiformis
  - Pubic lice: Scabies, anogenital pruritus, eczema

- **Treatment**
  - Head lice: Topical permethrins with interval removal of nits and retreatment in 1 week; malathion lotion also effective
  - Pyrethrins available over the counter; resistance common
  - Treat household contacts
  - Body lice: Launder all clothing and bedding (at least 30 minutes at 150°F in dryer, or iron pressing of wool garments); patient should then bathe; no pesticides required
  - Pubic lice: Treatment is same as for head lice; eyelash lesions treated with thick coating of petrolatum maintained for 1 week; recurrence is more common in HIV-infected patients

- **Pearl**

  Severe body lice infestation may cause iron deficiency; search for them if other sources of blood loss have been excluded.

Reference

Ko CJ, Elston DM. Pediculosis. J Am Acad Dermatol 2004;50:1. [PMID: 14699358]

Pemphigus Vulgaris

- ■ Essentials of Diagnosis
  - Typically presents in fifth or sixth decade
  - Caused by autoantibodies to desmogleins; occasionally drug-induced (penicillamine, captopril)
  - Thin-walled, fragile blisters; rupture to form painful erosions that crust and heal slowly without scarring
  - Often initially presents with oral involvement
  - Scalp, face, neck, axillae, and groin common sites; esophagus, trachea, conjunctiva, and other mucosal surfaces may also be involved
  - Lateral pressure applied to perilesional skin induces more blistering (Nikolsky's sign)
  - Diagnosis by lesional biopsy of intact blisters, perilesional direct immunofluorescence, indirect immunofluorescence

- ■ Differential Diagnosis
  - Paraneoplastic pemphigus (lymphomas/leukemias)
  - Pemphigus foliaceus
  - Fogo selvagem (endemic Brazilian pemphigus)
  - Bullous pemphigoid
  - Erythema multiforme, Stevens-Johnson syndrome, toxic epidermal necrolysis
  - Linear IgA dermatosis
  - Epidermolysis bullosa acquisita
  - Patients presenting with only oral lesions may be misdiagnosed with aphthous stomatitis, erythema multiforme, herpes simplex, lichen planus, or cicatricial pemphigoid

- ■ Treatment
  - Viscous lidocaine and antibiotic rinses for oral erosions
  - Early and aggressive systemic therapy required; mortality high in untreated patients
  - High doses of oral prednisone combined with another immunosuppressive (azathioprine or mycophenolate mofetil)
  - Monitor for side effects and infections
  - Plasmapheresis, intravenous immune globulin, rituximab, and tumor necrosis factor alpha inhibitors are alternatives

15

- ■ Pearl

Don't forget the oral presentation; it can sometimes resemble a less serious condition.

Reference

Prajapati V, Mydlarski PR. Advances in pemphigus therapy. Skin Therapy Lett 2008;13:4. [PMID: 18506357]

Photosensitive Drug Eruption

- ■ Essentials of Diagnosis
  - Morphology variable; photodistribution critical to diagnosis
  - Phototoxic reactions resemble sunburn; related to dose of both medication and UV radiation; doxycycline, amiodarone, fluoro-quinolones, and NSAIDs common causes
  - Photoallergic reactions typically red, scaly, pruritic; immune-related; often slow to develop and slow to improve; thiazides, sulfonamide antibiotics, sulfonylureas, and phenothiazines common causes
  - Pseudoporphyria with blistering caused by naproxen, tetracyclines, furosemide, dapsone, contraceptives, and other medications
  - Photodistributed lichenoid reactions most frequently due to thiazides, quinidine, NSAIDs, and captopril

- ■ Differential Diagnosis
  - Porphyria cutanea tarda or other porphyrias
  - Lupus erythematosus or dermatomyositis
  - Photoallergic or phototoxic contact dermatitis from fragrances, sunscreens, or furocoumarins in many plants
  - HIV-associated photosensitivity
  - Polymorphous light eruption or other idiopathic photosensitivity disorders
  - Pellagra
  - Xeroderma pigmentosum or other genetic photosensitivity disorders

- ■ Treatment
  - Avoidance of the causative agent
  - Sun avoidance, protection with broad-spectrum sunscreens containing physical blockers
  - Soothing local measures or topical corticosteroids

- ■ Pearl

UVA radiation is the most common trigger; make sure to recommend sunscreens with good UVA coverage.

Reference

Stein KR, Scheinfeld NS. Drug-induced photoallergic and phototoxic reactions. Expert Opin Drug Saf 2007;6:431. [PMID: 17688387]

Pityriasis Rosea

■ Essentials of Diagnosis

- Oval, salmon-colored, symmetric papules with long axis following cleavage lines
- Lesions show "collarette of scale" at periphery
- Trunk most frequently involved; sun-exposed areas often spared
- A "herald" patch precedes eruption by 1–2 weeks; some patients report prodrome of constitutional symptoms
- Typically lasts 6–10 weeks
- Pruritus common but usually mild
- Most common between ages of 10 and 35 years
- Variations in mode of onset, morphology, distribution, and course are common. Atypical forms include inverse distribution, mucosal, urticarial, vesicular, pustular, and purpuric variants
- Attempts to isolate infective agent have been disappointing

■ Differential Diagnosis

- Secondary syphilis
- Tinea corporis
- Seborrheic dermatitis
- Tinea versicolor
- Viral exanthem
- Drug eruption
- Psoriasis (guttate form)

■ Treatment

- Usually none required; most cases resolve spontaneously
- Topical steroids or oral antihistamines for pruritus
- UVB phototherapy may expedite involution of lesions
- Short course of systemic corticosteroids in selected severe cases
- One study showed oral erythromycin sped clearance, but this was not replicated in a subsequent trial

15

■ Pearl

Order a rapid plasma reagin in patients who are sexually active.

Reference

Drago F, Broccolo F, Rebora A. Pityriasis rosea: an update with a critical appraisal of its possible herpes viral etiology. J Am Acad Dermatol 2009;61:303. [PMID: 19615540]

Psoriasis

- **Essentials of Diagnosis**
  - Silvery scales on bright red, well-demarcated plaques most commonly on knees, elbows, and scalp
  - Pitted nails or onychodystrophy
  - Pinking of intergluteal folds
  - Lesions may be induced at sites of injury (Koebner's phenomenon)
  - Pruritus mild or absent
  - Associated with psoriatic arthritis in up to 25%
  - Increased risk of cardiovascular disease in severe psoriasis
  - Many variants (plaque, inverse, guttate, palmoplantar, pustular, erythrodermic, and others)

- **Differential Diagnosis**
  - Cutaneous candidiasis
  - Tinea corporis
  - Nummular eczema
  - Seborrheic dermatitis
  - Pityriasis rosea
  - Secondary syphilis
  - Pityriasis rubra pilaris
  - Squamous cell carcinoma in-situ (Bowen's disease)
  - Nail findings may mimic onychomycosis
  - Cutaneous features of reactive arthritis (Reiter's syndrome)
  - Plaque stage of cutaneous T-cell lymphoma

- **Treatment**
  - Topical steroids, calcipotriene, tar preparations, anthralin, calcineurin inhibitors, or tazarotene
  - Tar shampoos, topical steroids, calcipotriene, keratolytic agents, or intralesional steroids for scalp lesions
  - Phototherapy (UVB, psoralen plus UVA, Excimer laser, or the Goeckerman regimen) for widespread disease
  - In selected severe cases, systemic methotrexate, cyclosporine, acitretin, etanercept, infliximab, adalimumab, alefacept, golimumab, and ustekinumab

15

- **Pearl**

Be careful of systemic steroids in psoriasis; rebound or induction of pustular psoriasis may occur.

Reference

Nestle FO, Kaplan DH, Barker J. Psoriasis. N Engl J Med 2009;361:496. [PMID: 19641206]

Pyoderma Gangrenosum

- ■ Essentials of Diagnosis
  - Lesions begin as inflammatory pustules, sometimes at a trauma site
  - Erythematous halo enlarges, then necroses and ulcerates
  - Ulcers painful with ragged, undermined, violaceous borders; bases appear purulent
  - Ulcers heal slowly, forming atrophic scars
  - Often chronic and recurrent; may be accompanied by a polyarticular arthritis
  - Associated with inflammatory bowel disease, lymphoproliferative disorders, and arthritis; also seen with hepatitis B or C, HIV infection, lupus, pregnancy, PAPA syndrome, and others
  - Up to half of cases idiopathic
  - Diagnosis of exclusion; biopsies with special stains and cultures to rule out infections (bacterial, mycobacterial, fungal, tertiary syphilis, amebiasis)

- ■ Differential Diagnosis
  - Folliculitis, spider bites, or Sweet's syndrome (acute febrile neutrophilic dermatosis)
  - Ulcers secondary to underlying infection
  - Ulcers secondary to underlying neoplasm
  - Factitious ulcerations from injected substances
  - Vasculitis (especially Wegener's granulomatosis)
  - Coumadin necrosis

- ■ Treatment
  - Treat inflammatory bowel disease when present
  - Local compresses, occlusive dressings, potent topical steroids, intralesional steroids, or topical tacrolimus
  - High-dose systemic steroids in widespread disease; if control is not established or if a steroid taper is unsuccessful, a steroid-sparing agent (cyclosporine, mycophenolate mofetil, infliximab, etc.) is added
  - Dapsone, sulfasalazine, and clofazimine also steroid-sparing

15

- ■ Pearl

Its reappearance in inflammatory bowel disease may indicate an imminent enteric relapse.

Reference

Ruocco E, Sangiuliano S, Gravina AG, Miranda A, Nicoletti G. Pyoderma gangrenosum: an updated review. J Eur Acad Dermatol Venereol 2009;23:1008. [PMID: 19470075]

Rosacea

- ■ Essentials of Diagnosis
  - A chronic disorder of the mid-face in middle-aged and older people
  - History of flushing evoked by hot beverages, alcohol, spicy foods, or heat exposure; sometimes accompanied by burning or stinging
  - Erythema, sometimes persisting for hours or days after flushing episodes
  - Telangiectases become more prominent over time
  - Some patients have acneiform papules and pustules
  - Some advanced cases show large inflammatory nodules and nasal sebaceous hypertrophy (rhinophyma)

- ■ Differential Diagnosis
  - Acne vulgaris
  - Seborrheic dermatitis
  - Lupus erythematosus or dermatomyositis
  - Carcinoid syndrome, mastocytosis, or polycythemia vera
  - Topical steroid-induced rosacea
  - *Demodex* (mite) folliculitis in HIV-infected patients
  - Perioral dermatitis

- ■ Treatment
  - Treatment is suppressive and chronic
  - Topical metronidazole or sodium sulfacetamide and oral tetracyclines effective against papulopustular disease
  - Daily sunscreen use and avoidance of flushing triggers may slow progression
  - Oral isotretinoin can produce dramatic improvement in resistant cases, but relapse common
  - Laser therapy may obliterate telangiectases or erythema
  - Surgery in severe rhinophyma

- ■ Pearl

Watch for ocular symptoms—blepharitis, conjunctivitis, or even keratitis can occur in many rosacea patients.

Reference

van Zuuren EJ, Gupta AK, Gover MD, Graber M, Hollis S. Systematic review of rosacea treatments. J Am Acad Dermatol 2007;56:107. [PMID: 17190628]

Scabies

- ■ Essentials of Diagnosis
  - • Caused by *Sarcoptes scabiei* mite
  - • Pruritogenic papular eruption favoring finger webs, wrists, antecubital fossae, axillae, lower abdomen, genitals, buttocks, and nipples
  - • Itching usually worse at night
  - • Face and scalp are spared (except in children and the immunosuppressed)
  - • Burrows appear as short, slightly raised, wavy lines in skin, sometimes with vesicles
  - • Secondary eczematization, impetigo, and lichenification in longstanding infestation
  - • Red nodules on penis or scrotum
  - • A crusted form in institutionalized, HIV-infected, or malnourished individuals has high mite burden
  - • Burrow scrapings permit microscopic confirmation of mites, ova, or feces; many cases diagnosed on clinical grounds

- ■ Differential Diagnosis
  - • Atopic dermatitis
  - • Papular urticaria
  - • Insect bites
  - • Dermatitis herpetiformis

- ■ Treatment
  - • Permethrin 5% cream applied from the neck down for 8 hours; clothing and bed linens laundered thoroughly; repeat therapy in 1 week
  - • Lindane used infrequently because of potential CNS toxicity
  - • Oral ivermectin in refractory cases, institutional epidemics, or immunosuppressed patients
  - • Treat all household and sexual contacts (some may be asymptomatic carriers)
  - • Persistent postscabietic pruritic papules commonly last 1 month; may require topical corticosteroids

- ■ Pearl

Persistent pruritus for weeks after treatment is common; it does not invariably mean treatment failure.

Reference

Hicks MI, Elston DM. Scabies. Dermatol Ther 2009;22:279. [PMID: 19580575]

15

Seborrheic Dermatitis and Dandruff

- ■ Essentials of Diagnosis
  - Loose, dry, moist, or greasy scales with or without underlying crusted, pink or yellow-brown plaques
  - Predilection for scalp, eyebrows, eyelids, nasolabial creases, ears, and presternal area; may also occur in axillae, umbilicus, groin, and gluteal crease
  - May be accompanied by pruritus, especially on scalp
  - Typically chronic relapsing course
  - Infantile form on scalp known as cradle cap

- ■ Differential Diagnosis
  - Psoriasis
  - Impetigo
  - Atopic dermatitis
  - Contact dermatitis
  - Rosacea
  - Lupus erythematosus
  - Tinea versicolor
  - Pediculosis capitis (head lice)

- ■ Treatment
  - Selenium sulfide, tar, zinc, or ketoconazole shampoos
  - Topical corticosteroids or calcineurin inhibitors
  - Topical ketoconazole cream
  - Systemic corticosteroids and antibiotics in selected generalized or severe cases
  - Patient should be aware that chronic therapy is required; may taper frequency of topicals down to minimum frequency required to suppress symptoms

15

- ■ Pearl

Unusually severe seborrheic dermatitis may be a marker of Parkinson's disease or advanced HIV infection.

Reference

Naldi L, Rebora A. Clinical practice. Seborrheic dermatitis. N Engl J Med 2009;360:387. [PMID: 19164189]

Seborrheic Keratosis

- **Essentials of Diagnosis**
  - Oval, raised, brown to black, warty, "stuck on"-appearing, well-demarcated papules or plaques; greasy hyperkeratotic scale may be present
  - Usually multiple; some patients have hundreds
  - Chest and back most frequent sites; scalp, face, neck, and extremities also involved
  - Age at onset generally fourth to fifth decades
  - Familial predisposition with probable autosomal-dominant inheritance
  - Rapid eruptive appearance of numerous lesions (Leser-Trélat sign) may signify internal malignancy

- **Differential Diagnosis**
  - Melanoma
  - Actinic keratosis
  - Nevus
  - Verruca vulgaris
  - Solar lentigo
  - Basal cell carcinoma, pigmented type
  - Squamous cell carcinoma
  - Dermatosis papulosa nigra in dark-skinned patients; numerous small papules on face, neck, and upper chest
  - Stucco keratosis shows hyperkeratotic, gray, verrucous, exophytic papules on the extremities, can be easily scraped off

- **Treatment**
  - Seborrheic keratoses do not require therapy
  - Cryotherapy or curettage effective for removal, may leave dyspigmentation
  - Electrodesiccation and laser therapy

- **Pearl**

A public health menace this is not, but look closely at all such lesions to exclude cutaneous malignancies.

Reference

Noiles K, Vender R. Are all seborrheic keratoses benign? Review of the typical lesion and its variants. J Cutan Med Surg 2008;12:203. [PMID: 18845088]

15

Squamous Cell Carcinoma

- ■ Essentials of Diagnosis
  - Cumulative UV exposure is the major risk factor
  - Certain HPV infections, radiation, long-standing scars or wounds, HIV infection, and chronic immunosuppression also predispose (transplant patients have 250× risk)
  - Patients with albinism, xeroderma pigmentosum, and epidermodysplasia verruciformis at increased risk
  - Hyperkeratotic, firm, indurated, red or skin-colored papule, plaque, or nodule, most commonly in sun-damaged skin
  - May ulcerate and form crust
  - Lesions confined to the epidermis are squamous cell carcinoma in-situ or Bowen's disease; all others are considered invasive
  - Metastasis infrequent but devastating; lesions on lip or in scars and those with subcutaneous or perineural involvement are at higher risk
  - Regional lymphatics primary route of spread
  - Skin biopsies usually diagnostic

- ■ Differential Diagnosis
  - Keratoacanthoma (a rapidly growing and sometimes self-involuting variant of squamous cell carcinoma)
  - Actinic keratosis, hypertrophic form
  - Basal cell carcinoma
  - Verruca vulgaris
  - Chronic nonhealing ulcers due to other causes (venous stasis, infection, etc.)

- ■ Treatment
  - Excisional surgery with histologic examination of margins
  - Mohs microsurgery with immediate mapping of margins for high-risk lesions or in areas where tissue conservation is important
  - Curettage and electrodesiccation in small in-situ lesions
  - Radiation therapy as alternative treatment
  - Evaluate patients with aggressive lesions or perineural involvement on histologic examination for metastatic disease
  - Prophylactic radiotherapy in high-risk lesions
  - Regular screening examinations and sun protection

- ■ Pearl

This lesion is the main reason to treat all actinic keratoses; two-thirds of patients with this carcinoma have it arise at sites of previous AKs.

Reference

Garcia-Zuazaga J, Olbricht SM. Cutaneous squamous cell carcinoma. Adv Dermatol 2008;24:33. [PMID: 19256304]

Tinea Corporis (Ringworm, Dermatophytosis)

- ■ Essentials of Diagnosis
  - Single or multiple circular, sharply circumscribed, erythematous, scaly plaques with elevated borders and central clearing
  - Frequently involves neck, extremities, or trunk
  - A deep, papulopustular form affecting follicles (Majocchi's granuloma) may occur
  - Other types affect face (tinea faciei), hands (tinea manuum), feet (tinea pedis), groin (tinea cruris), and scalp (tinea capitis)
  - Skin scrapings for microscopic examination or culture establish diagnosis
  - May be acquired from contact with humans, soil, cats, dogs, rodents, or contaminated clothing
  - Widespread tinea may be presenting sign of HIV infection

- ■ Differential Diagnosis
  - Pityriasis rosea
  - Impetigo
  - Nummular dermatitis
  - Seborrheic dermatitis
  - Psoriasis
  - Granuloma annulare
  - Secondary syphilis
  - Subacute cutaneous lupus erythematosus

- ■ Treatment
  - One or two uncomplicated lesions usually respond to topical antifungals (allylamines or azoles)
  - A low-potency steroid cream during initial days of therapy may decrease inflammation
  - Oral griseofulvin, itraconazole, or terbinafine is effective in extensive disease, follicular involvement, or the immunocompromised host
  - Infected household pets (especially cats and dogs) may transmit and should be treated

15

- ■ Pearl

Be wary of combination products containing antifungals and potent steroids; skin atrophy and reduced efficacy may result.

Reference

Gupta AK, Chaudhry M, Elewski B. Tinea corporis, tinea cruris, tinea nigra, and piedra. Dermatol Clin 2003;21:395, v. [PMID: 12956194]

Tinea Versicolor (Pityriasis Versicolor)

- ■ Essentials of Diagnosis
  - Finely scaling patches on upper trunk and upper arms, usually asymptomatic
  - Lesions yellowish or brownish on pale skin, or hypopigmented on dark skin
  - Caused by yeast of the genus *Malassezia*
  - Short, thick hyphae and large numbers of spores on microscopic KOH examination
  - Wood's light helpful in defining extent of lesions

- ■ Differential Diagnosis
  - Seborrheic dermatitis
  - Pityriasis rosea
  - Pityriasis alba
  - Hansen's disease (leprosy)
  - Secondary syphilis (macular syphilid)
  - Vitiligo
  - Postinflammatory pigmentary alteration from another inflammatory dermatosis

- ■ Treatment
  - Topical agents in limited disease (selenium sulfide shampoos or lotions, zinc pyrithione shampoos, imidazole shampoos, topical allylamines)
  - Oral agents in more diffuse involvement (single-dose ketoconazole repeated once after 1 week, or 5–7 days of itraconazole)
  - Oral terbinafine not effective
  - Dyspigmentation may persist for months after effective treatment
  - Relapse likely if prophylactic measures not taken; a single monthly application of topical agent may be effective

- ■ Pearl

Oral ketoconazole works best if the patient exercises 1 hour after taking the medicine and avoids showering for a few hours; sweating helps!

Reference

Gupta AK, Batra R, Bluhm R, Boekhout T, Dawson TL Jr. Skin diseases associated with Malassezia species. J Am Acad Dermatol 2004;51:785. [PMID: 15523360]

15

Urticaria (Hives) and Angioedema

- ■ Essentials of Diagnosis
  - Pale or red, evanescent, edematous papules or plaques surrounded by red halo with severe itching or stinging; wheals appear suddenly and resolve in hours
  - Acute (complete remission within 6 weeks) or chronic
  - Subcutaneous swelling (angioedema) occurs alone or with urticaria; eyelids and lips often affected; respiratory involvement may produce airway obstruction, and gastrointestinal involvement may cause abdominal pain; anaphylaxis possible
  - Can be induced by drugs (penicillins, aspirin, NSAIDs, opioids, radiocontrast dyes, ACEAC inhibitors)
  - Foods may cause acute (but rarely chronic) urticaria
  - Infections also a cause (streptococcal upper respiratory infections, viral hepatitis, helminthic infections, or infections of the tonsils, a tooth, sinuses, gallbladder, prostate)
  - Also associated with other autoimmune diseases, especially thyroid

- ■ Differential Diagnosis
  - Hereditary or acquired complement-mediated angioedema
  - Physical urticarias (pressure, cold, heat, solar, vibratory, cholinergic, aquagenic)
  - Urticarial hypersensitivity reactions to insect bites
  - Urticarial vasculitis
  - Bullous pemphigoid (urticarial phase)
  - Cutaneous mastocytosis
  - Erythema multiforme
  - Cryopyrin-associated periodic syndromes

- ■ Treatment
  - Treat acute urticaria with antihistamines and avoid identified triggers; short course of prednisone in selected cases
  - Chronic urticaria treated with high-dose antihistamines (sedating at night, nonsedating during waking hours) on a regular rather than as-needed basis; chronic prednisone discouraged
  - Symptom-directed work-up to rule out triggers

15

- ■ Pearl

Angiotensin-converting enzyme inhibitor–induced angioedema may occur at any time—even years—after beginning the medicine.

Reference

Kaplan AP, Greaves MW. Angioedema. J Am Acad Dermatol. 2005;53:373.
[PMID: 16112343]

Vitiligo

■ Essentials of Diagnosis

- Depigmented white patches surrounded by a normal, hyperpigmented, or occasionally inflamed border
- Hairs in affected area usually turn white
- Localized form may be focal, segmental, or mucosal
- Generalized form most common; vulgaris subtype has widely scattered patches; acrofacial subtype affects distal fingers and facial orifices
- Universal form depigments entire body surface
- Ocular abnormalities (iritis, uveitis, and retinal pigmentary abnormalities) may occur
- Associated with autoimmune thyroiditis; possibly other autoimmune diseases

■ Differential Diagnosis

- Leukoderma associated with metastatic melanoma
- Occupational vitiligo from phenols or other chemicals
- Lichen sclerosus
- Tinea versicolor
- Pityriasis alba
- Postinflammatory hypopigmentation
- Hansen's disease (leprosy)
- Cutaneous T-cell lymphoma
- Piebaldism
- Tuberous sclerosis

■ Treatment

- Spontaneous repigmentation infrequently occurs
- Cosmetic camouflage for treatment-resistant cases
- Sunscreens to prevent burns of involved skin
- Potent topical steroids in focal lesions may help repigment; topical tacrolimus and pimecrolimus sometimes effective on the face or genitals
- Psoralen plus UVA or narrow-band UVB phototherapy
- Total permanent depigmentation with monobenzone an option in extensive disease in highly selected patients

■ Pearl

An under-appreciated part of the endocrine immunopathies; consider thyroid or other autoimmune diseases in symptomatic patients.

Reference

Whitton ME, Ashcroft DM, González U. Therapeutic interventions for vitiligo. J Am Acad Dermatol 2008;59:713. [PMID: 18793940]

Zoster (Herpes Zoster, Shingles)

- **Essentials of Diagnosis**
  - Occurs unilaterally within the distribution of a sensory nerve with some spillover into neighboring dermatomes
  - Prodrome of pain and paresthesias followed by papules and plaques of erythema that quickly develop vesicles
  - Vesicles become pustular, crust over, and heal
  - May disseminate (≥ 20 lesions outside the primary dermatome) in the elderly, debilitated, or immunosuppressed; visceral involvement (lungs, liver, or brain) may follow
  - Involvement of the nasal tip (Hutchinson's sign) a harbinger of ophthalmic zoster
  - Ramsay-Hunt syndrome (ipsilateral facial paralysis, zoster of the ear, and auditory symptoms) from facial and auditory nerve involvement
  - Postherpetic neuralgia more common in older patients
  - Direct fluorescent antibody test rapid and specific

- **Differential Diagnosis**
  - Herpes simplex infection
  - Prodromal pain can mimic the pain of angina, duodenal ulcer, appendicitis, and biliary or renal colic
  - Zoster 30 times more common in the HIV-infected; ascertain HIV risk factors

- **Treatment**
  - Oral acyclovir, famciclovir, or valacyclovir
  - Intravenous acyclovir for disseminated or ocular zoster
  - Bed rest to reduce risk of neuralgia in the elderly
  - Prednisone does not prevent neuralgia
  - Topical capsaicin, local anesthetics, nerve blocks, analgesics, tricyclic antidepressants, or gabapentin for postherpetic neuralgia
  - Patients with active lesions should avoid contact with neonates and immunosuppressed individuals

- **Pearl**

  "Shingles"—the word—is a linguistic corruption from Latin cingulum ("girdle"), reflecting the common thoracic presentation of this disorder.

15

Reference

Tyring SK. Management of herpes zoster and postherpetic neuralgia. J Am Acad Dermatol 2007;57(suppl):S136. [PMID: 18021865]

16

Gynecologic, Obstetric, and Breast Disorders

Abnormal Uterine Bleeding

- **Essentials of Diagnosis**
  - Excessive menses, intermenstrual bleeding, or both; post-menopausal bleeding
  - Common soon after menarche, 4–6 years premenopause
  - Papanicolaou smear (all ages) and endometrial biopsy (all post-menopausal women and those over age 35 with chronic anovulation or more than 6 months of bleeding)

- **Differential Diagnosis**
  - Pregnancy (especially ectopic), spontaneous abortion
  - Anovulation (eg, polycystic ovaries, hypothyroidism, perimenopause)
  - Uterine myoma or carcinoma, adenomyosis, polyp
  - Cervicitis, carcinoma of the cervix, trauma
  - Exogenous hormones (eg, unopposed estrogen, progestin only contraceptives), or Copper T IUD
  - Coagulation disorders (eg, von Willebrand's disease)

- **Treatment**
  - Papanicolaou smear (all ages) and endometrial biopsy (all post-menopausal women and those over age 35 with chronic anovulation or more than 6 months of bleeding)
  - Active bleeding with significant anemia: High-dose estrogen (25 mg intravenously or oral contraceptive taper: two pills twice daily for 3 days tapering over 2 weeks to one daily); high-dose progestin when high-dose estrogen contraindicated
  - Chronic bleeding: NSAIDs (any type, around the clock for 5 days) plus oral contraceptives, levonorgestrel intrauterine system, or cyclic progestin
  - Hysterectomy, uterine artery embolization, or endometrial ablation for bleeding refractory to hormonal therapy
  - Hysterectomy if endometrial cancer, hyperplasia with atypia

- **Pearl**

If a reproductive-aged woman has abnormal bleeding, a pregnancy test is the obligatory first test.

Reference

Ely JW, Kennedy CM, Clark EC, Bowdler NC. Abnormal uterine bleeding: a management algorithm. J Am Board Fam Med 2006;19:590. [PMID: 17090792]

Amenorrhea

■ Essentials of Diagnosis

- Absence of menses for more than three cycles in women with past menses (secondary); absence of menarche by age 16 years (primary)
- May be anatomic, ovarian, or hypothalamic-pituitary-ovarian
- Anatomic causes: Congenital anomalies of the uterus, imperforate hymen, cervical stenosis, Asherman's syndrome.
- Ovarian failure: Autoimmune diseases, Turner's syndrome, ovarian dysgenesis, premature ovarian failure, radiation, chemotherapy
- Hypothalamic-pituitary-ovarian: hyperandrogenic disorders, anorexia, hyperprolactinemia, hypothyroidism, hypothalamic or pituitary lesions
- Exclude pregnancy; measure thyroid-stimulating hormone, prolactin
- Withdrawal bleed: Give 10 mg of medroxy-progesterone acetate for 10 days. Bleeding indicates ovaries are producing estrogen, uterus and outflow tract are intact. No bleeding suggests hypothalamic-pituitary causes, premature ovarian failure, Asherman's syndrome
- Follicle-stimulating hormone (FSH) and luteinizing hormone (LH) to evaluate for premature ovarian failure
- Polycystic ovary syndrome is a diagnosis of exclusion; irregular menses, hirsutism, acne, insulin resistance. Check androgen levels only in women with clitoromegaly, other signs of masculinization

■ Differential Diagnosis

- Pregnancy
- Physiologic (adolescence, perimenopause)
- Causes as outlined above

■ Treatment

- Polycystic ovarian syndrome: Oral contraceptives or levonorgestrel intrauterine system (IUS) for cycle regularity and to decrease the risk of endometrial cancer; weight loss to induce spontaneous ovulation
- Hypoestrogenic causes: Treat underlying disorder (eg, anorexia); estrogen treatment to prevent osteoporosis
- Hyperprolactinemia: Surgery for macroadenoma, otherwise treat with bromocriptine or expectant management

16

■ Pearl

Despite an extensive differential, three processes top the list: pregnancy, pregnancy, and pregnancy.

Reference

Rothman MS, Wierman ME. Female hypogonadism: evaluation of the hypothalamic-pituitary-ovarian axis. Pituitary 2008;11:163. [PMID: 18404388]

Cervical Dysplasia

- ■ Essentials of Diagnosis
  - • Caused by HPV infection; risk factors: Early intercourse, multiple partners, smoking, HIV
  - • Includes low- and high-grade squamous intraepithelial lesions (LSIL, HSIL) or cervical intraepithelial neoplasia (CIN 1–3)
  - • Seventy-five percent of low-grade (CIN 1) lesions regress spontaneously; only 35% of high-grade (CIN 2–3) regress
  - • Atypical squamous cells of undetermined significance (ASCUS, ASC) associated with biopsy-proven dysplasia in 10%
  - • Atypical glandular cells of undetermined significance (AGUS, AGC) associated with endometrial hyperplasia, adenocarcinoma, or high-grade dysplasia in 40%
  - • Colposcopy confirms and excludes invasive cancer

- ■ Differential Diagnosis
  - • Inflammation due to vaginitis, cervicitis, or atrophy
  - • Inaccurate interpretation of cytology or histology

- ■ Treatment
  - • Advise smoking cessation
  - • ASCUS: Three options acceptable: repeat Pap at 6 and 12 months with colposcopy for any repeat abnormality; HPV test in women > 20 years and if positive perform colposcopy (repeat Pap 1 year if negative) or immediate colposcopy
  - • Low-grade lesions: Colposcopy with biopsy confirms diagnosis; expectant management versus ablation or excision; for women < 20 years, repeat Pap 1 year
  - • High-grade lesions including ASCUS favor high grade (ASC-H): Colposcopy with biopsy to confirm diagnosis; treat with ablation or excision
  - • Atypical glandular cells: Colposcopy, endocervical curettage, and if abnormal bleeding is present, endometrial biopsy

- ■ Pearl

Do not confuse atypical glandular cells with atypical squamous cells: the former are much more likely to indicate neoplasia or cancer.

Reference

Wright TC Jr, Massad LS, Dunton CJ, Spitzer M, Wilkinson EJ, Solomon D; 2006 American Society for Colposcopy and Cervical Pathology-sponsored Consensus Conference. 2006 consensus guidelines for the management of women with abnormal cervical cancer screening tests. Am J Obstet Gynecol 2007;197:346. [PMID: 17904957]

16

Chronic Pelvic Pain

- ■ Essentials of Diagnosis
  - Subacute pelvic pain of more than 6 months duration
  - Etiology often multifactorial
  - Up to 40% have been physically or sexually abused
  - Up to 30% with pelvic inflammatory disease (PID) go on to have chronic pelvic pain
  - Pain that resolves with ovulation suppression suggests gynecologic cause
  - Concomitant depression very common
  - Ultrasound and physical exam often not diagnostic
  - Half of women who undergo laparoscopy for chronic pelvic pain have no visible pathology

- ■ Differential Diagnosis
  - Gynecologic: Endometriosis, adenomyosis, pelvic adhesions, chronic PID or endometritis, mittelschmerz; leiomyomas can cause pelvic heaviness but rarely cause pain.
  - Gastrointestinal: Irritable bowel syndrome, inflammatory bowel disease, diverticular disease, constipation, neoplasia, hernia
  - Urologic: Detrusor overactivity, interstitial cystitis, urinary calculi, urethral syndrome, bladder carcinoma
  - Musculoskeletal: Myofascial pain, low back pain, disk problems, nerve entrapment, muscle strain or spasm
  - Psychiatric: Somatization, depression, abuse, anxiety

- ■ Treatment
  - Evaluate for and treat the above causes, especially psychiatric
  - NSAIDs; avoid opioids
  - Ovulation suppression with oral contraceptives, depomedroxy-progesterone acetate, levonorgestrel IUS, or a short course of leuprolide acetate can be both diagnostic and therapeutic.
  - Pelvic floor physical therapy or biofeedback for pelvic floor muscle spasm
  - Diagnostic laparoscopy if gynecologic cause is suspected, medical management fails, or diagnosis remains in question
  - Hysterectomy with bilateral oophorectomy for refractory gynecologic pain in women who have completed childbearing

16

- ■ Pearl
  One of the most challenging conditions in all of gynecology; therapy is quite commonly not gratifying.

Reference

Levy BS. The complex nature of chronic pelvic pain. J Fam Pract 2007;56(suppl diagnosis):S16. [PMID: 18671924]

Dysmenorrhea

- ■ Essentials of Diagnosis
  - • Occurs in 50% of menstruating women
  - • Low, midline, cramping pelvic pain radiating to back or legs; pain starting before or with menses, peaking after 24 hours, and subsiding after 2 days; often associated with nausea, diarrhea, headache, and flushing
  - • Primary dysmenorrhea: Pain without pelvic pathology and beginning within 1–2 years after menarche
  - • Secondary dysmenorrhea: Pain with underlying pathology such as endometriosis or adenomyosis, developing years after menarche

- ■ Differential Diagnosis
  - • Endometriosis
  - • Adenomyosis
  - • Uterine myoma
  - • Cervical stenosis, uterine anomalies
  - • Chronic endometritis or pelvic inflammatory disease
  - • Copper T intrauterine device

- ■ Treatment
  - • NSAIDs or COX-2 inhibitors before the onset of bleeding, continued for 2–3 days taken around the clock.
  - • Suppression of ovulation with oral contraceptives, depomedroxy-progesterone acetate, or levonorgestrel intrauterine system
  - • In secondary dysmenorrhea, laparoscopy may be indicated to diagnose endometriosis
  - • Hysterectomy with or without bilateral salpingo-oophorectomy for severe refractory dysmenorrhea

- ■ Pearl

16

Endometriosis is the most important cause in younger women; think adenomyosis with increasing age.

Reference

Harel Z. Dysmenorrhea in adolescents and young adults: from pathophysiology to pharmacological treatments and management strategies. Expert Opin Pharmacother 2008;9:2661. [PMID: 18803452]

Ectopic Pregnancy

■ Essentials of Diagnosis

- Pregnancy implantation outside uterine cavity
- Most commonly presents 6–8 weeks after last menstrual period
- Classic triad: Pregnant, bleeding or spotting, pelvic pain.
- Rupture causes sudden increase in pain, dizziness, and anemia leading to shock and cardiovascular collapse
- Transvaginal ultrasound to identify intrauterine gestation when beta human chorionic gonadotropin (β-hCG) is above approximately 2000 mU/mL; an empty uterine cavity when β-hCG > 2000 is highly suspicious; transvaginal ultrasound often cannot demonstrate an extrauterine pregnancy
- Diagnosis confirmed by lack of placental villi after suction curettage or by laparoscopy
- In patients with a desired pregnancy who are hemodynamically stable, serum β-hCG can be obtained every 48 hours and should approximately double; failure to double indicates either ectopic or abnormal intrauterine gestation

■ Differential Diagnosis

- Intrauterine pregnancy (threatened abortion, early pregnancy failure, gestational trophoblastic neoplasia)
- Ruptured corpus luteum cyst
- Other GI, GU and gynecologic causes of acute abdomino-pelvic pain

■ Treatment

- Suction curettage to confirm diagnosis
- Surgical removal of the Fallopian tube is definitive and is recommended for larger or complicated ectopic pregnancies and in those who do not desire future fertility
- Methotrexate can be offered as an alternative for patients with small, unruptured ectopic pregnancies who can be compliant with multiple follow-up visits and laboratory work; 6% have tubal rupture after methotrexate.
- Emergent surgery if hemodynamically unstable
- Rh_o immune globulin to Rh-negative patients
- Effective contraception to prevent future ectopic pregnancy

16

■ Pearl

Shock of inapparent cause in a reproductive-aged woman is ruptured ectopic pregnancy until proven otherwise.

Reference

Barnhart KT. Clinical practice. Ectopic pregnancy. N Engl J Med 2009;361:379. [PMID: 19625718]

Endometriosis

■ Essentials of Diagnosis

- Seen in 10% of all menstruating women, 25% of infertile women
- Progressive, recurrent, characterized by aberrant growth of endometrium outside the uterus
- Classic triad: Cyclic pelvic pain, dysmenorrhea, and dyspareunia
- May be associated with infertility or pelvic mass (endometrioma)
- Pelvic examination may or may not be normal. Abnormalities can include a fixed retroverted uterus, tender or nodular uterosacral ligaments, or an adnexal mass.
- Hematochezia, painful defecation, or hematuria if bowel or bladder invaded
- Ultrasound often normal but useful for diagnosis of endometrioma.
- Laparoscopy with biopsy of endometriotic lesions confirms diagnosis

■ Differential Diagnosis

- Other causes of chronic pelvic pain
- Primary dysmenorrhea
- Adenomyosis

■ Treatment

- NSAIDs
- Ovulation suppression with continuous oral contraceptives until fertility is desired; levonorgestrel IUS also effective; depomedroxy-progesterone acetate also effective but associated with 9-month delay in return to fertility
- If OCPs ineffective, gonadotropin-releasing hormone (GnRH) analogs (eg, leuprolide) with add-back estrogen can be used for up to 6 months followed by continuous OCPs
- Laparoscopy with ablation of lesions for refractory pain is temporarily helpful in up to two-thirds of patients; 50% recur. Laparoscopic ablation of lesions also results in temporary improvement in fertility rates.
- Hysterectomy with bilateral salpingo-oophorectomy for those who have completed childbearing

■ Pearl

Endometriosis can occur anywhere in the body, including fingers, lungs, and other organs, behaving like a metastatic tumor, but without the cellular atypia or invasion.

Reference

Ozkan S, Arici A. Advances in treatment options of endometriosis. Gynecol Obstet Invest 2009;67:81. [PMID: 18931504]

16

Mammary Dysplasia (Fibrocystic Changes of the Breast)

■ Essentials of Diagnosis

- Common age 20–50 years
- Presents with cyclic breast pain with maximal pain during the premenstrual phase and resolution during menses.
- On exam, tender, often multiple, usually bilateral masses in the breasts; excessive nodularity, generalized lumpiness.
- Rapid fluctuation in size of masses
- Rare in postmenopausal women not on hormonal therapy
- Eighty percent of women have histologic fibrocystic changes

■ Differential Diagnosis

- Breast carcinoma
- Fibroadenoma
- Fat necrosis
- Intraductal papilloma

■ Treatment

- A diagnostic work-up of any discrete mass or asymmetric area is necessary
- Biopsy (fine-needle aspiration or core-needle biopsy) to exclude carcinoma and determine whether cystic or solid
- In women younger than 35 years, ultrasound can be used instead of biopsy to differentiate cystic from solid masses
- Mammography in women older than 40 years
- Frequent follow-up of all women with breast masses even if work-up is negative given possibility of false-negative testing.
- For breast thickening or ill-defined masses, follow-up breast exam in different stage of menstrual cycle
- For mastalgia: Supportive brassiere (night and day), NSAIDs, oral contraceptives; for severe pain, danazol (100–200 mg bid), bromocriptine (2.5 mg bid), or tamoxifen (10 mg/day)

16

■ Pearl

All women with this condition fear breast cancer: psychological management is an important adjunct to medical therapy.

Reference

Santen RJ, Mansel R. Benign breast disorders. N Engl J Med 2005;353:275. [PMID: 16034013]

Menopausal Syndrome

- **Essentials of Diagnosis**
    - Cessation of menses without other cause, usually due to aging or bilateral oophorectomy
    - Average age is 51 years; earlier in women who smoke
    - Perimenopause: Declining ovarian function over 4–6 years
    - Menstrual irregularity, hot flushes, night sweats, mood fluctuation, sleep disturbance, vaginal dryness
    - Elevated serum FSH and LH

- **Differential Diagnosis**
    - Other causes of amenorrhea, especially pregnancy
    - Hyperthyroidism or hypothyroidism
    - Pheochromocytoma
    - Uterine neoplasm
    - Sjögren's syndrome
    - Depression
    - Anorexia

- **Treatment**
    - The most effective treatment for hot flashes and other menopausal symptoms is oral estrogen therapy. However, estrogen therapy has been shown to increase the risk of breast cancer in randomized controlled trials and so should be reserved for those with severe symptoms and after a thorough discussion. Other therapies such as megestrol acetate, clonidine, selective serotonin reuptake inhibitors (SSRIs), and gabapentin are modestly effective.
    - Hot flashes often resolve by 2–4 years after menopause
    - For irregular bleeding in the perimenopause, oral contraceptives, levonorgestrel intrauterine system, cyclic or combined continuous estrogen plus progestin, or progestins alone
    - Estrogen cream and nonhormonal lubricants for vaginal dryness
    - Although long-term use of combined hormonal therapy decreases osteoporosis and colon cancer, it increases the risk of breast cancer and thromboembolism

- **Pearl**

The role of hormonal therapy in older women remains a controversy despite years of studying.

Reference

Nelson HD, Vesco KK, Haney E, et al. Nonhormonal therapies for menopausal hot flashes: systematic review and meta-analysis. JAMA 2006;295:2057. [PMID: 16670414]

Mucopurulent Cervicitis

- ■ Essentials of Diagnosis
  - A sexually transmitted infection most commonly caused by *Neisseria gonorrhoeae* or *Chlamydia*
  - Cervical inflammation can also result from herpesvirus, or vaginitis due to *Trichomonas* or *Candida*
  - Usually asymptomatic but may have abnormal vaginal discharge, or postcoital bleeding
  - Red, friable cervix with purulent, often blood-streaked endocervical discharge
  - Must be distinguished from physiologic ectopy of columnar epithelium common in young women

- ■ Differential Diagnosis
  - Pelvic inflammatory disease
  - Cervical carcinoma or dysplasia
  - Cervical ulcer secondary to syphilis, chancroid, or granuloma inguinale
  - Normal epithelial ectopy
  - Cervical inflammation due to vaginitis

- ■ Treatment
  - In general, treat only if tests are positive for *N. gonorrhoeae* or *Chlamydia;* empirically in a high-risk or noncompliant patient
  - Gonorrhea: Ceftriaxone 125 mg IM or cefixime 400 mg PO, single dose
  - Chlamydia: Azithromycin 1 g PO single dose or doxycycline 100 mg bid for 7 days (once pregnancy excluded)
  - Sexual abstinence until treatment completed; provide or refer partner for therapy

- ■ Pearl

All patients with cervicitis should be tested for HIV, syphilis, and hepatitis C, and partners should be offered treatment.

Reference

Sheeder J, Stevens-Simon C, Lezotte D, Glazner J, Scott S. Cervicitis: to treat or not to treat? The role of patient preferences and decision analysis. J Adolesc Health 2006;39:887. [PMID: 17116520]

16

Myoma of the Uterus
(Fibroid Tumor, Leiomyoma, Fibromyoma)

- ■ Essentials of Diagnosis
  - Irregular enlargement of uterus caused by benign smooth muscle tumors
  - Occurs in 40–50% of women over age 40 years
  - Often asymptomatic or can cause heavy or irregular vaginal bleeding, anemia, urinary frequency, pelvic pressure, dysmenorrhea
  - Acute pelvic pain rare and due to torsion of pedunculated myoma or degeneration of very large myoma
  - May be intramural, submucosal, subserosal, cervical, or parasitic (ie, deriving its blood supply from an adjacent organ)
  - Pelvic ultrasound confirms diagnosis

- ■ Differential Diagnosis
  - Pregnancy
  - Adenomyosis
  - Ovarian or adnexal mass
  - Abnormal uterine bleeding due to other causes
  - Leiomyosarcoma
  - Other abdominal/pelvic mass

- ■ Treatment
  - Exclude pregnancy
  - Papanicolaou smear and endometrial biopsy (if > 35 years and irregular bleeding)
  - NSAIDs to reduce blood loss; hormonal therapy to reduce endometrial volume (oral contraceptives, depomedroxyprogesterone acetate, levonorgestrel intrauterine system)
  - GnRH agonists for 3–6 months for women planning surgery or nearing menopause
  - Medical therapies often ineffective for large or submucosal myomas; myomectomy, hysterectomy, or uterine fibroid embolization may be necessary

16

- ■ Pearl
  Always try hormonal therapy first before blaming irregular postmenopausal bleeding on fibroids.

Reference

Levy BS. Modern management of uterine fibroids. Acta Obstet Gynecol Scand 2008;87:812. [PMID: 18607823]

Pelvic Inflammatory Disease (PID, Salpingitis, Endometritis, Tubo-Ovarian Abscess)

■ Essentials of Diagnosis

- Most common in young, sexually active women with multiple partners or a new sexual partner
- Upper genital tract infection associated with *Neisseria gonorrhoeae* and *Chlamydia trachomatis,* anaerobes, *Haemophilus influenzae,* enteric gram-negative rods, and streptococci
- Difficult to diagnose because severity varies from asymptomatic to toxic
- Sequelae: Chronic pelvic pain, infertility, pelvic adhesions
- Delay in diagnosis and treatment probably contributes to sequelae. Maintain a low threshold for diagnosis.
- Minimum diagnostic criteria per CDC: pelvic/abdominal pain AND one of the following: Cervical motion, uterine, or adnexal tenderness AND absence of competing diagnosis
- Diagnostic specificity improved by presence of fever, cervical mucopus, leukocytosis, elevated erythrocyte sedimentation rate
- Pelvic ultrasound may reveal a tubo-ovarian abscess
- Laparoscopy for cases with uncertain diagnosis or no improvement despite antibiotic therapy

■ Differential Diagnosis

- Any cause of acute abdominal-pelvic pain or peritonitis (eg. appendicitis, diverticulitis, acute cystitis, urinary calculi)
- Ruptured ovarian cyst, ovarian torsion, ectopic pregnancy

■ Treatment

- Oral antibiotics for mild cases (14-day course) covering *N. gonorrhoeae* and *Chlamydia* (ceftriaxone 250 mg IM plus doxycycline 100 mg bid for 14 days)
- Hospitalization and intravenous antibiotics for toxic, adolescent, HIV-infected, or pregnant patients
- Surgical or percutaneous drainage of tubo-ovarian abscess
- Screen for HIV, hepatitis, syphilis
- Sexual abstinence until treatment completed; partner should be treated

16

■ Pearl

Do not rely on cervical cultures; often negative, they should not be used to guide management.

Reference

Sweet RL. Treatment strategies for pelvic inflammatory disease. Expert Opin Pharmacother 2009;10:823. [PMID: 19351231]

Pelvic Organ Prolapse

- ■ Essentials of Diagnosis
  - • Common in older multiparous women as a delayed result of child-birth injury to pelvic floor
  - • Includes prolapse of the uterus, bladder (cystocele), rectum (rectocele), small bowel (enterocele), or vaginal cuff
  - • Often asymptomatic; may have pelvic pressure or pulling, vaginal bulge, low back pain; difficulties with sexual function, defecation, or voiding
  - • Pelvic examination confirms the diagnosis. Ask the patient to perform Valsalva's to see the severity of the prolapse.
  - • Prolapse may be slight, moderate, or marked
  - • Attenuation of pelvic structures with aging can accelerate development

- ■ Differential Diagnosis
  - • Vaginal or cervical neoplasm
  - • Rectal prolapse
  - • Rectal carcinoma

- ■ Treatment
  - • Supportive measures (eg, Kegel exercises), limit straining and lifting
  - • Treat predisposing factors such as obesity, obstructive airway disease, constipation, and pelvic masses
  - • Conjugated estrogen creams to decrease vaginal irritation
  - • Pessaries may reduce prolapse and its symptoms; ineffective for very large prolapse
  - • Corrective surgery for symptomatic prolapse that significantly affects quality of life

16

- ■ Pearl

Ulcerations of the protruding organ, while appearing to be traumatic, should all be biopsied; malignancy may occur in them, especially of the cervix and vagina.

Reference

Hampton BS. Pelvic organ prolapse. Med Health R I 2009;92:5. [PMID: 19248418]

Pre-eclampsia–Eclampsia

- Essentials of Diagnosis
  - Progressive, multisystem condition affecting 5–10% of pregnant women
  - Pre-eclampsia is hypertension plus proteinuria after 20 weeks of gestation; addition of seizures means eclampsia
  - Mild pre-eclampsia defined as blood pressure > 140/90, proteinuria > 300 mg/24 hours, and absence of criteria for severe shown below.
  - Severe pre-eclampsia defined as blood pressure > 160/110 or proteinuria > 5 g/24 hours or hematologic, neurologic, cardiopulmonary, hepatorenal, or fetal complications listed below.
  - Neurologic: Headache, blurred vision or scotomas, altered mental status, seizure
  - Fetal: Intrauterine growth restriction, oligohydramnios
  - Hematologic: Thrombocytopenia, hemolysis, disseminated intravascular coagulopathy
  - Cardiopulmonary: Pulmonary edema
  - Hepato/renal: Oliguria, anuria, elevated serum creatinine, elevated AST or ALT, right upper quadrant tenderness
  - HELLP syndrome: Hemolysis, elevated liver enzymes, and low platelets
  - Risk factors: first pregnancy, older age, twins, prior preeclampsia, hypertension, diabetes, renal or autoimmune disease

- Differential Diagnosis
  - Hypertension or renal disease due to other cause
  - Primary seizure disorder
  - Hemolytic-uremic syndrome
  - Thrombotic thrombocytopenic purpura

- Treatment
  - The only treatment is delivery of the fetus
  - Prior to term, severe cases should have labor induced; mild cases can be observed in the hospital with induction of labor for worsening disease. At term, mild cases should have labor induced
  - Antihypertensives if blood pressure > 180/110 mm Hg
  - Magnesium sulfate can be given to women to prevent development of seizures and to prevent recurrent seizures in those with eclampsia.

- Pearl

Deliver the baby, cure the disease.

Reference

Cudihy D, Lee RV. The pathophysiology of pre-eclampsia: current clinical concepts. J Obstet Gynaecol 2009;29:576. [PMID: 19757258]

16

Puerperal Mastitis

- ■ Essentials of Diagnosis
  - Occurs in nursing mothers within 3 months after delivery
  - Unilateral inflammation and redness of breast or one quadrant of breast with tenderness, induration, warmth, fever, malaise
  - Sore or fissured nipple may be present
  - Increased incidence in first-time mothers
  - *Staphylococcus aureus* and streptococci are usual causative agents; community-acquired MRSA increasingly common
  - May progress to breast abscess
  - Ultrasound can confirm abscess diagnosis

- ■ Differential Diagnosis
  - Local irritation or trauma
  - Nondraining duct
  - Benign or malignant tumors (inflammatory carcinoma)
  - Subareolar abscess (occurs in nonlactating women)
  - Fat necrosis

- ■ Treatment
  - For very mild cases, warm compresses and increased frequency of breastfeeding
  - Oral dicloxacillin or first-generation cephalosporin
  - If suspect community-acquired MRSA, culture milk and use Septra or clindamycin
  - Hospitalize for intravenous antibiotics if no improvement in 48 hours or in toxic patients
  - Increase frequency of breastfeeding
  - Incision and drainage for abscess; stop breastfeeding from affected breast (may pump milk and discard)

16

- ■ Pearl

Patients with this mastitis may appear surprisingly toxic, diverting attention from the correct diagnosis.

Reference

Jahanfar S, Ng CJ, Teng CL. Antibiotics for mastitis in breastfeeding women. Cochrane Database Syst Rev 2009:CD005458. [PMID: 19160255]

Spontaneous Abortion

■ Essentials of Diagnosis

- Vaginal bleeding, pelvic pain, and cramping before the 20th week of pregnancy occurring in up to 20% of pregnancies
- Threatened abortion: Pregnancy may continue or abortion may ensue; cervix closed, bleeding and cramping mild, intrauterine pregnancy confirmed
- Inevitable or incomplete abortion: Cervix dilated and products of conception may or may not be partially expelled; brisk bleeding
- Completed abortion: Products of conception completely expelled; cervix closed, cramping and bleeding decreased
- Early pregnancy failure (embryonic demise, missed abortion): Failed pregnancy detected by ultrasound; cervix closed, absent or minimal bleeding and cramping
- Serum β-hCG fails to rise appropriately (except in threatened abortion)
- Pelvic ultrasonography contraindicated when bleeding heavy or cervix open because it delays treatment

■ Differential Diagnosis

- Ectopic pregnancy
- Gestational trophoblastic neoplasia
- Cervical neoplasm or lesion, trauma

■ Treatment

- Follow hematocrit and bleeding quantity closely as women with spontaneous abortion can have rapid blood loss
- Confirm intrauterine pregnancy with ultrasound; if unable to confirm intrauterine location, follow closely until ectopic pregnancy is ruled out
- Threatened abortion: β-hCG in 2–3 days; immediate follow-up if brisk bleeding develops. Limiting activity is ineffective.
- Inevitable or incomplete abortion: Suction curettage to immediately stop the bleeding
- Missed abortion: Suction curettage, methotrexate, or wait for spontaneous abortion
- Rh_o immune globulin to Rh-negative mothers
- Follow-up to ensure patient is no longer pregnant

16

■ Pearl

Over-the-counter pregnancy testing by hopeful potential mothers has indicated this condition to be far more common than was once suspected.

Reference

El-Sayed MM, Mohamed SA, Jones MH. Expectant management of first-trimester miscarriage. J Obstet Gynaecol 2009;29:681. [PMID: 19821656]

Urinary Incontinence

- **Essentials of Diagnosis**
  - Uncontrolled loss of urine; classified as stress, urge, mixed, or overflow
  - Stress incontinence: Urine loss during coughing or exercising; leakage observed on examination during cough or with Valsalva's maneuver
  - Urge incontinence due to spontaneous bladder contractions; accompanied by urgency, associated with frequency and nocturia, normal examination
  - Overflow incontinence is very unusual in women and is caused by overdistention of bladder due to neurologic lesion or outflow obstruction; postvoid residual markedly elevated
  - Urinary tract infections commonly cause transient incontinence or worsening of preexisting incontinence
  - Urodynamic evaluation indicated when diagnosis is uncertain or before surgical correction

- **Differential Diagnosis**
  - Urinary tract infection
  - Mobility disorders affecting ability to get to the toilet
  - Neurologic causes as outlined above
  - Urinary fistula, urethral diverticulum
  - Medications: Diuretics, anticholinergics, antihistamines, α-adrenergic blockers

- **Treatment**
  - Exclude urinary tract infection
  - A diary of voiding aids in diagnosis and guides therapy
  - Kegel exercises, formal training of the pelvic muscles (biofeedback)
  - For urge incontinence: Timed voids, limit fluid intake and caffeine, anticholinergic medications (oxybutynin chloride, tolterodine)
  - Surgical treatment is effective in up to 85% for stress incontinence refractory to conservative management

- **Pearl**

Socially isolating and depressing, but treatment is simple and quality of life thus enhanced.

Reference

Sassani P, Aboseif SR. Stress urinary incontinence in women. Curr Urol Rep 2009;10:333. [PMID: 19709478]

Vaginitis

- **Essentials of Diagnosis**
  - Vaginal burning, pain, pruritus, discharge
  - Results from atrophy, infection, or allergic reaction
  - Common infectious causes include *Candida albicans, Trichomonas vaginalis,* bacterial vaginosis (*Gardnerella* and other anaerobes)
  - *Trichomonas* is sexually transmitted and causes profuse, frothy, malodorous discharge and vaginal irritation
  - Bacterial vaginosis may be asymptomatic or associated with a thin, gray, "fishy" discharge
  - *C. albicans* associated with pruritus, burning, and a thick, white, nonmalodorous discharge
  - Wet mount with KOH, saline, and pH are usually diagnostic: Trichomonads are motile, pH > 4.5; bacterial vaginosis reveals clue cells, pH > 4.5; hyphae and spores with a normal pH (< 4.5) mean *Candida*

- **Differential Diagnosis**
  - Physiologic discharge, ovulation
  - Atrophic vaginitis, vulvar dystrophies (lichen sclerosis), and vulvar neoplasia in older women
  - Cervicitis, syphilis, herpesvirus outbreak
  - Cervical carcinoma
  - Foreign body (retained tampon)
  - Contact dermatitis (eg, condoms, perfumed products, soap)
  - Pubic lice, scabies

- **Treatment**
  - Limit vaginal irritants
  - Culture cervix for *N-eisseria gonorrhoeae* and *Chlamydia* if no other cause for symptoms
  - For *T. vaginalis:* Metronidazole (2 g as a single dose) for both patient and partner
  - For *C. albicans:* Antifungal (eg, clotrimazole) vaginal cream or suppository or single-dose oral fluconazole (150 mg)
  - For bacterial vaginosis: Metronidazole (500 mg twice daily for 7 days or vaginal gel twice daily for 5 days)
  - For atrophic vaginitis, estrogen cream per vagina twice per week

16

- **Pearl**

Symptoms alone do not diagnose this condition; it is essential to perform a wet mount in all patients with this symptom complex.

Reference

Mac Bride MB, Rhodes DJ, Shuster LT. Vulvovaginal atrophy. Mayo Clin Proc 2010;85:87. [PMID: 20042564]

17

Common Surgical Disorders

Abdominal Aortic Aneurysm

- **Essentials of Diagnosis**
  - More than 90% originate below the renal arteries
  - Most asymptomatic, discovered incidentally
  - Back or abdominal pain often precedes rupture
  - Diameter is the most important predictor of aneurysm rupture (up to a 40% risk of rupture over 5 years for aneurysms > 5 cm)
  - Four-fold higher incidence in men, but risk of rupture is two to four times more common in women
  - Most rupture leftward and posteriorly; left knee jerk disappears
  - Frequently associated with aneurysms in other locations, and all patients with abdominal aortic aneurysms should be assessed for concomitant femoral and popliteal aneurysms
  - Ultrasound ideal for screening; CT for operative planning
  - One-time ultrasound screening is recommended for men ≥ 65 years of age, and as early as 55 years of age if family history positive; one-time screening ultrasound recommended for women ≥ 65 if family history is positive, or history of tobacco use

- **Differential Diagnosis**
  - Pancreatic pseudocyst, pancreatitis, renal colic
  - Penetrating (posterior) duodenal ulcer

- **Treatment**
  - In asymptomatic healthy patients, surgery recommended for aneurysms > 5.0 cm
  - Resection may be beneficial even for aneurysms as small as 4 cm (women, ulcerated or saccular aneurysms)
  - In symptomatic patients, immediate repair regardless of size
  - Endovascular repair (transfemoral insertion of a prosthetic graft) considered if the anatomy of aneurysm is suitable and can be performed using local or epidural anesthesia for high-risk patients
  - Smoking cessation important

- **Pearl**

A pulsatile mass left of the midline is often a tortuous aorta; if it is to the right of the midline, investigate for aneurysm.

Reference

Chaikof EL, Brewster DC, Dalman RL, et al; Society for Vascular Surgery. The care of patients with an abdominal aortic aneurysm: the Society for Vascular Surgery practice guidelines. J Vasc Surg 2009;50(4 suppl):S2. [PMID: 19786250]

Acute Appendicitis

- ■ Essentials of Diagnosis
  - Lifetime risk is 7%; 70% present before 30 years of age
  - Perforations associated with a 20% mortality risk in the elderly
  - Non-abrupt abdominal pain initially poorly localized or periumbilical, then focal in right lower quadrant over 4–48 hours
  - Pain followed by nausea with or without vomiting; anorexia
  - Low-grade fever, right lower quadrant tenderness at McBurney's point with or without peritoneal signs
  - Prolonged symptoms, high fever, rigors, localized pain, and marked leukocytosis often seen in perforation
  - Pelvic and rectal exam may reveal tenderness, particularly in retrocecal appendicitis; microscopic hematuria or pyuria common
  - Mild leukocytosis with neutrophil predominance; if WBC > 18,000/mL, consider rupture with localized abscess

- ■ Differential Diagnosis
  - Gynecologic or urologic pathology (eg, ectopic pregnancy, pelvic inflammatory disease, ovarian or testicular torsion)
  - Gastroenteritis (idiopathic, cytomegalovirus, *Yersinia* enterocolitis)
  - Cecal or sigmoid colon diverticulitis; pancreatitis; cholecystitis
  - Bowel obstruction; intussusception; mesenteric adenitis
  - Perforated peptic ulcer; Crohn's; Meckel's diverticulitis; pneumonia

- ■ Treatment
  - Patients with clinical manifestations consistent with nonruptured appendicitis should undergo urgent appendectomy
  - Patients in whom the evaluation is not entirely consistent with appendicitis should undergo either ultrasound or CT scan
  - For ruptured appendicitis, CT-guided drainage of localized abscess with later appendectomy; follow-up colonoscopy or CT imaging recommended after resolution of acute episode
  - Up to 30% of patients have a normal appendix at operation
  - When diagnosis unclear, observe with serial examinations

- ■ Pearl

Modern imaging techniques have made surgeons more reluctant to explore for this condition; it is not bad medicine to resect a normal appendix when the clinical picture is suggestive.

Reference

Andersson RE, Petzold MG. Nonsurgical treatment of appendiceal abscess or phlegmon: a systematic review and meta-analysis. Ann Surg 2007;246:741. [PMID: 17968164]

17

Acute Cholecystitis

- ■ Essentials of Diagnosis
  - • Caused by obstruction of the gallbladder, typically by gallstones, but also due to malignancy, polyps, lymph nodes, and parasites
  - • Gallstones are present in up to 35% of the adult population; only 1–3% of these patients will develop cholecystitis
  - • Acalculous cholecystitis, which comprises 2–15% of patients with cholecystitis, is caused by bile stasis, sludge formation, and bacterial overgrowth resulting in gallbladder obstruction
  - • Escalating right upper quadrant or epigastric pain over 12–24 hours that may be colicky in nature, but never completely resolves; malaise, nausea, fever, and vomiting are typical
  - • Classic finding is Murphy's sign (an inspiratory arrest with palpation in the right upper quadrant)
  - • Signs and symptoms of common bile duct obstruction, including tea-colored urine, clay-colored stools, scleral icterus
  - • Fever, leukocytosis, slight elevation in liver function studies, and occasionally an elevation in amylase and lipase; bilirubin elevation > 3 mg/dL concerning for common bile duct obstruction
  - • Ultrasound is useful and may reveal stones, ductal dilation (common bile duct > 8 mm concerning for obstruction), and inflammation (thickened gallbladder wall, pericholecystic fluid)
  - • Radionuclide hepatobiliary iminodiacetic acid (HIDA) scan is the most accurate test (97% sensitive and 87% specific)

- ■ Differential Diagnosis
  - • Acute appendicitis; pancreatitis; hepatitis; pneumonia
  - • Gastroenteritis; peptic ulcer; myocardial infarction
  - • Radicular pain in thoracic dermatome (eg, preeruptive zoster)

- ■ Treatment
  - • Bowel rest, fluids, analgesics, and antibiotics
  - • Early laparoscopic cholecystectomy (within 48 hours of onset of symptoms) leads to reduced morbidity and mortality
  - • Immediate cholecystectomy for gallbladder ischemia, perforation, emphysematous cholecystitis
  - • Endoscopic retrograde cholangiopancreatography (ERCP) with sphincterotomy should be performed when there is evidence of common bile duct stones, pancreatitis, or cholangitis

- ■ Pearl

In cholecystitis, the patient generally knows the exact time of onset of symptoms; this is seldom the case in typical appendicitis.

Reference

Elwood DR. Cholecystitis. Surg Clin North Am 2008;88:1241, viii. [PMID: 18992593]

17

Acute Lower-Extremity Arterial Occlusion

- ■ Essentials of Diagnosis
    - Important to discern whether the patient has embolic, thrombotic, or traumatic etiology resulting in lower-extremity ischemia
    - Most common source of emboli is cardiac (80–90%); 60–70% of these patients have underlying cardiac disease such as myocardial infarction, valvular disease, arrhythmia, endocarditis
    - Traumatic causes include posterior knee dislocation, iatrogenic catheter injury, penetrating trauma (gunshot wound or stab injury)
    - Thrombotic occlusion occurs most commonly in underlying atherosclerotic disease with a new acute insult (low-flow state, injury)
    - Classic manifestations of ischemia are the 6 P's: pain, pallor, paresthesias, paralysis, poikilothermia, and pulselessness; pain is first and most common, paralysis is late
    - Signs of ischemia are most pronounced at the next joint distal to the level of occlusion
    - Embolic events typically present with the sudden onset of pain in the setting of an arrhythmia; contralateral vascular examination is normal
    - Thrombotic events typically present with a slower onset of less severe symptoms, a history of claudication, rest pain, and peripheral vascular disease; exam may reveal stigmata of chronic bilateral vascular disease

- ■ Differential Diagnosis
    - Neuropathic pain; reflex sympathetic dystrophy
    - Deep venous thrombosis
    - Systemic vasculitis; cholesterol atheroemboli

- ■ Treatment
    - Heparin should be given in patients without a contraindication in order to prevent propagation of the embolus or thrombosis and maintain patency of collateral vessels; aspirin also given
    - Re-establish blood flow via surgical embolectomy or catheter-directed thrombolysis
    - Fasciotomy is indicated if ischemia is estimated to be longer than 4 hours to prevent the development of compartment syndrome
    - Monitor electrolytes and renal function closely

- ■ Pearl

In the patient with an intra-arterial femoral line in the ICU on a ventilator, there will be no history, rather only nonspecific clinical deterioration; check distal pulses frequently in such patients.

Reference

O'Connell JB, Quiñones-Baldrich WJ. Proper evaluation and management of acute embolic versus thrombotic limb ischemia. Semin Vasc Surg 2009;22:10. [PMID: 19298930]

Cerebral Vascular Occlusive Disease

- **Essentials of Diagnosis**
  - Most common in patients with standard risk factors for atherosclerosis (eg, hypertension, hypercholesterolemia, diabetes, smoking)
  - Majority of patients asymptomatic
  - Symptoms: Transient monocular blindness (amaurosis fugax), transient hemiparesis with or without aphasia or sensory changes lasting < 20 minutes (transient ischemic attack)
  - Bruit may be present but correlates poorly with degree of stenosis
  - Duplex ultrasound useful in assessing stenosis; gadolinium angiography is indicated only when the anatomy is not clearly delineated on ultrasound

- **Differential Diagnosis**
  - Carotid artery dissection
  - Steal syndromes
  - Giant cell arteritis
  - Takayasu's arteritis
  - Lipohyalinosis
  - Radiation fibrosis
  - Cardiac emboli
  - Brain tumor or abscess (in patient with stroke)
  - Fibromuscular dysplasia

- **Treatment**
  - Thrombolytic agents in carefully selected patients with cerebral ischemia: Less than 3 hours of symptoms, no hemorrhage on CT
  - Carotid endarterectomy is appropriate for those patients with carotid stenosis > 80% without symptoms or stenosis > 60% with symptoms (based on duplex ultrasound evaluation)
  - Indications for carotid angioplasty and stenting are controversial; asymptomatic patients with multiple comorbidities and contralateral occlusion may be most appropriate, but long-term data unavailable
  - Long-term antiplatelet therapy, antihypertensive agents, angiotensin-converting inhibitors, and statin therapy are important adjuncts to surgical revascularization

- **Pearl**

Only one in four untreated patients with > 70% stenosis will have a stroke; of patients found to have 100% occlusion, only half will have suffered a neurologic event historically.

Reference

Howell GM, Makaroun MS, Chaer RA. Current management of extracranial carotid occlusive disease. J Am Coll Surg 2009;208:442. [PMID: 19318007]

Diverticulitis

- **Essentials of Diagnosis**
  - Approximately 10–25% of patients with diverticula develop diverticulitis over their lifetime
  - Acute, intermittent cramping left lower abdominal pain with change in bowel habits (often constipation alternating with diarrhea), low-grade fever, and leukocytosis
  - A tender, palpable abdominal mass may be present on examination
  - Abdominal distension with nausea and vomiting may be present due to associated ileus or obstruction from inflammation
  - Symptoms of fistulization to bladder (pneumaturia, fecaluria) or vagina (foul-smelling drainage or passage of stool from vagina) may be present in long-standing disease
  - CT scan is diagnostic method of choice; water-soluble contrast should be used instead of barium if perforation suspected
  - Consider cystography or cystoscopy if concern for urinary fistula
  - Endoscopy not useful in the acute setting

- **Differential Diagnosis**
  - Colorectal carcinoma; appendicitis; urinary tract infection
  - Colonic obstruction; ischemic or infectious colitis
  - Pelvic inflammatory disease
  - Ruptured ectopic pregnancy or ovarian cyst
  - Inflammatory bowel disease; nephrolithiasis

- **Treatment**
  - Liquid diet (10 days) and 7- to 10-day course of oral antibiotics (metronidazole plus fluoroquinolone) for mild first attack
  - Nasogastric suction and broad-spectrum intravenous antibiotics for patients requiring hospitalization
  - Percutaneous catheter drainage for intra-abdominal abscess
  - Emergent laparotomy with colonic resection and diversion for generalized peritonitis, perforation, clinical deterioration
  - High-residue diet, stool softener, psyllium for chronic therapy
  - Elective sigmoid colectomy for recurrent attacks or complicated diverticulitis treated with drainage and intravenous antibiotics
  - Elective colonoscopy after resolution of inflammation to ensure no underlying mass or inflammatory bowel disease

17

- **Pearl**

A disease of low-fiber diet; this condition, as well as appendicitis, is seldom encountered in societies ingesting large amounts of fiber.

Reference

Touzios JG, Dozois EJ. Diverticulosis and acute diverticulitis. Gastroenterol Clin North Am 2009;38:513. [PMID: 19699411]

Functional Intestinal Obstruction (Adynamic Ileus, Paralytic Ileus)

- ■ Essentials of Diagnosis
  - Severely impaired transit of intestinal contents due to decreased peristalsis in the absence of mechanical obstruction
  - Most commonly occurs after surgery, but also in the setting of peritonitis, intra-abdominal infection or inflammation (eg, pancreatitis), critical illness, electrolyte derangements, narcotic use, anticholinergic drugs, pneumonia, uremia
  - Progressive abdominal pain, anorexia, vomiting, and obstipation
  - Minimal abdominal tenderness; decreased to absent bowel sounds
  - Radiographic images show diffuse gastrointestinal distention, no obvious transition point, and air in the rectum; consider CT if plain films are equivocal

- ■ Differential Diagnosis
  - Mechanical obstruction due to any cause
  - Perforated viscus; intra-abdominal abscess
  - Colonic pseudo-obstruction (Ogilvie's syndrome)

- ■ Treatment
  - Resolution may not occur for 7–10 days
  - Restriction of oral intake including oral medications; nasogastric suction in those with protracted vomiting or gastric distension
  - Minimize narcotics and anticholinergic drugs; prokinetic drugs (metoclopramide, erythromycin) if no evidence of obstruction
  - Early ambulation and gum chewing may shorten course
  - Attention to electrolyte disorders (eg, hypokalemia) and dehydration; consider parenteral nutrition
  - For Ogilvie's syndrome, decompressive colonoscopy or intravenous neostigmine can be considered; however, neostigmine should only be administered in an intensive care unit
  - Serial abdominal radiographs to measure intestinal distension (risk of cecal perforation significantly increased when > 11 cm)
  - Surgical intervention indicated if evidence of obstruction, perforation, or bowel ischemia

- ■ Pearl

In any ileus, look at the chest film carefully; lower lobe pneumonia may be the cause.

Reference

Batke M, Cappell MS. Adynamic ileus and acute colonic pseudo-obstruction. Med Clin North Am 2008;92:649, ix. [PMID: 18387380]

Inguinal Hernia

■ Essentials of Diagnosis

- A weakness in the abdominal wall results in the protrusion of structures (ie, adipose tissue, viscus) through the defect
- Usually presents as a mass or swelling in the groin; can be associated with sudden pain and bulging during heavy lifting or straining
- 95% of groin hernias involve the inguinal canal; 5% involve the femoral canal; typically asymptomatic and found on routine screening; discomfort worse at end of the day, relieved when patient reclines and hernia reduces
- Indirect hernias, which develop through the internal inguinal ring and lie lateral to the inferior epigastric vessels, are likely congenital
- Direct hernias are more common, lie medial to the inferior epigastric vessels, and result from weakness in the inguinal floor
- Femoral hernias, the least common, are most likely to present as surgical emergencies
- Early symptoms of incarceration are those of partial bowel obstruction (vomiting, distention, obstipation)
- Incarcerated hernias cannot be reduced and may be tender; strangulated hernias are warm and erythematous due to underlying ischemia
- Always examine patients in the standing position as well as supine to allow the hernia sac to fill

■ Differential Diagnosis

- Hydrocele; varicocele; inguinal lymphadenopathy
- Testicular torsion; femoral artery aneurysm

■ Treatment

- Most should be repaired unless various conditions preclude
- Elective outpatient surgical repair for reducible hernias
- Attempt reduction of incarcerated (irreducible) hernias when peritoneal signs are absent with conscious sedation, Trendelenburg position, and steady, gentle pressure; if reduction unsuccessful, operation within 6–12 hours of presentation is usually necessary
- Strangulated hernias require immediate operation and broad-spectrum antibiotic coverage

■ Pearl

In inguinal hernia, incarceration or strangulation occurs in 1% per year; this fact may guide a patient's preference for elective repair.

Reference

Amato B, et al. Shouldice technique versus other open techniques for inguinal hernia repair. Cochrane Database Syst Rev 2009:CD001543. [PMID: 19821279]

17

Malignant Tumors of the Esophagus

- ■ Essentials of Diagnosis
  - Early cancers rarely present with symptoms
  - Progressive dysphagia—initially during ingestion of solid foods, later with liquids with retrosternal pain; weight loss ominous; hoarseness and productive cough may indicate invasion into the laryngeal nerves or tracheobronchial tree
  - Smoking and alcohol associated with squamous cell carcinoma (proximal and mid-esophagus); obesity, Barrett's esophagus, and gastroesophageal reflux associated with adenocarcinoma (distal esophagus and gastroesophageal junction); adenocarcinoma more common
  - Barium esophagram is diagnostic procedure of choice and typically shows irregular mucosal pattern or concentrically narrowed esophageal lumen
  - Endoscopy can allow for tumor visualization, biopsy, and endoscopic ultrasound to determine the depth of the lesion
  - CT scan with positron emission tomography (PET) delineates extent of disease and distant metastases

- ■ Differential Diagnosis
  - Benign esophageal tumor or stricture
  - Esophageal diverticulum or web; achalasia; globus hystericus

- ■ Treatment
  - Tumor invasion or metastasis at time of presentation precludes cure in most
  - Open surgical approaches, either transthoracic (Ivor-Lewis) or transhiatal, are most commonly used, but minimally invasive techniques are gaining favor; endoscopic mucosal resection may be an option for very early disease
  - Chemoradiation followed by surgical resection indicated for advanced disease (T2–4, N1), but 5-year survival remains 40%
  - Therapies focused on reducing dysphagia and maintaining oral intake include expandable metallic stent placement, laser fulguration, feeding tube placement, and radiation therapy.

- ■ Pearl

Food sticking upon swallowing is nearly always associated with an anatomic explanation, often a tumor: take this symptom seriously.

Reference
Quiros RM, Bui CL. Multidisciplinary approach to esophageal and gastric cancer. Surg Clin North Am 2009;89:79, viii. [PMID: 19186232]

Mesenteric Ischemia

- **Essentials of Diagnosis**

    Acute:
    - Emboli commonly due to atrial fibrillation, myocardial infarction; often lodges in the superior mesenteric artery
    - Nonocclusive insufficiency is due to a low flow state, frequently seen with heart failure, hypovolemia, and vasopressor use
    - Venous occlusion leading to arterial insufficiency is associated with hypercoagulable states, pancreatitis, and portal hypertension
    - Pain out of proportion to exam present in 95%
    - Usually history of atherosclerotic vascular disease with stigmata of vascular disease present on exam (eg, diminished pulses)
    - Labs normal early; leukocytosis and elevated lactate occur later
    - CT scan confirms the diagnosis in 90%; angiography is more accurate and may allow for catheter-based thrombolytic therapy

    Chronic:
    - Results from atherosclerotic plaques of superior mesenteric, celiac axis, and inferior mesenteric; more than one of these major arteries must be involved because of collateral circulation
    - Epigastric or periumbilical postprandial pain; patients limit intake to avoid pain, with weight loss and less pain
    - Patients typically have a history of smoking, peripheral vascular disease, and hypertension; 50% have abdominal bruit

    Ischemic colitis:
    - Colonic ischemia due to inferior mesenteric artery or hypogastric arterial insufficiency secondary to a low flow state; episodic bouts of crampy lower abdominal pain and mild, often bloody diarrhea

- **Differential Diagnosis**

    - Diverticulitis; appendicitis; pancreatitis; cholecystitis
    - Inflammatory bowel disease and colitis due to other causes
    - Visceral malignancy; polyarteritis nodosa; renal colic
    - Expanding aortic aneurysm; aortic dissection

- **Treatment**

    - Goals of laparotomy: removal of necrotic bowel, salvage remaining bowel, and preserve intestinal length
    - Surgical embolectomy or bypass of the occluded portion of the superior mesenteric artery
    - Intra-arterial papaverine in some with nonocclusive ischemia

17

- **Pearl**

Chronic nonocclusive mesenteric ischemia is a commonly overlooked cause of weight loss in patients with peripheral vascular disease.

Reference

Herbert GS, Steele SR. Acute and chronic mesenteric ischemia. Surg Clin North Am 2007;87:1115, ix. [PMID: 17936478]

Pancreatic Pseudocyst

- ■ Essentials of Diagnosis
  - • Organized collection of pancreatic fluid in or around the pancreas; may complicate acute or chronic pancreatitis
  - • The majority (80%) of pancreatic fluid collections that occur < 8 weeks after the inciting event will resolve spontaneously
  - • Symptomatic Pseudocysts are typically 6 cm and present for more than 6 weeks
  - • Symptoms are associated with local mass effect and local inflammation and include occasional fever, epigastric pain with back radiation, early satiety
  - • Leukocytosis, persistent serum amylase elevation may be present; however, laboratory studies can be normal
  - • Pancreatic cyst demonstrated by sonography or CT scan
  - • Complications include hemorrhage (erosion into pancreatic vessels), infection, rupture, fistula formation, pancreatic ascites, obstruction of adjacent structures (gastric outlet, bowel)

- ■ Differential Diagnosis
  - • Pancreatic phlegmon or abscess; aortic aneurysm
  - • Sterile pancreatic necrosis; resolving pancreatitis
  - • Pancreatic carcinoma and cystic neoplasms

- ■ Treatment
  - • Up to two-thirds spontaneously resolve; no intervention for uncomplicated acute fluid collections or asymptomatic pseudocysts
  - • Avoidance of alcohol; treatment of other causes of the initial pancreatitis (eg, hypertriglyceridemia, medications, gallstones)
  - • Percutaneous catheter drainage associated with complications; only consider in patients with symptomatic pseudocysts who cannot undergo endoscopic or surgical intervention due to comorbidities and with normal ductal anatomy
  - • ERCP with sphincterotomy and pancreatic duct stent for proximal decompression can aid in spontaneous resolution
  - • Decompression into an adjacent hollow viscus (stomach, duodenum, jejunum) may be necessary and can be performed via endoscopic or surgical (laparoscopic or open) techniques
  - • Octreotide to inhibit pancreatic secretion not of benefit

17

- ■ Pearl

There are only two pathologic causes of pulsatile abdominal masses: transmission through a pancreatic pseudocyst and aortic aneurysm.

Reference

Cannon JW, Callery MP, Vollmer CM Jr. Diagnosis and management of pancreatic pseudocysts: what is the evidence? J Am Coll Surg 2009;209:385. [PMID: 19717045]

Pharyngoesophageal Diverticulum (Zenker's Diverticulum)

- ■ Essentials of Diagnosis
  - • Most prevalent in the fifth to eighth decades of life
  - • Results from herniation of the mucosa through a weak point in the muscle layer between the oblique fibers of the thyropharyngeus and the horizontal fibers of the cricopharyngeus (Killian's triangle)
  - • Dysphagia is present in 90% of patients and worsens as the pouch enlarges; other symptoms include regurgitation of undigested food, halitosis, hoarseness, chronic cough, malnutrition, and weight loss
  - • Gurgling sounds in the neck on auscultation are pathognomonic; cervical crepitus occasionally present
  - • Barium swallow confirms diagnosis by demonstrating the sac

- ■ Differential Diagnosis
  - • Esophageal, mediastinal, or neck tumor
  - • Esophageal duplication cyst
  - • Cricopharyngeal achalasia (occasionally associated)
  - • Esophageal web
  - • Achalasia or lower esophageal stricture
  - • Epiphrenic diverticulum (lower esophagus)
  - • Cervical osteophyte
  - • Thyroid mass

- ■ Treatment
  - • Untreated Zenker's diverticula can lead to bezoar, tracheal fistula, vocal cord paralysis, fistula to the paravertebral ligament leading to cervical osteomyelitis, peptic ulceration, and hemorrhage
  - • There is no medical therapy; all patients should be considered candidates for cricopharyngeal myotomy extending onto the esophagus with either a diverticulopexy (< 2 cm) or a diverticular resection (> 2 cm)
  - • Endoscopic techniques can be used in a subset of patients and include division of the septum between the diverticulum and the esophagus and the underlying cricopharyngeal muscle

17

- ■ Pearl

Unsuspected Zenker's diverticulum may be inadvertently perforated at upper endoscopy, a reason to consider contrast radiography before elective esophagoduodenostomy.

Reference

Ferreira LE, Simmons DT, Baron TH. Zenker's diverticula: pathophysiology, clinical presentation, and flexible endoscopic management. Dis Esophagus 2008;21:1. [PMID: 18197932]

Small Bowel Obstruction (SBO)

- ■ Essentials of Diagnosis
  - • Partial or complete obstruction of the intestinal lumen by an intrinsic or extrinsic lesion
  - • Etiology: Adhesions (eg, from prior surgery or pelvic inflammatory disease) 60%, malignancy 20%, hernia 10%, inflammatory bowel disease 5%, volvulus 3%, other (eg, gallstone ileus) 2%
  - • Crampy or colicky abdominal pain, vomiting (often feculent in complete obstruction), abdominal distention, constipation, or obstipation; absence of flatus may indicate complete obstruction
  - • Distended, tender abdomen with or without peritoneal signs; high-pitched tinkling or peristaltic rushes audible
  - • Patients often intravascularly volume-depleted secondary to emesis, decreased oral intake, and sequestration of fluid into the bowel wall, bowel lumen, and the peritoneal cavity
  - • Plain films of the abdomen show dilated small bowel with more than three air-fluid levels; contrast-enhanced CT scan can reveal evidence of bowel ischemia (thickened walls, pneumatosis, mesenteric inflammation)

- ■ Differential Diagnosis
  - • Adynamic ileus due to any cause (eg, hypokalemia, pancreatitis, nephrolithiasis, recent operation or trauma)
  - • Colonic obstruction
  - • Intestinal pseudo-obstruction
  - • Spontaneous bacterial peritonitis

- ■ Treatment
  - • Nasogastric suction
  - • Fluid and electrolyte (potassium, magnesium, phosphorus) replacement with isotonic crystalloid, and close monitoring of urine output
  - • The decision for surgical intervention based on the degree of obstruction (partial vs. complete), etiology of obstruction (50% of adhesion-related obstructions resolve spontaneously), and concern for bowel strangulation and necrosis
  - • Surgical exploration indicated for suspected strangulated hernia, obstruction not responsive to conservative therapy, or the development of peritoneal signs

- ■ Pearl

  Although Osler referred to adhesions as "the refuge of the diagnostically destitute," they remain the most common cause of small bowel obstruction.

Reference

Cappell MS, Batke M. Mechanical obstruction of the small bowel and colon. Med Clin North Am 2008;92:575, viii. [PMID: 18387377]

17

18

Common Pediatric Disorders[*]

Acute Lymphoblastic Leukemia (ALL)

- Essentials of Diagnosis
  - Cause of childhood leukemias; peak at ages 2–6 years
  - Chromosomal abnormalities (eg, Down's syndrome)
  - Intermittent fever, bone pain, petechiae, purpura, pallor, mild splenomegaly without hepatomegaly, and lymphadenopathy
  - Anemia and thrombocytopenia are common; leukocyte counts often less than 10,000/μL; lymphocytes described as atypical
  - Bone marrow shows homogeneous infiltration of more than 25% of leukemic blasts; most express common ALL antigen (CALLA)

- Differential Diagnosis
  - Epstein-Barr virus (EBV) or cytomegalovirus infection
  - Immune thrombocytopenic purpura
  - Aplastic anemia

- Treatment
  - Induction with prednisone, vincristine, asparaginase, and occasionally daunorubicin; intrathecal methotrexate and/or cytarabine if at high risk for relapse
  - CNS therapy (intrathecal chemotherapy, sometimes cranial irradiation) to treat lymphoblasts present in meninges and to prevent CNS relapse
  - Maintenance therapy with mercaptopurine, weekly methotrexate, and monthly vincristine or prednisone
  - Bone marrow transplant considered in selected patients
  - Younger children, WBC > 100,000 have worse prognosis; likewise t(9;22) and t(4;11) translocations

- Pearl

Back pain with bilateral leg radiation may be the presenting feature of acute leukemia; there should be a high index of suspicion for this curable condition if there are systemic symptoms.

Reference

Pui CH, Robison LL, Look AT. Acute lymphoblastic leukaemia. Lancet 2008;371:1030. [PMID: 18358930]

* The following common childhood diseases are discussed in other chapters: aspiration of foreign body and cystic fibrosis, Chapter 2; pharyngitis, mumps, poliomyelitis, varicella and zoster, infectious mononucleosis, rabies, and rubella, Chapter 8; appendicitis, Chapter 17; otitis media and otitis externa, Chapter 21.

Bacterial Meningitis

- **Essentials of Diagnosis**
    - Signs of systemic illness (fever, malaise, poor feeding); headache, stiff neck, and altered mental status in older children
    - In infants and young children, signs of meningeal irritation (Kernig's and Brudzinski's signs) may be absent
    - Predisposing factors include ear infection, sinusitis, recent neurosurgical procedures, and skull fracture
    - No symptom or sign reliably distinguishes bacterial cause from meningitis due to viruses, fungi, or other pathogens
    - Organisms depend upon the age
    - Age less than 2 months: Group B or D streptococci, gram-negative bacilli, *Listeria*
    - Ages 2 months to 12 years: *Haemophilus influenzae, Streptococcus pneumoniae,* and *Neisseria meningitidis*
    - Cerebrospinal fluid shows elevated protein, low glucose, elevated WBC (> 1000/μL) with a high percent of neutrophils (> 50%)
    - Gram stain and culture often lead to the definitive diagnosis

- **Differential Diagnosis**
    - Meningitis due to nonbacterial organisms
    - Brain abscess; encephalitis
    - Sepsis without meningitis; intracranial mass or hemorrhage

- **Treatment**
    - Prompt empiric antibiotics can be life-saving; exact regimen depends on patient's age; therapy narrowed once susceptibilities known
    - Concomitant dexamethasone decreases morbidity and mortality in patients with meningitis secondary to *H. influenzae;* unclear benefit if meningitis is due to other bacterial causes
    - Patients monitored for acidosis, syndrome of inappropriate secretion of antidiuretic hormone, and hypoglycemia
    - Coagulopathies may require platelets and fresh-frozen plasma
    - Mortality can be up to 10% in neonates; severe neurologic sequelae may occur in 10–25% of affected patients

18

- **Pearl**

In an ill-appearing child with fever and headache, lumbar puncture, blood culture, and antibiotics should precede a CT scan; modern imaging techniques have made this sequence as much the exception as the rule.

Reference

Mongelluzzo J, et al. Corticosteroids and mortality in children with bacterial meningitis. JAMA 2008;299:2048. [PMID: 18460665]

Colic

- ## Essentials of Diagnosis
    - A syndrome characterized by severe and paroxysmal crying that usually worsens in the late afternoon and evening
    - Abdomen sometimes distended, the facies pained, fists often clenched; infant unresponsive to soothing
    - An abnormal sensitivity of the gastrointestinal tract to stimuli may contribute to its pathogenesis, but its exact etiology is unknown
    - Most cases present between the ages of 1–3 months

- ## Differential Diagnosis
    - Normal crying in an infant
    - Intussusception
    - Volvulus
    - Gastroenteritis
    - Constipation
    - Any illness in the infant causing distress (eg, otitis media, corneal abrasion)
    - Food allergy

- ## Treatment
    - Reassurance to parents; education regarding the baby's cues
    - Elimination of cow's milk from formula (or from the mother's diet if she is nursing) in refractory cases to rule out milk protein allergy
    - Soothing with massage, creating a comfortable environment (eg, playing soothing music), avoidance of overfeeding may be useful adjuncts
    - Hypoallergenic diet and soy formula have not been demonstrated to have clear benefit, but may be helpful in difficult cases
    - Phenobarbital elixir and dicyclomine not recommended

- ## Pearl

Rule of Threes: during the first 3 months, a healthy infant cries more than 3 hours a day, for more than 3 days a week, for more than 3 weeks—though to first-time parents this seems a gross underestimation.

18

Reference

Cohen-Silver J, Ratnapalan S. Management of infantile colic: a review. Clin Pediatr (Phila) 2009;48(1):14. [PMID: 18832537]

Constipation

- **Essentials of Diagnosis**
  - Defined as infrequent bowel movements associated with difficulty passing; stools are often hard in consistency
  - Can lead to painful defecation and eventually stool withholding and encopresis
  - May be caused by anatomic abnormalities, neurologic problems, or endocrine disorders; in most cases, however, no cause is identified
  - A positive family history may be elicited
  - Rectal examination to evaluate fissures and assess rectal tone
  - Abdominal radiograph may confirm the diagnosis

- **Differential Diagnosis**
  - Hirschsprung's disease
  - Hypothyroidism
  - Hyperparathyroidism
  - Congenital gastrointestinal malformation
  - Infantile botulism
  - Lead intoxication

- **Treatment**
  - Impacted children will usually require a clean-out; although enemas are sometimes used, severe impaction may require oral polyethylene glycol electrolyte solution
  - Mainstay of therapy is behavioral; long course of toilet sitting and positive feedback necessary; biofeedback may be helpful
  - Close follow-up with families for support is critical
  - Dietary changes (increased fiber and lower milk and caffeine intake) usually beneficial
  - Mineral oil titrated to one or two soft stools per day is a recommended first-line agent
  - Lactulose or docusate sodium may be useful in difficult cases
  - Laxatives should not be used as a long-term solution
  - Families need to be reassured that functional constipation is difficult to cure and that months to years of treatment may be necessary

18

- **Pearl**

Regarding constipation and diarrhea, children complain of these symptoms far less often than adults; it may result in overlooking a systemic cause for either condition.

Reference

Pijpers MA, Tabbers MM, Benninga MA, Berger MY. Currently recommended treatments of childhood constipation are not evidence based: a systematic literature review on the effect of laxative treatment and dietary measures. Arch Dis Child 2009;94:117. [PMID: 18713795]

Croup

- **Essentials of Diagnosis**
    - Affects children predominantly between ages 3 months and 5 years; more common during fall and winter
    - Children often febrile, but not toxic appearing
    - Barking cough, stridor, and hoarseness following upper respiratory infection symptoms, typically worse at night
    - Lateral neck films can be useful; viral croup may show subglottic narrowing (steeple sign), normal epiglottis
    - Direct laryngoscopy may cause airway obstruction if bacterial epiglottitis present
    - Croup may recur, but usually lessens in severity with age as airway diameter increases

- **Differential Diagnosis**
    - Foreign body in the esophagus or larynx
    - Retropharyngeal abscess
    - Epiglottitis

- **Treatment**
    - Mist therapy utility is anecdotal
    - Corticosteroids reduce the number of return visits to the emergency department, but may not shorten course of disease
    - Oxygen and racemic epinephrine are accepted therapy

- **Pearl**

Every mother knows that a walk with a child in the cool night air is the treatment of choice.

Reference

Bjornson CL, Johnson DW. Croup. Lancet 2008;371:329. [PMID: 18295000]

18

Down's Syndrome

- ■ Essentials of Diagnosis
  - • Occurs in 1:600–800 newborns, with increasing incidence in children of mothers over 35 years of age
  - • Ninety-five percent of patients have 47 chromosomes with trisomy 21
  - • Characteristic findings include small, broad head; upward slanting palpebral fissures; inner epicanthal folds; speckled irides (Brushfield's spots); flat nasal bridge; transverse palmar crease (simian crease); and short hands
  - • One-third to one-half have congenital heart disease (AV canal defects most common)
  - • Atlantoaxial subluxation and sensorineural hearing loss more frequent than in the general population
  - • Leukemia is 20 times more common, and there is an increased susceptibility to infections

- ■ Differential Diagnosis
  - • There is none; the combination of phenotypic abnormalities and chromosomal analysis confirms the diagnosis

- ■ Treatment
  - • Goal of therapy is to help affected patients develop full potential
  - • Therapy directed toward correction of specific problems (eg, cardiac surgery, antibiotics)
  - • No evidence exists to support use of megadoses of vitamins or intensive exercise programs
  - • Electrocardiography and echocardiography in the neonatal period to evaluate for congenital heart disease
  - • Cervical spine radiography recommended once during the preschool years to evaluate for atlantoaxial instability
  - • Patients with Down's syndrome should have annual vision and hearing examinations and thyroid screening

- ■ Pearl

  Chromosome 21 codes the beta-amyloid seen ubiquitously in small vessels in Down's patients' brains and in those adults with amyloid angiopathy; it is also responsible for the plaque in Alzheimer's disease.

18

Reference

Davidson MA. Primary care for children and adolescents with Down syndrome. Pediatr Clin North Am 2008;55:1099. [PMID: 18929054]

Enuresis

- ■ Essentials of Diagnosis
  - Involuntary urination at an age at which control is expected (cognitive age of approximately 5 years), mostly occurring at night
  - Primary enuresis occurs in children who have never had control and accounts for nearly 90% of cases; secondary in children with at least 6 months of prior control
  - Symptoms must be present at least twice per week for at least 6 months to make the diagnosis
  - Approximately 75% of children with enuresis have at least one parent who had similar difficulties as a child
  - Affects 7% of boys and 3% of girls at age 5; decreasing to 3% of boys and 2% of girls by age 10
  - Secondary enuresis often caused by psychosocial stressors
  - Medical problems, including urinary tract infection and diabetes mellitus, must be excluded

- ■ Differential Diagnosis
  - Urinary tract infection
  - Diabetes mellitus
  - Congenital genitourinary anomalies
  - Constipation
  - Child abuse
  - Behavioral difficulties

- ■ Treatment
  - Therapy for causative medical problems
  - Support and positive reinforcement for children and families
  - Fluid restriction and bladder emptying before bedtime
  - Alarm systems effective, but may take weeks to work
  - Desmopressin works quickly but does not provide long-term control
  - Imipramine not recommended due to side effects and overdose potential

- ■ Pearl

Clinical, developmental, and family histories, as well as awareness of the environment of the family, are crucial to help patients deal with this disorder.

18

Reference

van Dommelen P, Kamphuis M, van Leerdam FJ, de Wilde JA, Rijpstra A, Campagne AE, Verkerk PH. The short- and long-term effects of simple behavioral interventions for nocturnal enuresis in young children: a randomized controlled trial. J Pediatr 2009;154:662. [PMID: 19167725]

Febrile Seizures

- ### Essentials of Diagnosis
  - Occur in 2–5% of children
  - Peak between 14 and 18 months of age; most common between age 9 months and 5 years
  - Last less than 15 minutes, are generalized, and occur in developmentally normal children
  - Seizures lasting more than 15 minutes, persistent neurologic deficits, or recurrent seizures are considered complex
  - The development of a febrile seizure is associated with the rate of rise of the child's temperature, not the temperature's peak
  - Risk factors include positive family history or previous personal history of febrile seizures
  - One in three will have a recurrent seizure, 75% within a year
  - Risk of developing epilepsy is approximately 1% in children without risk factors; up to 9% of children with risk factors (eg, positive family history, atypical seizure type or duration, underlying neurologic disease) will develop epilepsy

- ### Differential Diagnosis
  - Meningitis
  - Encephalitis
  - Intracranial hemorrhage
  - Intracranial tumor
  - Trauma

- ### Treatment
  - No treatment for simple febrile seizures
  - Electroencephalography not recommended in the initial evaluation
  - Lumbar puncture indicated in children under 12 months of age if no source of infection can be found
  - Prophylactic anticonvulsants may lower the risk of recurrence, but are not recommended routinely

- ### Pearl

18

Though seen in a relatively small number of children, it is always reasonable to obtain a CT or MRI of the brain after any first-time seizure.

Reference

Steering Committee on Quality Improvement and Management, Subcommittee on Febrile Seizures American Academy of Pediatrics. Febrile seizures: clinical practice guideline for the long-term management of the child with simple febrile seizures. Pediatrics 2008;121:1281. [PMID: 18519501]

Henoch-Schönlein Purpura (Anaphylactoid Purpura)

- ■ Essentials of Diagnosis
  - • A small-vessel vasculitis affecting skin, gastrointestinal tract, and kidney
  - • Typically occurs between ages 2 and 8 years; boys affected more often than girls (2:1); occasionally observed in adults
  - • Two-thirds of patients have a preceding upper respiratory tract infection
  - • Skin lesions often begin as urticaria and progress to a maculopapular eruption, finally becoming a symmetric purpuric rash that often begins on the buttocks and lower extremities
  - • Eighty percent develop migratory polyarthralgias or polyarthritis; edema of the hands, feet, scalp, and periorbital areas occurs commonly
  - • Colicky abdominal pain occurs in two-thirds, and it may be complicated by intussusception
  - • Renal involvement in 25–50%
  - • Platelet count, prothrombin time, and partial thromboplastin time normal; urinalysis may reveal hematuria and proteinuria; serum IgA often elevated

- ■ Differential Diagnosis
  - • Immune thrombocytopenic purpura
  - • Meningococcemia
  - • Rocky Mountain spotted fever
  - • Other hypersensitivity vasculitides
  - • Juvenile rheumatoid arthritis
  - • Kawasaki's disease
  - • Child abuse

- ■ Treatment
  - • Pain medications and NSAIDs to treat joint pain and inflammation
  - • Corticosteroid therapy may decrease duration of abdominal pain, but does not appear to alter skin or renal manifestations
  - • No satisfactory specific treatment
  - • Prognosis is generally good; less than 1% of patients have residual renal disease

18

- ■ Pearl

  Although superficially confused with thrombocytopenic purpura, when palpable, it is always vasculitis, at any age.

Reference

Ronkainen J, Koskimies O, Ala-Houhala M, et al. Early prednisone therapy in Henoch-Schönlein purpura: a randomized, double-blind, placebo-controlled trial. J Pediatr 2006;149:241. [PMID: 16887443]

Intussusception

- **Essentials of Diagnosis**
  - Telescoping of one part of the bowel into another, leading to edema, hemorrhage, ischemia, and eventually infarction
  - The most common cause of intestinal obstruction in the first 6 years of life; boys are affected more commonly than girls (4:1)
  - Majority (80%) of cases occur before 2 years of age
  - Lead points include hypertrophied Peyer's patches, intestinal polyps, lymphoma, or other tumors; in children over 6, lymphoma most common lesion
  - Most (90%) are ileocolic; ileoileal or colocolic may occur
  - Symptoms include intermittent colicky abdominal pain, vomiting, and bloody stool (currant jelly stools); children are often asymptomatic between bouts of pain
  - Plain films may show signs of obstruction, but a barium or air-barium enema is the standard for diagnosis

- **Differential Diagnosis**
  - Volvulus
  - Incarcerated hernia
  - Acute appendicitis
  - Acute gastroenteritis
  - Urinary tract infection
  - Small bowel obstruction due to other cause
  - Henoch-Schönlein purpura

- **Treatment**
  - Patients stabilized with fluid; decompressed with a nasogastric tube
  - Surgical consultation to exclude perforation
  - Air-barium enema has a reduction rate of up to 90%, but it is never performed if perforation is suspected; reduction by enema may result in perforation in 1%
  - If perforation occurs or if enema fails, surgical decompression may be necessary
  - Recurs in up to 10% of cases if reduced via enema, usually in the first day after reduction; recurrence rate after surgical reduction is between 2% and 5%

- **Pearl**

At first resembling colic, increasing lethargy and blood in the stool suggests this as the explanation.

Reference

McCollough M, Sharieff GQ. Abdominal pain in children. Pediatr Clin North Am 2006;53:107. [PMID: 16487787]

Juvenile Rheumatoid Arthritis (Still's Disease)

- ■ Essentials of Diagnosis
  - • Useful diagnostic criteria: Age of onset less than 16 years; duration greater than 6 weeks; true arthritis must be present; other etiologies that cause arthritis must be excluded
  - • Three types: Oligoarticular, polyarticular, and systemic
  - • Oligoarticular: Fewer than five joints involved, predominantly large joints in the lower extremities
  - • Polyarticular: More than five joints involved; affects both large and small joints; rheumatoid nodules are often present
  - • Systemic: Arthritis characterized by quotidian fever; fevers may be accompanied by evanescent salmon-colored rash; pervasive visceral involvement including hepatosplenomegaly, lymphadenopathy, and serositis
  - • Erythrocyte sedimentation rate, C-reactive protein often elevated but nonspecific; antinuclear antibody elevated in 40–85% of cases, more commonly in oligo- and polyarthritis

- ■ Differential Diagnosis
  - • Rheumatic fever; infective arthritis; Lyme disease
  - • Reactive arthritis due to various causes
  - • Systemic lupus erythematosus; dermatomyositis; leukemia
  - • Inflammatory bowel disease; bone tumors; osteomyelitis

- ■ Treatment
  - • Stepwise approach to therapy is essential; goals of treatment are to restore joint function and relieve pain
  - • NSAIDs and physical therapy are the mainstays
  - • Methotrexate, hydroxychloroquine, sulfasalazine, and local corticosteroid injections for those symptomatic after NSAIDs
  - • Azathioprine, cyclophosphamide, and systemic steroids may be necessary for treatment of refractory cases

- ■ Pearl

Articular disease is more commonly found in children; in adults, the presentation may be that of fever of unknown origin and is elusive to diagnose.

18

Reference

Frosch M, Roth J. New insights in systemic juvenile idiopathic arthritis—from pathophysiology to treatment. Rheumatology (Oxford) 2008;47:121. [PMID: 17971384]

Kawasaki's Disease
(Mucocutaneous Lymph Node Syndrome)

- ■ Essentials of Diagnosis
  - Illness of unknown etiology characterized by sometimes severe vasculitis primarily of medium-sized arteries; 80% of cases occur before the age of 5 years
  - Criteria for diagnosis include fever for 5 days and at least four of the following: Bilateral nonexudative conjunctivitis; involvement of mucous membranes (eg, fissuring of lips, strawberry tongue); cervical lymphadenopathy of at least 1.5 cm; rash; and changes in extremities (edema, desquamation)
  - Arthritis common
  - Cardiovascular complications include myocarditis, pericarditis, and arteritis predisposing to coronary artery aneurysm formation
  - Acute myocardial infarction may occur; 1–2% of patients die from this complication during the initial phase of the disease
  - Thrombocytosis, elevated sedimentation rate typical
  - Patients require echocardiogram to evaluate for coronary aneurysms
  - No specific test is yet available; the diagnosis of Kawasaki's disease is based on clinical criteria and exclusion of other possibilities

- ■ Differential Diagnosis
  - Acute rheumatic fever
  - Juvenile rheumatoid arthritis
  - Viral exanthems
  - Infectious mononucleosis
  - Streptococcal pharyngitis
  - Measles
  - Toxic shock syndrome

- ■ Treatment
  - Intravenous immune globulin and high-dose aspirin are the mainstays of therapy
  - Role of corticosteroids is controversial and is not considered first-line therapy

- ■ Pearl

Kawasaki's disease and anomalous origin of the left coronary artery from the pulmonary artery are the most likely causes of Q-wave infarction in childhood; the latter is more likely to be found on an incidental ECG.

Reference

Son MB, Gauvreau K, Ma L, Baker AL, Sundel RP, Fulton DR, Newburger JW. Treatment of Kawasaki disease: analysis of 27 US pediatric hospitals from 2001 to 2006. Pediatrics 2009;124:1. [PMID: 19564276]

18

Otitis Media

- ■ Essentials of Diagnosis
  - • Peak incidence between the ages of 6 months and 3 years
  - • History may include fever, ear pain, and other nonspecific systemic symptoms (eg, vomiting, poor feeding)
  - • Tympanometry shows an opaque, bulging, hyperemic tympanic membrane with a loss of landmarks; pneumatic otoscopy shows loss of mobility
  - • Breastfeeding probably protective
  - • Exposure to tobacco smoke and pacifier use thought to increase incidence; other risk factors include craniofacial or congenital anomalies (eg, cleft palate)
  - • Although caused by viruses, most cases assumed to be bacterial
  - • Bacterial causes are (1) *Streptococcus pneumoniae,* 40–50%; (2) *Haemophilus influenzae,* 20–30%; (3) *Moraxella catarrhalis,* 10–15%

- ■ Differential Diagnosis
  - • Otitis externa
  - • Cholesteatoma
  - • Foreign body

- ■ Treatment
  - • Treatment controversial; most children with otitis media not treated in Europe
  - • CDC recommendations: (1) Children > 2 years not in day care and not exposed to antibiotics in the last 3 months, amoxicillin 40–45 mg/kg per day for 5 days; (2) children < 2 years in day care or with recent antibiotic exposure, high-dose amoxicillin 80–100 mg/kg per day for 10 days; (3) second-line therapy includes amoxicillin clavulanate, cefuroxime, or intramuscular ceftriaxone
  - • Three or more episodes in 6 months or four episodes in a year warrant prophylactic antibiotics; tympanostomy tubes considered with persistent infection

- ■ Pearl

Nasotracheal intubation is an overlooked cause of otitis media—it is caused by obstruction of the eustachian tube.

18

Reference

Ramakrishnan K, Sparks RA, Berryhill WE. Diagnosis and treatment of otitis media. Am Fam Physician 2007;76:1650. [PMID: 18092706]

Pyloric Stenosis

- **Essentials of Diagnosis**
  - Increase in size of the muscular layer of the pylorus of unknown etiology
  - Occurs in approximately 3 per 1000 births; boys: girls 4:1; Caucasians more commonly affected than African-Americans or Asians
  - Vomiting usually begins between 2 and 8 weeks of age but may occur as early as 1 week of age or as late as 5 months
  - Emesis often described by parents as projectile; rarely bilious
  - Infant is hungry and nurses avidly, but weight gain is poor and growth retardation occurs
  - Dehydration and hypokalemic hypochloremic alkalosis are characteristic
  - Palpable olive-sized mass in the subhepatic region best felt after the child has vomited
  - Ultrasound is 90% sensitive
  - Barium studies, not commonly performed, demonstrate increased pyloric channel and bulge of pyloric muscle into antrum (shoulder sign)

- **Differential Diagnosis**
  - Gastroesophageal reflux disease
  - Esophageal stenosis or achalasia
  - Duodenal stenosis
  - Small bowel obstruction due to other causes
  - Antral web
  - Adrenal insufficiency
  - Pylorospasm
  - Inborn errors of metabolism

- **Treatment**
  - Ramstedt's pyloromyotomy is curative and the treatment of choice
  - Dehydration and electrolyte abnormalities should be corrected before surgery
  - Excellent prognosis after surgery

18

- **Pearl**

Pyloric stenosis: an epigastric mass in a vomiting infant with metabolic alkalosis? Game, set, match for this diagnosis.

Reference

Hall NJ, Pacilli M, Eaton S, et al. Recovery after open versus laparoscopic pyloromyotomy for pyloric stenosis: a double-blind multicentre randomised controlled trial. Lancet 2009;373:390. [PMID: 19155060]

Respiratory Syncytial Virus (RSV) Bronchiolitis

- **Essentials of Diagnosis**
  - The major cause of bronchiolitis and pneumonia in children less than 1 year of age
  - Epidemics with seasonal variability most common from late fall to early spring
  - Clinical presentation of bronchiolitis is characterized by variable fever, cough, tachypnea, diffuse wheezing, inspiratory retractions, and difficulty feeding
  - Apnea may be the presenting symptom, especially in newborns and infants
  - Chest x-ray shows hyperinflation and peribronchiolar thickening with occasional atelectasis
  - RSV antigen detected in nasal or pulmonary secretions is diagnostic
  - Diagnosis often made clinically

- **Differential Diagnosis**
  - Bronchiolitis due to other viruses or bacteria
  - Asthma
  - Community-acquired pneumonia
  - Pertussis
  - Foreign body aspiration
  - Chlamydial pneumonitis
  - Laryngomalacia

- **Treatment**
  - Severely ill children should be hospitalized, given humidified oxygen, and kept in respiratory isolation to prevent spread to other patients
  - Bronchodilator therapy, although usually instituted, has not been demonstrated to reduce the severity of symptoms or shorten the course of disease
  - Corticosteroids considered in hospitalized patients, though they may not reduce symptom severity or shorten disease course
  - Ribavirin may be given to selected patients at very high risk for complications (eg, those with complex congenital heart disease)

18

- **Pearl**

When croup lasts for more than a week, think RSV.

Reference

Yanney M, Vyas H. The treatment of bronchiolitis. Arch Dis Child 2008;93:793. [PMID: 18539685]

Roseola Infantum (Exanthema Subitum)

- ■ Essentials of Diagnosis
  - • A benign illness typically caused by human herpes virus 6, occurring with a peak incidence between 6 and 15 months of age; 95% of cases occur before the third year
  - • Abrupt onset of fever (as high as 40°C) lasting from 3 to 5 days in an otherwise mildly ill child; dissociation between systemic symptoms and febrile course
  - • No conjunctivitis or pharyngeal exudate; mild cough or coryza occasionally present
  - • Fever ceases abruptly; a characteristic rash develops within 12–24 hours after becoming afebrile in 20%, consisting of rose-pink maculopapules beginning on the trunk and spreading outward with disappearance in 1–2 days
  - • Rash may occur without fever

- ■ Differential Diagnosis
  - • Erythema infectiosum
  - • EBV
  - • Measles
  - • Rubella
  - • Enterovirus infection
  - • Scarlet fever
  - • Drug allergy
  - • Kawasaki's disease

- ■ Treatment
  - • Supportive care only; antipyretics for fever control
  - • Reassurance for parents
  - • Febrile seizures occur, but no more commonly than with other self-limited infections
  - • Children are no longer infectious once afebrile

- ■ Pearl

Fever comes, rash comes, fever goes? The diagnosis is roseola.

18

Reference

Caselli E, Di Luca D. Molecular biology and clinical associations of Roseoloviruses human herpesvirus 6 and human herpesvirus 7. New Microbiol 2007;30:173. [PMID: 17802896]

Tetralogy of Fallot

■ Essentials of Diagnosis

- Most common cause of cyanotic heart disease after 1 week of age
- Components include right ventricular outflow tract obstruction, overriding aorta, ventricular septal defect, and right ventricular hypertrophy
- Varying cyanosis after the neonatal period, dyspnea on exertion, easy fatigability, growth retardation
- Exam may be notable for right ventricular lift, harsh systolic ejection murmur maximal at the left sternal border, single loud S_2
- Studies may demonstrate an elevated hematocrit, boot-shaped heart with diminished pulmonary vascularity on chest x-ray
- Echocardiography, cardiac catheterization, and angiocardiography all useful in confirming the diagnosis

■ Differential Diagnosis

Other cyanotic heart diseases:
- Pulmonary atresia with intact ventricular septum
- Tricuspid atresia
- Hypoplastic left heart syndrome
- Complete transposition of the great arteries
- Total anomalous pulmonary venous return
- Persistent truncus arteriosus

■ Treatment

- Acute treatment of cyanotic episodes ("tet" spells) includes supplemental oxygen, placing the patient in the knee-chest position; consideration of intravenous propranolol, morphine
- Palliation with oral beta-blockers or surgical anastomosis between the subclavian and pulmonary artery (Blalock-Taussig shunt) recommended for very small infants with severe symptoms and in those who are not candidates for complete correction
- Surgical correction (closure of ventricular septal defect and right ventricular outflow tract reconstruction) is the treatment of choice in selected patients; patients are still at risk for sudden death because of arrhythmias
- Complete repair in childhood has a 10-year survival rate of more than 90% and a 30-year survival rate of 85%

■ Pearl

The combination of right ventricular hypertrophy, small pulmonary arteries, and pulmonary oligemia is seen in no other condition.

Reference

Apitz C, Webb GD, Redington AN. Tetralogy of Fallot. Lancet 2009;374:1462. [PMID: 19683809]

Urinary Tract Infection

- **Essentials of Diagnosis**
  - Girls at higher risk than boys
  - Circumcision decreases rates of urinary tract infection only during the first year of life
  - Bacterial infection of the urinary tract, defined as $> 10^3$ colony-forming units/mL by suprapubic aspiration, $> 10^4$ CFU/mL by catheter, or $> 10^5$ CFU/mL by clean catch
  - Most common pathogens are *E. coli, Klebsiella,* enterococci, and *Proteus mirabilis*
  - Urinalysis usually positive for leukocytes and bacteria
  - Symptoms may be nonspecific in younger children and infants (eg, intermittent fever, poor feeding, emesis, diarrhea)
  - Difficult to differentiate lower tract infections from pyelonephritis
  - Risk factors include uncircumcised boys (during first year of life), female sex, presence of vesicoureteral reflux or obstructive uropathy, constipation, genitourinary anatomic abnormality

- **Differential Diagnosis**
  - Appendicitis
  - Gastroenteritis
  - Pelvic inflammatory disease (adolescents)
  - Diabetes mellitus
  - Urethral irritation

- **Treatment**
  - Empiric antibiotics such as penicillins or cephalosporins are first-line therapies; trimethoprim-sulfamethoxazole may be used in older children
  - Voiding cystourethrogram for infants and children once free of infection to exclude vesicoureteral reflux
  - Prophylactic antibiotics continued until voiding cystourethrogram performed

- **Pearl**

18

Urinary tract infections in boys and men are inevitably all due to anatomic abnormalities—all should be investigated thoroughly with appropriate imaging.

Reference

Quigley R. Diagnosis of urinary tract infections in children. Curr Opin Pediatr 2009;21:194. [PMID: 19663036]

Wilms' Tumor (Nephroblastoma)

- ■ Essentials of Diagnosis
  - Second most common abdominal tumor in children
  - Presents between ages 2 and 5 years; occasionally may be seen in neonates or adolescents
  - Occurs sporadically or as part of a malformation syndrome or cytogenic abnormality (eg, Beckwith-Wiedemann)
  - Often discovered incidentally as an asymptomatic abdominal mass; occasionally presents with intermittent fever, abdominal pain, hematuria
  - Abdominal ultrasound or CT reveals a solid intrarenal mass; 5–10% are bilateral
  - Metastatic lesions in lung often present on chest x-ray

- ■ Differential Diagnosis
  - Neuroblastoma
  - Rhabdomyosarcoma
  - Germ cell tumor/teratoma
  - Lymphoma
  - Polycystic kidneys
  - Renal abscess
  - Hydronephrosis

- ■ Treatment
  - Once the diagnosis is made, almost all patients undergo surgical exploration of the abdomen with attempted excision of the tumor and possible nephrectomy
  - Vincristine, dactinomycin, and doxorubicin are mainstays of chemotherapy
  - Irradiation to sites of known disease prevent recurrence

- ■ Pearl

This is the diagnosis in a toddler with a nontender, large abdominal mass found incidentally.

Reference

Davidoff AM. Wilms' tumor. Curr Opin Pediatr 2009;21:357. [PMID: 19417665]

18

19

Selected Genetic Disorders[*]

Acute Intermittent Porphyria

- **Essentials of Diagnosis**
  - Autosomal dominant with variable expressivity and low penetrance
  - Caused by deficiency of porphobilinogen deaminase activity, with increased urinary δ-aminolevulinic acid and porphobilinogen
  - Unexplained abdominal pain, peripheral or central nervous system dysfunction, psychiatric illness; no skin photosensitivity
  - Symptoms begin in the teens or twenties, usually in young women
  - Attacks precipitated by drugs (eg, steroids, sulfonamides, estrogens), infections, reduced caloric intake, smoking, alcohol
  - Absence of fever and leukocytosis, occasional profound hyponatremia; port-wine color of urine may be present
  - Diagnosis confirmed by demonstrating increased porphobilinogen in urine during acute attack

- **Differential Diagnosis**
  - Other causes of acute abdominal pain
  - Polyneuropathy due to other causes (eg, Guillain-Barré)
  - Heavy metal poisoning (eg, lead)
  - Psychosis and hyponatremia due to other causes

- **Treatment**
  - High-carbohydrate diet may prevent attacks; periodic hepatic imaging to monitor for hepatocellular carcinoma
  - Flares require stopping exacerbating medications, analgesics, intravenous glucose, and hematin
  - Closely monitor respiratory status due to bulbar paralysis

- **Pearl**

  In a young woman with abdominal pain and multiple surgical scars, remember this disease before worsening the scar burden.

References

Badminton MN, Elder GH. Management of acute and cutaneous porphyrias. Int J Clin Pract 2002;56:272. [PMID: 12074210]

Thunell S. GeneReviews: Hydroxymethylbilane synthase deficiency. AIP 2005. http://www.ncbi.nlm.nih.gov/bookshelf/br.fcgi?book=gene&part=aip

[*] The following genetic disorders are discussed in other chapters: cystic fibrosis, Chapter 2; sickle cell anemia, thalassemia, von Willebrand's disease, Chapter 5; Huntington's chorea, Chapter 12; Down's syndrome, Chapter 18.

Alkaptonuria

- ## Essentials of Diagnosis
  - Rare, autosomal-recessive disorder with 100% penetrance
  - Caused by deficiency of homogentisate 1,2-dioxygenase; leads to accumulation of an oxidation product in cartilage, large joints, and spine
  - Predominant symptom is often early back and joint pain (in 20- and 30-year-olds) with radiographic features consistent with spondylitis; joint disease tends to start earlier and progress more rapidly in men than women
  - After age 30, a slight, darkish blue color below the skin in areas overlying cartilage such as ears ("ochronosis") develops; some have more hyperpigmentation in sclerae and conjunctivae
  - After age 40, aortic or mitral stenosis due to accumulation of metabolites in heart valves; predisposition to coronary artery disease occasionally
  - Renal and prostate stones common
  - Diagnosed by demonstrating homogentisic acid in the urine, which turns black on air exposure (may not occur for several hours after voiding)

- ## Differential Diagnosis
  - Ankylosing spondylitis or other spondyloarthropathies
  - Osteoarthritis
  - Amiodarone toxicity
  - Argyria
  - Rheumatic heart disease

- ## Treatment
  - Similar to that for other arthropathies
  - Rigid dietary restriction may be used but of unproven benefit
  - Cardiac surveillance with echocardiography every 2 years after age 40 recommended

- ## Pearl

The only disease in medicine causing black cartilage.

References

Phornphutkul C, Introne WJ, Perry BM, et al. Natural history of alkaptonuria. N Engl J Med 2002;347:2111. [PMID: 12501223]

Introne W. GeneReviews: Alkaptonuria. July 2, 2009. http://www.ncbi.nlm.nih.gov/bookshelf/br.fcgi?book=gene&part=alkap

19

Alpha₁-Antitrypsin Deficiency

■ Essentials of Diagnosis

- Common and unrecognized disorder that may lead to chronic obstructive pulmonary disease and severe liver disease
- Autosomal recessive, some heterozygotes who smoke have increased risk of respiratory manifestations
- Caused by genetic defects in the *PI* gene resulting in deficiency (*null* or *S* allele) or entrapment (*Z* allele) of alpha₁-antitrypsin (AAT), leading to unabated neutrophil elastase damage in the lungs and harmful AAT accumulation in the liver
- Basilar predominant panacinar emphysema at age 40–50 in smokers or above age 50 in nonsmokers
- Liver disease occurs in a subset of patients (*Z* allele) and manifests as cirrhosis and fibrosis
- Less commonly presents with bronchiectasis, necrotizing panniculitis, and Wegener's granulomatosis
- Low plasma alpha₁-antitrypsin level followed by confirmatory variant protein phenotype or genetic testing

■ Differential Diagnosis

- Other causes of emphysema or cirrhosis

■ Treatment

- Diagnostic testing recommended for all patients < 45 years of age with irreversible airflow obstruction, unexplained liver disease, or necrotizing panniculitis; genetic screening of siblings
- Smoking cessation and avoidance of passive smoking are crucial
- Alpha₁-antitrypsin augmentation therapy intravenously to slow the decline of lung function; major drawback is exceptional cost, limited efficacy in lung disease; liver dysfunction does not improve with enzyme replacement
- Treat manifestations of liver disease, avoid alcohol
- Surgical options include lung-volume reduction, lung transplantation, and liver transplantation

■ Pearl

In a young patient with dyspnea and irreversible obstructive airflow obstruction, test for alpha₁-antitrypsin deficiency.

References

Silverman EK, Sandhaus RA. Clinical practice. Alpha₁-antitrypsin deficiency. N Engl J Med 2009;360:2749. [PMID: 19553648]

Schlade-Bartusiak, K. GeneReviews. Alpha₁-Antrypsin Deficiency. February 6, 2008. http://www.ncbi.nlm.nih.gov/bookshelf/br.fcgi?book=gene&part=alpha1-a

19

Gaucher's Disease

- ## Essentials of Diagnosis
  - Autosomal recessive inheritance with three major clinical subtypes; most common in patients of Ashkenazi Jewish heritage
  - Deficiency of beta-glucocerebrosidase causes accumulation of sphingolipid within phagocytic cells throughout the body
  - In type I Gaucher's disease, infiltration primarily involves the liver, spleen, bone marrow, and lymph nodes
  - Anemia, thrombocytopenia, and splenomegaly are common; erosion of bones due to local infarction with bone pain
  - Bone marrow aspirates reveal typical "Gaucher cells" (lipid-engorged macrophages), with eccentric nucleus, periodic acid-Schiff–positive inclusions; elevated serum acid phosphatase
  - Less common forms of Gaucher's disease, type II and type III, involve sphingolipid accumulation in neurologic tissue and lead to various neurologic problems
  - Definitive diagnosis requires demonstration of deficient glucocerebrosidase activity in leukocytes

- ## Differential Diagnosis
  - Other causes of heptosplenomegaly or lymphadenopathy
  - Bone malignancy; avascular necrosis

- ## Treatment
  - First-line management with recombinant form of the enzyme glucocerebrosidase (imiglucerase); given intravenously on a regular basis improves orthopedic and hematologic problems; major drawback is exceptional cost; neurologic abnormalities seen in type II and type III disease do not improve with enzyme replacement
  - For those not responding to enzyme replacement, a glucosylceramide synthase inhibitor (miglustat) can be used
  - Bone marrow transplantation can benefit patients with chronic neurologic involvement
  - Splenectomy for those with bleeding problems due to platelet sequestration

- ## Pearl

In a Jewish patient with hip fracture and splenomegaly, the diagnosis is Gaucher's disease until proven otherwise.

19

References

Chen M, Wang J. Gaucher disease: review of the literature. Arch Pathol Lab Med 2008;132:851. [PMID: 18466035]

Pastores G. GeneReviews: Gaucher Disease. March 13, 2008. http://www.ncbi.nlm.nih.gov/bookshelf/br.fcgi?book=gene&part=gaucher

Hemochromatosis

■ Essentials of Diagnosis

- The most common genetic disease among white North Americans
- Autosomal-recessive inheritance caused by *C282Y* mutation
- Low penetrance of iron-overload–related disease, affecting approximately 28% male and only 1% female homozygotes
- Hyperabsorption of iron and its parenchymal storage results in tissue injury with symptoms and signs of hepatic, pancreatic, cardiac, articular, and gonadal dysfunction
- Symptoms typically occur between age 40 and 60 years in men and after menopause in women; depend on affected organs
- Clinical manifestations may include cirrhosis, hepatocellular carcinoma, heart failure, diabetes mellitus, arthropathy, hypopituitarism
- Elevated serum iron, normal transferrin, percentage saturation of iron > 50%, and increased ferritin
- Liver biopsy characteristic, with iron stain identifying accumulation in parenchymal cells

■ Differential Diagnosis

- Other causes of cirrhosis or heart failure or hypopituitarism
- Other causes of iron overload, especially multiple transfusions (> 100 units) as in homozygous beta-thalassemia or sickle cell disease

■ Treatment

- Genetic screening recommended for all first-order relatives
- Early recognition and diagnosis (precirrhotic state) is crucial
- Low-iron diet; avoid uncooked seafood due to increased susceptibility to bacterial infection; avoid alcohol
- Weekly phlebotomy to deplete iron stores, followed by maintenance phlebotomy or intramuscular deferoxamine, is usually indicated
- Liver transplantation for decompensated cirrhosis

■ Pearl

Hemochromatosis is a genetic disorder, hemosiderosis is acquired; the two are clinically similar, but the history distinguishes them.

References

Allen KJ, Gurrin LC, Constantine CC, et al. Iron-overload-related disease in HFE hereditary hemochromatosis. N Engl J Med 2008;358;221. [PMID: 18199861]

Kowdley K. GeneReviews: HFE-Associated Hereditary Hemochromatosis. December 4, 2006. http://www.ncbi.nlm.nih.gov/bookshelf/br.fcgi?book=gene&part=hemochromatosis

19

Homocystinuria

- **Essentials of Diagnosis**
  - Autosomal-recessive disorder with variable expressivity that can manifest in infancy or adulthood
  - Caused by cystathionine β-synthase deficiency resulting in extreme elevations of plasma and urinary homocystine levels and is characterized by involvement of the eye, skeletal system, vascular system, and central nervous system
  - Patients often present in second and third decades of life with evidence of arterial or venous thromboses without underlying risk factors for hypercoagulability
  - Repeated venous and arterial thromboses common; reduced life expectancy from myocardial infarction, stroke, and pulmonary embolism
  - Ectopia lentis almost always present; mental retardation and asthenic habitus common
  - Diagnosis established by extremely elevated plasma and urinary homocystine levels

- **Differential Diagnosis**
  - Marfan's syndrome
  - Other causes of mental retardation
  - Other causes of hypercoagulability

- **Treatment**
  - Treatment in infancy with pyridoxine and folate helps some
  - Pyridoxine nonresponders treated with dietary reduction in methionine and supplementation of cysteine, also from infancy
  - Betaine may also be useful
  - Surgery for ectopia lentis
  - Anticoagulation as appropriate for thrombosis

- **Pearl**

In a young person with pulmonary embolism, thick eyeglasses, and an ill-characterized psychiatric disorder, remember homocystinemia; the thick glasses result from ectopia lentis.

References

Ramakrishnan S, Sulochana KN, Lakshmi S, Selvi R, Angayarkanni N. Biochemistry of homocysteine in health and diseases. Indian J Biochem Biophys 2006;43:275. [PMID: 17133733]

Picker J. GeneReviews: Homocystinuria Caused by Cystathionine Beta-Synthase Deficiency. March 29, 2006. http://www.ncbi.nlm.nih.gov/bookshelf/br.fcgi?book=gene&part=homocystinuria

19

Marfan's Syndrome

- **Essentials of Diagnosis**
  - Autosomal-dominant disorder; 25% de novo gene mutation
  - A systemic connective tissue disease due to mutations in the fibrillin gene; characterized by abnormalities of the skeletal system, eye, cardiovascular system
  - Spontaneous pneumothorax, ectopia lentis, myopia are characteristic; patients are tall with long extremities and arachnodactyly, thoracic deformity, and joint laxity
  - Aortic dilation and dissection most feared complication; mitral valve prolapse seen 85%; mitral regurgitation in some
  - Clinical diagnosis based on family history and observation of characteristic findings in multiple organ systems

- **Differential Diagnosis**
  - Homocystinuria; Ehler's-Danlos syndrome; Klinefelter's syndrome; Fragile X syndrome
  - Aortic dissection due to other causes
  - Mitral or aortic regurgitation due to other causes

- **Treatment**
  - Patients of all ages require echocardiography—often annually—to monitor aortic diameter and mitral valve function
  - Endocarditis prophylaxis required
  - Beta-blockade may retard the rate of aortic dilation; vigorous exercise avoidance protects some from aortic dissection
  - Replacement of aortic root recommended when diameter exceeds 50 mm (normal is less than 40 mm), or rate of increase approaches 10 mm/year
  - Most untreated patients die in their fourth or fifth decade from dissection or heart failure (due to aortic regurgitation); with treatment, life expectancy approximates that of the general population

- **Pearl**

Another disorder proving the axiom that the first minute of inspection is the most important time the physician spends with the patient.

References

Keane MG, Pyeritz RE. Medical management of Marfan syndrome. Circulation 2008;117:2802. [PMID: 18506019]

Dietz HC. GeneReviews: Marfan Syndrome. June, 30, 2009. http://www.ncbi.nlm.nih.gov/bookshelf/br.fcgi?book=gene&part=marfan

19

Neurofibromatosis

- **Essentials of Diagnosis**
  - Sporadic or autosomal dominant with variable expressivity
  - Two genetically and clinically distinct forms: Type 1 (von Recklinghausen's disease), more common and characterized by multiple hyperpigmented macules and neurofibromas; type 2, characterized by eighth cranial nerve tumors and occasionally other intracranial or intraspinal tumors
  - Type 1 associated with cutaneous lesions (neurofibromas), axillary freckling, iris hamartomas (Lisch's nodules), and patches of cutaneous pigmentation (café au lait spots) that begin in childhood; ocular gliomas may occur
  - In adolescence and adulthood, malignant degeneration of neurofibromas possible, leading to peripheral sarcoma (neurofibrosarcomas); also associated with meningioma, bone cysts, pheochromocytomas, and scoliosis
  - Type 2 often presents in early adulthood with symptoms and signs of tumor of the spinal or cranial nerves, most commonly bilateral vestibular schwannomas; tumors usually not malignant but delicate anatomical location and high tumor burden lead to early mortality
  - Clinical criteria for diagnosis in both type 1 and type 2

- **Differential Diagnosis**
  - Intracranial or intraspinal tumor due to other causes
  - McCune-Albright syndrome
  - Multiple endocrine neoplasia type 2B

- **Treatment**
  - Genetic counseling important
  - Disfigurement may be corrected by plastic surgery
  - Intraspinal or intracranial tumors and tumors of peripheral nerves treated surgically if symptomatic

- **Pearl**

Up to six café au lait spots are normal; more suggests a consideration of von Recklinghausen's disease.

References

Gerber PA, Antal AS, Neumann NJ, et al. Neurofibromatosis. Eur J Med Res 2009;14:102. [PMID: 19380279]

Friedman JM. GeneReviews: Neurofibromatosis 1. June 2, 2009. http://www.ncbi.nlm.nih.gov/bookshelf/br.fcgi?book=gene&part=nf1

Evans DG. GeneReviews: Neurofibromatosis 2. May 19, 2009. http://www.ncbi.nlm.nih.gov/bookshelf/br.fcgi?book=gene&part=nf2

19

Wilson's Disease (Hepatolenticular Degeneration)

- ■ Essentials of Diagnosis
  - Rare autosomal-recessive disorder with variable onset between first and sixth decades; genetic defect in copper-transporting enzyme (P-type ATPase) prevents copper excretion into bile resulting in excessive copper deposition in liver and brain
  - Genetic defect in copper-transporting enzyme (P-type ATPase) prevents copper excretion into the bile and results in excessive deposition of copper in the liver and brain
  - Presentation usually includes symptoms of hepatic and/or neuropsychiatric dysfunction including cirrhosis, jaundice, liver failure, and basal ganglia dysfunction
  - Kayser-Fleischer rings in the cornea (in almost all cases of neurologic Wilson's disease), hepatomegaly, parkinsonian tremor and rigidity, psychiatric abnormalities
  - Diagnosis based on biochemical tests often followed by confirmatory genetic testing of the *ATP7B* gene: Elevated urinary copper excretion (> 100 μg/24 h), elevated hepatic copper concentration (> 250 μg/g of dry liver), decreased serum ceruloplasmin (< 20 μg/dL)

- ■ Differential Diagnosis
  - Other causes of liver dysfunction
  - Other causes of psychiatric and neurologic disturbances, especially Parkinson's disease

- ■ Treatment
  - Early treatment to remove excess copper crucial; in asymptomatic patients, oral zinc acetate promotes fecal copper excretion
  - Restrict dietary copper (shellfish, organ foods, legumes)
  - For symptomatic patients, oral copper chelation with penicillamine or trientine facilitates urinary excretion of chelated copper; pyridoxine supplementation necessary
  - Ammonium tetrathiomolybdate promising as initial therapy for neurologic Wilson's disease
  - Liver transplantation liver failure, intractable neurologic disease
  - Family members (especially siblings) require screening tests (serum ceruloplasmin, liver tests, slit lamp eye examination)

- ■ Pearl

The only disease in medicine with an alkaline phosphatase which may be zero.

References

Ala A, Walker AP, Ashkan K, Dooley JS, Schilsky ML. Wilson's disease. Lancet 2007;369:397. [PMID: 17276780]

Cox DW. GeneReviews: Wilson Disease. January 24, 2006.
http://www.ncbi.nlm.nih.gov/bookshelf/br.fcgi?book=gene&part=Wilson

20

Common Disorders of the Eye

Acute Conjunctivitis

- **Essentials of Diagnosis**
  - Acute onset of red, itchy, burning eyes with tearing, eyelid crusting, foreign body sensation, and discharge
  - Conjunctival injection and edema, mucoid or purulent discharge, lid edema, and possible preauricular lymph node enlargement
  - Vision may be normal or slightly decreased
  - Causes include bacterial and viral (including herpetic) infections and allergy

- **Differential Diagnosis**
  - Acute anterior uveitis
  - Acute angle-closure glaucoma
  - Corneal abrasion or infection
  - Dacryocystitis
  - Nasolacrimal duct obstruction
  - Chronic conjunctivitis
  - Scleritis in autoimmune disease

- **Treatment**
  - Topical broad-spectrum ophthalmic antibiotic (eg, fluoroquinolone), cool compresses, artificial tears
  - Ophthalmology follow-up for persistent symptoms or decreased visual acuity

- **Pearl**

There are many causes of the red eye; be careful with potentially damaging empiric topical steroid therapy.

Reference

O'Brien TP, Jeng BH, McDonald M, Raizman MB. Acute conjunctivitis: truth and misconceptions. Curr Med Res Opin 2009;25:1953. [PMID: 19552618]

Acute (Angle-Closure) Glaucoma

- ■ Essentials of Diagnosis
  - Less than 5% of all glaucoma
  - Acute onset of eye pain and redness, photophobia, blurred vision with colored halos around lights, headaches, nausea, or abdominal pain
  - Decreased vision, conjunctival injection, steamy cornea, mid-dilated and nonreactive pupil, and elevated intraocular pressure by tonometry
  - Preexisting narrow anterior chamber angle predisposes; older patients, hyperopes, Asians, and Inuits more susceptible
  - Precipitated by pupillary dilation caused by stress, pharmacologic mydriasis, dark environment (eg, movie theater)

- ■ Differential Diagnosis
  - Acute conjunctivitis
  - Acute anterior uveitis
  - Corneal abrasion or infection
  - Other types of glaucoma

- ■ Treatment
  - Prompt ophthalmologic referral
  - Pharmacotherapy includes: Topical beta-blocker (timolol), alpha-agonist (brimonidine), carbonic anhydrase inhibitor (dorzolamide); if elevated intraocular pressure does not respond to topical therapy, systemic carbonic anhydrase inhibitor (acetazolamide) or hyperosmotic agent (eg, glycerol or mannitol)
  - Laser peripheral iridotomy usually curative

- ■ Pearl

Acute angle closure is a cause of the nonsurgical acute abdomen; acute elevation of intraocular pressure stimulates the vagus nerve nucleus, located directly posterior to the globe, and causes gastrointestinal symptoms.

Reference

Tarongoy P, Ho CL, Walton DS. Angle-closure glaucoma: the role of the lens in the pathogenesis, prevention, and treatment. Surv Ophthalmol 2009;54:211. [PMID: 19298900]

Age-Related Macular Degeneration

■ Essentials of Diagnosis

- Non-neovascular ("dry") form: Central or paracentral blind spot and gradual loss of central vision; may be asymptomatic
- Small and hard or large and soft drusen, geographic atrophy of the retinal pigment epithelium, and pigment clumping
- Neovascular ("wet") form: Distortion of straight lines or edges, central or paracentral blind spot, and rapid loss of central vision
- Gray-green choroidal neovascular membrane, lipid exudates, subretinal hemorrhage or fluid, pigment epithelial detachment, and fibrovascular disciform scars
- Risk factors include age, positive family history, cigarette smoking, hyperopia, light iris color, hypertension, and cardiovascular disease

■ Differential Diagnosis

- Dominant drusen
- Choroidal neovascularization from other causes (eg, ocular histoplasmosis, angioid streaks, myopic degeneration, traumatic choroidal rupture, optic disk drusen, choroidal tumors, laser scars, and inflammatory chorioretinal lesions)

■ Treatment

- Prompt ophthalmologic referral
- Micronutrient supplementation with Age Related Eye Disease Study formulation (eg, Preservision AREDS) slows progression in patients with moderate to severe dry AMD
- Intravitreal injection of antiangiogenesis drugs (eg, Lucentis or Avastin) by a retina specialist has become the standard of care for wet AMD

■ Pearl

Age-related macular degeneration is the leading cause of blindness in America for patients over 65.

Reference

Bressler SB. Introduction: understanding the role of angiogenesis and antiangiogenic agents in age-related macular degeneration. Ophthalmology 2009;116(suppl):S1. [PMID: 19800534]

20

Blepharitis and Meibomitis

- ■ Essentials of Diagnosis
  - Chronic itching, burning, mild pain, foreign body sensation, tearing, and crusting around the eyes on awakening
  - Crusty, red, thickened eyelids with prominent blood vessels or inspissated oil glands in the eyelid margins, conjunctival injection, mild mucoid discharge, and acne rosacea

- ■ Differential Diagnosis
  - Sebaceous gland carcinoma

- ■ Treatment
  - Warm compresses for at least 5 minutes, followed by lid massage at least once daily
  - Artificial tears for ocular surface irritation
  - Topical antibiotic ointment at bedtime
  - Recurrent or persistent meibomitis may be treated with:
    - Pulse therapy with topical azithromycin eyedrop daily for 2 to 4 weeks
    - Oral doxycycline for 6–8 weeks, followed by slow taper; in women, negative pregnancy test before and contraception during treatment are essential

- ■ Pearl

Contact lens intolerance is often clue to meibomitis.

Reference

Gilbard JP. Dry eye and blepharitis: approaching the patient with chronic eye irritation. Geriatrics 2009;64:22. [PMID: 19572764]

20

Cataract

- ■ Essentials of Diagnosis
  - Slowly progressive, painless visual loss or blurring, with glare from oncoming headlights, reduced color perception, and decreased contrast sensitivity
  - Lens opacification grossly visible or seen by ophthalmoscopy
  - Causes include aging, trauma, drugs (steroids, anticholinesterases, antipsychotics), uveitis, radiation, tumor, retinitis pigmentosa, systemic diseases (diabetes mellitus, hypoparathyroidism, Wilson's disease, myotonic dystrophy, galactosemia, Down's syndrome, atopic dermatitis), congenital

- ■ Differential Diagnosis
  - Generally unmistakable
  - Ectopia lentis may cause some diagnostic confusion

- ■ Treatment
  - Surgical removal of the cataract with concurrent intraocular lens implantation for visual impairment or occupational requirement

- ■ Pearl

An unexpected benefit, to the delight of patients, is the return of excellent color vision when the cataracts are removed.

Reference

Vrensen GF. Early cortical lens opacities: a short overview. Acta Ophthalmol 2009;87:602. [PMID: 19719805]

20

Chronic (Open-Angle) Glaucoma

- **Essentials of Diagnosis**
  - Ninety-five percent or more of glaucoma in United States
  - Insidious onset resulting in eventual complete loss of vision; asymptomatic early; common in blacks, elderly, and myopic patients
  - Tonometry may reveal elevated intraocular pressure (> 21 mm Hg) but highly variable
  - Pathologic cupping of optic disk seen funduscopically, can be asymmetric
  - Loss of peripheral visual field

- **Differential Diagnosis**
  - Normal diurnal variation of intraocular pressure
  - Other types of glaucoma; congenital optic nerve abnormalities; ischemic, compressive, or toxic optic neuropathy
  - Bilateral retinal disorders (chorioretinitis, retinoschisis, retinitis pigmentosa)

- **Treatment**
  - Prostaglandin analog (latanoprost, travoprost, bimatoprost)
  - Beta-blocking agents (timolol)
  - α-Adrenergic agents (brimonidine)
  - Carbonic anhydrase inhibitors (dorzolamide, brinzolamide)
  - Miotics (pilocarpine)
  - Surgery: Laser trabeculoplasty, trabeculectomy, or aqueous shunt procedure

- **Pearl**

If an ophthalmologist calls you in consultation for dyspnea, check the med list; asthma or congestive cardiac failure may be the result of topical beta-blockers in some patients.

Reference
Schwartz GF, Quigley HA. Adherence and persistence with glaucoma therapy. Surv Ophthalmol 2008;53(suppl 1):S57. [PMID: 19038625]

Corneal Ulceration

- ■ Essentials of Diagnosis
  - Acute eye pain, photophobia, redness, tearing, discharge, and blurred vision
  - Upper eyelid edema, conjunctival injection, mucopurulent discharge, white corneal infiltrate with overlying epithelial defect that stains with fluorescein dye, hypopyon (if severe)
  - Causes include trauma, contact lens wear, infection (bacterial, herpetic, fungal, *Acanthamoeba*)

- ■ Differential Diagnosis
  - Acute anterior uveitis
  - Acute angle-closure glaucoma
  - Acute conjunctivitis
  - Sterile or immunologic ulcer
  - Corneal abrasion or foreign body

- ■ Treatment
  - Frequent topical broad-spectrum antibiotics and daily ophthalmologic follow-up
  - Prompt ophthalmologic referral for any central ulcer or a peripheral ulcer > 2 mm in diameter

- ■ Pearl

Never patch a corneal ulcer.

Reference

Tuli SS, Schultz GS, Downer DM. Science and strategy for preventing and managing corneal ulceration. Ocul Surf 2007;5:23. [PMID: 17252163]

20

Diabetic Retinopathy

- **Essentials of Diagnosis**
  - May have decreased or fluctuating vision or floaters; often asymptomatic early in the course of the disease
  - Nonproliferative: Dot and blot hemorrhages, microaneurysms, hard exudates, cotton-wool spots, venous beading, and intraretinal microvascular abnormalities
  - Proliferative: Neovascularization of optic disk, retina, or iris; preretinal or vitreous hemorrhages; tractional retinal detachment

- **Differential Diagnosis**
  - Hypertensive retinopathy
  - HIV retinopathy
  - Radiation retinopathy
  - Central or branch retinal vein occlusion
  - Ocular ischemic syndrome
  - Sickle cell retinopathy
  - Retinopathy of severe anemia
  - Embolization from intravenous drug abuse (talc retinopathy)
  - Collagen vascular disease
  - Sarcoidosis
  - Eales' disease

- **Treatment**
  - Ophthalmologic referral and regular follow-up in all diabetics
  - Laser photocoagulation, intravitreal Kenalog, intravitreal antiangiogenesis drugs (eg, Lucentis or Avastin) for macular edema and proliferative disease
  - Pars plana vitrectomy for nonclearing vitreous hemorrhage and tractional retinal detachment involving or threatening the macula

- **Pearl**

Though a debate about this has lasted decades, it appears that aggressive glycemic control prevents progression; be sure your patients understand and know their A1c.

Reference

El-Asrar AM, Al-Mezaine HS, Ola MS. Changing paradigms in the treatment of diabetic retinopathy. Curr Opin Ophthalmol 2009;20:532. [PMID: 19644368]

Giant Cell (Temporal) Arteritis

- ■ Essentials of Diagnosis
  - • Sudden painless unilateral loss of vision in a patient over 50 years of age in association with ipsilateral temporal headache; may also have diplopia, visual field deficits
  - • Review of systems positive for any or all of the following: jaw claudication, ear pain, scalp tenderness, proximal muscle and joint aches (polymyalgia rheumatica), fever, anorexia, weight loss
  - • Palpable, tender, nonpulsatile temporal artery may be present
  - • Afferent pupillary defect (Marcus-Gunn pupil), pale swollen optic nerve, and possibly a macular cherry-red spot
  - • Erythrocyte sedimentation rate (ESR) and C-reactive protein (CRP) often significantly elevated

- ■ Differential Diagnosis
  - • Nonarteritic ischemic optic neuropathy
  - • Optic neuritis
  - • Compressive optic nerve tumor
  - • Central retinal artery occlusion

- ■ Treatment
  - • High-dose IV or oral steroids should be started immediately to prevent vision loss in the contralateral eye
  - • Prompt ophthalmologic referral for temporal artery biopsy (but start the steroids while making these arrangements)

- ■ Pearl

An elderly woman with a headache and ophthalmic symptoms has giant cell (temporal) arteritis until proven otherwise.

Reference

Chew SS, Kerr NM, Danesh-Meyer HV. Giant cell arteritis. J Clin Neurosci 2009;16:1263. [PMID: 19586772]

HIV Retinopathy

- ■ Essentials of Diagnosis
  - Cotton-wool spots, intraretinal hemorrhages, microaneurysms seen on funduscopic examination in a patient with known or suspected HIV infection
  - Typically asymptomatic unless accompanied by other HIV-related retinal pathology (eg, cytomegalovirus retinitis)

- ■ Differential Diagnosis
  - Diabetic retinopathy
  - Hypertensive retinopathy
  - Radiation retinopathy
  - Retinopathy of severe anemia
  - Central or branch retinal vein occlusion
  - Sickle cell retinopathy
  - Embolization from intravenous drug abuse (talc retinopathy)
  - Sarcoidosis
  - Eales' disease

- ■ Treatment
  - Treat the underlying HIV disease
  - Ophthalmologic referral is appropriate for any patient with HIV, especially with a low CD4 count and/or visual symptoms

- ■ Pearl

HIV retinopathy is the most common ophthalmologic manifestation of HIV infection; it usually indicates a low CD4 count.

Reference

Holland GN. AIDS and ophthalmology: the first quarter century. Am J Ophthalmol 2008;145:397. [PMID: 18282490]

Hordeolum and Chalazion

- ■ Essentials of Diagnosis
  - • Eyelid lump, swelling, pain, and redness
  - • Visible or palpable, well-defined subcutaneous nodule within the eyelid; eyelid edema, erythema, and point tenderness with or without preauricular node
  - • Hordeolum: Acute obstruction and infection of eyelid gland (meibomian gland—internal hordeolum; gland of Zeis or Moll—external hordeolum), associated with *Staphylococcus aureus*
  - • Chalazion: Chronic obstruction and inflammation of meibomian gland with leakage of sebum into surrounding tissue and resultant lipogranuloma; rosacea may be associated

- ■ Differential Diagnosis
  - • Preseptal cellulitis
  - • Sebaceous cell carcinoma
  - • Pyogenic granuloma

- ■ Treatment
  - • Warm compresses for 10 minutes at least four times daily
  - • Topical antibiotic/steroid (eg, Maxitrol) ointment twice daily
  - • Incision and curettage for persistent chalazion (> 6–8 weeks)
  - • Intralesional steroid injection for chalazion near the nasolacrimal drainage system

- ■ Pearl

Avoid early surgical treatment with its risk of scarring; most will resolve with conservative treatment.

Reference

Mueller JB, McStay CM. Ocular infection and inflammation. Emerg Med Clin North Am 2008;26:57. [PMID: 18249257]

Hypertensive Retinopathy

- ■ Essentials of Diagnosis
    - Usually asymptomatic; may have decreased vision
    - Generalized or localized retinal arteriolar narrowing, almost always bilateral
    - Arteriovenous crossing changes (AV nicking), retinal arteriolar sclerosis (copper or silver wiring), cotton-wool spots, hard exudates, flame-shaped hemorrhages, retinal edema, arterial macroaneurysms, chorioretinal atrophy
    - Optic disk edema in malignant hypertension

- ■ Differential Diagnosis
    - Diabetic retinopathy
    - Radiation retinopathy
    - HIV retinopathy
    - Central or branch retinal vein occlusion
    - Sickle cell retinopathy
    - Retinopathy of severe anemia
    - Embolization from intravenous drug abuse (talc retinopathy)
    - Autoimmune disease
    - Sarcoidosis
    - Eales' disease

- ■ Treatment
    - Treat the hypertension
    - Ophthalmologic referral

- ■ Pearl

The only pathognomonic funduscopic change of hypertension is focal arteriolar narrowing due to spasm, and it is typically seen in hypertensive crisis.

Reference

DellaCroce JT, Vitale AT. Hypertension and the eye. Curr Opin Ophthalmol 2008;19:493. [PMID: 18854694]

Pingueculum and Pterygium

- **Essentials of Diagnosis**
  - Pingueculum: Yellow-white flat or slightly raised conjunctival lesion in the interpalpebral fissure adjacent to the limbus but not involving the cornea
  - Pterygium: Wing-shaped fold of fibrovascular tissue arising from the interpalpebral conjunctiva, extending onto and into the cornea
  - Irritation, redness, decreased vision; may be asymptomatic
  - Both lesions can be highly vascularized and injected; their growth is associated with sunlight, windy and dry conditions, and chronic irritation

- **Differential Diagnosis**
  - Ocular surface squamous neoplasia
  - Dermoid
  - Pannus

- **Treatment**
  - Protect the eyes from sun, dust, and wind with sunglasses or goggles
  - Reduce ocular irritation with artificial tears
  - Topical NSAIDs or mild topical steroids can help control flare-ups of inflammation
  - Surgical removal for extreme irritation not relieved with above treatments or extension of pterygium toward the pupil causing irregular astigmatism and blurred vision

- **Pearl**

Xanthomas are always, xanthelasma is sometimes, and pterygium and pingueculum are never associated with hyperlipidemia except coincidentally.

Reference

Detorakis ET, Spandidos DA. Pathogenetic mechanisms and treatment options for ophthalmic pterygium: trends and perspectives (Review). Int J Mol Med 2009;23:439. [PMID: 19288018]

Postseptal (Orbital) Cellulitis

- ■ Essentials of Diagnosis
    - • Inflammation and infection of the orbital tissues posterior to the orbital septum; the globe is often involved
    - • Causes: (1) Extension of infection from paranasal sinuses (90% of cases), face or teeth, nasolacrimal sac, or globe; (2) direct inoculation of orbit from trauma or surgery; (3) hematogenous spread from bacteremia
    - • Fever and leukocytosis (75% of cases)
    - • Proptosis, ophthalmoplegia, pain with eye movement
    - • Decreased vision and/or pupillary abnormality in severe cases
    - • CT scan should be obtained in all suspected cases

- ■ Differential Diagnosis
    - • Preseptal cellulitis
    - • Mucormycosis
    - • Inflammatory orbital pseudotumor or Wegener's granulomatosis
    - • Thyroid ophthalmopathy
    - • Insect or animal bite
    - • Tumor

- ■ Treatment
    - • ENT consult for cases arising from sinusitis
    - • IV antibiotics (eg, ticarcillin-clavulanate, ceftriaxone, vancomycin, metronidazole)
    - • Daily assessment with repeat CT scan if worsening despite appropriate therapy
    - • Surgical drainage of abscess may be required

- ■ Pearl

A poorly controlled diabetic or immunocompromised patient with orbital cellulitis has mucormycosis, a life-threatening condition, until proven otherwise.

Reference

Bilyk JR. Periocular infection. Curr Opin Ophthalmol 2007;18:414. [PMID: 17700236]

20

Preseptal Cellulitis

■ Essentials of Diagnosis

- Inflammation and infection confined to the eyelids and peri-orbital structures anterior to the orbital septum; the globe is typically uninvolved
- In children, underlying sinusitis is often the cause. In adults, trauma or a cutaneous source (eg, infected chalazion) is more typical
- Eyelid pain, tenderness, redness, warmth and swelling
- Visual acuity is unaffected, and there is *no* proptosis or restriction of eye motility
- CT scan can distinguish from orbital cellulitis, detect sinusitis, and exclude other causes

■ Differential Diagnosis

- Orbital cellulitis
- Insect or animal bite
- Retained foreign body
- Allergic reaction
- Inflammatory orbital pseudotumor
- Tumor

■ Treatment

- Antibiotics:
  - Children—intravenous (eg, ceftriaxone and vancomycin)
  - Teens and adults—oral (eg, amoxicillin-clavulanate or trimethoprim-sulfamethoxazole) for 10 days
- Surgical drainage if progresses to localized abscess

■ Pearl

In children this condition can be explosive and progress rapidly to orbital cellulitis; you will never be faulted for obtaining a CT scan and admitting for IV antibiotics if this is in the differential.

Reference

Chaudhry IA, Shamsi FA, Elzaridi E, Al-Rashed W, Al-Amri A, Arat YO. Inpatient preseptal cellulitis: experience from a tertiary eye care centre. Br J Ophthalmol 2008;92:1337. [PMID: 18697809]

20

Retinal Artery Occlusion (Branch or Central)

- ■ Essentials of Diagnosis
  - • Sudden unilateral and painless loss of vision or visual field defect
  - • Focal wedge-shaped area of retinal whitening or edema within the distribution of a branch arteriole or diffuse retinal whitening with a cherry-red spot at the fovea; arteriolar constriction with segmentation of blood column; visible emboli
  - • Central vision may be spared by a cilioretinal artery (present in up to 30% of individuals)
  - • Associated underlying diseases include carotid plaque or cardiac-source emboli; giant cell (temporal) arteritis
  - • Less common than vein occlusion in hypercoagulable states

- ■ Differential Diagnosis
  - • Ophthalmic artery occlusion
  - • Inherited metabolic or lysosomal storage disease (cherry-red spot)
  - • Ocular migraine

- ■ Treatment
  - • Medical emergency calling for immediate ophthalmologic referral
  - • Digital ocular massage, systemic acetazolamide or topical beta-blocker to lower intraocular pressure, anterior chamber paracentesis, and carbogen by facemask
  - • Check ESR and CRP to rule out giant cell (temporal) arteritis as an underlying etiology
  - • Consider ophthalmic artery thrombolysis if within 6–12 hours of onset of symptoms and no contraindications

- ■ Pearl

The retina is part of the central nervous system, and when rendered ischemic, the approach is that of any other transient ischemic attacks or stroke.

Reference

Haymore JG, Mejico LJ. Retinal vascular occlusion syndromes. Int Ophthalmol Clin 2009;49:63. [PMID: 19584622]

Retinal Detachment

- **Essentials of Diagnosis**
  - Risk factors include lattice vitreoretinal degeneration, posterior vitreous separation (especially with vitreous hemorrhage), high myopia, trauma, and previous ocular surgery (especially with vitreous loss)
  - Acute onset of photopsias (flashes of light), floaters ("cobwebs"), or shadow ("curtain") across the visual field, with peripheral or central visual loss
  - Elevation of the retina with a flap tear or break in the retina, vitreous pigmented cells or hemorrhage seen by ophthalmoscopy

- **Differential Diagnosis**
  - Retinoschisis
  - Choroidal detachment
  - Posterior vitreous separation

- **Treatment**
  - Immediate ophthalmologic referral
  - Repair of small tears by laser photocoagulation or cryopexy
  - Repair of retinal detachment by pneumatic retinopexy, scleral buckling, pars plana vitrectomy with drainage of subretinal fluid, endolaser, cryopexy, gas or silicone oil injection

- **Pearl**

Beware of flashers, floaters and visual field abnormalities in any patient with marked myopia and a history of eye trauma. This is a retinal detachment until proven otherwise.

Reference

D'Amico DJ. Clinical practice. Primary retinal detachment. N Engl J Med 2008;359:2346. [PMID: 19038880]

20

Retinal Vein Occlusion
(Branch, Hemiretinal, or Central)

- ■ Essentials of Diagnosis
  - Sudden, unilateral, and painless visual loss or field defect
  - Local or diffuse venous dilation and tortuosity, retinal hemorrhages, cotton-wool spots, and edema; optic disk edema and hemorrhages; neovascularization of disk, retina, or iris by funduscopy and slit lamp examination
  - Associated underlying diseases include atherosclerosis and hypertension, glaucoma, hypercoagulable state including factor V Leiden or natural anticoagulant deficiency (AT-III, protein S, protein C), lupus anticoagulant; hyperviscosity (polycythemia or Waldenström's), Behçet's disease, lupus
  - Retrobulbar external venous compression (thyroid disease, orbital tumor) and migraine also may be responsible

- ■ Differential Diagnosis
  - Venous stasis
  - Ocular ischemic syndrome
  - Diabetic retinopathy
  - Papilledema
  - Radiation retinopathy
  - Hypertensive retinopathy
  - Retinopathy of anemia
  - Leukemic retinopathy

- ■ Treatment
  - Prompt ophthalmologic referral
  - Laser photocoagulation, intravitreal steroids, intravitreal anti-angiogenesis drugs for iris or retinal neovascularization or persistent macular edema
  - Surveillance and treatment of underlying diseases

- ■ Pearl

Check for an elevated homocysteine level since this is a modifiable risk factor.

Reference

Haymore JG, Mejico LJ. Retinal vascular occlusion syndromes. Int Ophthalmol Clin 2009;49:63. [PMID: 19584622]

Subconjunctival Hemorrhage

- ■ Essentials of Diagnosis
  - • Acute painless onset of bright red blood in the white part of the eye; striking appearance, but painless with minimal to no effect on vision
  - • Most often occurs in patients on aspirin or anticoagulation who have a recent history of severe coughing, sneezing, heavy lifting, or constipation (Valsalva)
  - • Often seen in eye trauma, even a minor finger poke or aggressive eye rubbing
  - • Can have associated conjunctival edema (chemosis)

- ■ Differential Diagnosis
  - • Kaposi's sarcoma
  - • Conjunctival neoplasms such as lymphoma

- ■ Treatment
  - • None: Just like a bruise, the blood will change color and eventually be absorbed within a month; artificial tears if irritation present
  - • Hold aspirin, other NSAIDs, anticoagulation if possible
  - • Cough suppressant
  - • Stool softener
  - • Hematologic work-up and ophthalmologic referral if recurrent

- ■ Pearl

If a patient presents with this unilaterally, supportive care is fine; if he returns the next day with the same problem on the other side, evaluate for a hematologic cause such as leukemia.

Reference

Mimura T, Usui T, Yamagami S, Funatsu H, Noma H, Honda N, Amano S. Recent causes of subconjunctival hemorrhage. Ophthalmologica 2009;224:133. [PMID: 19738393]

20

Uveitis

- **Essentials of Diagnosis**
  - Inflammation of the uveal tract, including the iris (iritis), ciliary body (cyclitis), and choroid (choroiditis); categorized as anterior (iridocyclitis), posterior (chorioretinitis), or diffuse (panuveitis)
  - Acute onset of eye pain, redness, photophobia, and blurred vision (anterior uveitis); gradual visual loss with floaters, but otherwise asymptomatic (posterior uveitis); may be unilateral or bilateral
  - Injected conjunctiva or sclera with flare and inflammatory cells on slit lamp examination, white cells on corneal endothelium, and iris nodules (anterior uveitis); white cells and opacities in the vitreous, retinal, or choroidal infiltrates, edema, and vascular sheathing (posterior uveitis)
  - Multiple causes: Post-trauma or surgery, lens-induced, HLAB27–associated (ankylosing spondylitis, Reiter's syndrome, psoriatic arthritis, inflammatory bowel disease), infectious (herpes simplex or zoster, syphilis, tuberculosis, toxoplasmosis, toxocariasis, histoplasmosis, leprosy, Lyme disease, CMV, Candida), sarcoidosis, Behçet's disease, Vogt-Koyanagi-Harada syndrome

- **Differential Diagnosis**
  - Acute conjunctivitis
  - Corneal abrasion or infection
  - Retinal detachment
  - Retinitis pigmentosa
  - Intraocular tumor (eg, retinoblastoma, leukemia, melanoma, lymphoma)
  - Retained intraocular foreign body
  - Scleritis

- **Treatment**
  - Prompt ophthalmologic referral in all cases
  - Anterior disease: Frequent topical steroids, periocular steroid injection, dilation of the pupil with cycloplegic agent
  - Posterior disease: More commonly requires systemic steroids and immunosuppressive agents

- **Pearl**

The acute red eye in a patient with many systemic diseases is difficult for primary providers to evaluate; refer such patients promptly to ophthalmology given the plethora of causes of this problem.

20

Reference

Lyon F, Gale RP, Lightman S. Recent developments in the treatment of uveitis: an update. Expert Opin Investig Drugs 2009;18:609. [PMID: 19388878]

21

Common Disorders of the Ear, Nose, and Throat

Acute Otitis Externa

- **Essentials of Diagnosis**
  - Often a history of water exposure or trauma to the ear canal
  - Presents with otalgia, often accompanied by pruritus and purulent discharge
  - Usually caused by *Pseudomonas aeruginosa, Staphylococcus aureus,* or fungi (*Candida, Aspergillus*)
  - Movement of the auricle and tragus elicits pain; erythema and edema of the ear canal with a purulent exudate on examination
  - Tympanic membrane (TM) is red but moves normally with pneumatic otoscopy, but often not seen due to ear canal edema

- **Differential Diagnosis**
  - Malignant otitis externa (external otitis in an immunocompromised or diabetic patient, or one with osteomyelitis of the temporal bone); *Pseudomonas* causative in diabetes
  - Acute suppurative otitis media with tympanic membrane rupture

- **Treatment**
  - Prevent additional moisture and mechanical injury to the ear canal
  - Otic drops containing a mixture of an aminoglycoside or quinolones as well as a corticosteroid
  - Purulent debris filling the canal should be removed; occasionally, a wick is needed to facilitate entry of the otic drops
  - Analgesics

- **Pearl**

A painful red ear in a toxic-appearing diabetic is assumed to be malignant otitis externa until proved otherwise.

Reference

Drehobl M, Guerrero JL, Lacarte PR, Goldstein G, Mata FS, Luber S. Comparison of efficacy and safety of ciprofloxacin otic solution 0.2% versus polymyxin B-neomycin-hydrocortisone in the treatment of acute diffuse otitis externa. Curr Med Res Opin 2008;24:3531. [PMID: 19032135]

Acute Otitis Media

- **Essentials of Diagnosis**
    - Bacterial infection resulting in accumulation of purulent fluid in the middle ear and mastoid space
    - Ear pain, with aural fullness and hearing loss; fever and chills; onset often follows upper respiratory syndrome or barotrauma
    - Dullness and hyperemia of eardrum with loss of landmarks and light reflex
    - Bulging eardrum, eardrum rupture, and drainage can occur in severe cases
    - Most common organisms in both children and adults include *Streptococcus pneumoniae, Haemophilus influenzae, Moraxella catarrhalis,* and group A streptococcus
    - Complications include mastoiditis, facial paralysis, petrous apicitis, sigmoid sinus thromboses, meningitis, brain abscess

- **Differential Diagnosis**
    - Bullous myringitis
    - Acute external otitis
    - Otalgia referred from other sources (especially pharynx)
    - Serous otitis media

- **Treatment**
    - Antibiotics (first-line treatment is amoxicillin or erythromycin plus sulfonamide) versus supportive care controversial; oral and/or nasal decongestants and analgesics
    - Surgical drainage and tympanostomy tubes for refractory cases, with audiology and otolaryngology referral
    - Prophylactic antibiotics for recurrent acute otitis media

- **Pearl**

Recurrent otitis media remains one of the few indications for tonsillectomy; when they are markedly enlarged, tonsils may obstruct the eustachian tube and cause the problem.

Reference

Wilkinson EP, Friedman RA. Acute suppurative otitis media. Ear Nose Throat J 2008;87:250. [PMID: 18572776]

21

Acute Sialadenitis
(Parotitis, Submandibular Gland Adenitis)

■ Essentials of Diagnosis

- Inflammation of parotid or submandibular gland due to salivary stasis from obstruction or decreased production
- Predisposing conditions include sialolithiasis, duct stricture, and dehydration
- Diffuse swelling and pain overlying the parotid or submandibular gland
- Examination shows erythema and edema over affected gland and pus from affected duct
- May be confused with rapidly enlarging lymph node
- Causative organism usually *Staphylococcus aureus*
- Complications: Parotid or submandibular space abscess

■ Differential Diagnosis

- Salivary gland tumor
- Facial cellulitis or dental abscess
- Sjögren's syndrome
- Mumps
- Lymphoepithelial cysts or Burkitt's lymphoma in immunocompromised patients

■ Treatment

- Antibiotics with gram-positive coverage
- Warm compresses and massage
- Sialogogues (eg, lemon wedges or lemon drops)
- Hydration
- Oral hygiene

■ Pearl

In patients presenting with unilateral anterior cervical "lymphadenopathy," ask about recent vigorous exercise on warm days; the "node" may be a salivary gland, and hyperamylasemia may save you a costly and painful evaluation.

Reference

Arduino PG, Carrozzo M, Pentenero M, Bertolusso G, Gandolfo S. Non-neoplastic salivary gland diseases. Minerva Stomatol 2006;55:249. [PMID: 16688102]

21

Acute Sinusitis

- **Essentials of Diagnosis**
  - Nasal congestion, purulent nasal discharge, facial pain, and headache; facial pain or pressure over the affect sinus or sinuses
  - Teeth may hurt or feel abnormal in maxillary sinusitis
  - History of allergic rhinitis, acute upper respiratory infection, or dental infection often present
  - Acute onset of symptoms (between 1–4 week duration)
  - Coronal CT scans have become the diagnostic study of choice; opacification of affected sinus or sinuses seen.
  - Typical pathogens include *Streptococcus pneumoniae,* other streptococci, *Haemophilus influenzae, Staphylococcus aureus, Moraxella catarrhalis; Aspergillus* in immunocompromised patients and anaerobes in chronic sinusitis
  - Complications: Orbital cellulitis or abscess, meningitis, brain abscess, cavernous sinus thrombosis

- **Differential Diagnosis**
  - Viral or allergic rhinitis
  - Dental abscess
  - Dacryocystitis
  - Carcinoma of sinus or inverting papilloma
  - Cephalalgia due to other causes, especially cluster headache

- **Treatment**
  - Oral and nasal decongestants, antibiotics (first-line therapy amoxicillin or macrolide), nasal saline
  - Functional endoscopic sinus surgery or external sinus procedures for medically resistant sinusitis, nasal polyposis, sinusitis complications

- **Pearl**

Sphenoid sinusitis is the only cause in medicine of a nasal ridge headache radiating to the top of the skull.

Reference

Ahovuo-Saloranta A, Borisenko OV, Kovanen N, Varonen H, Rautakorpi UM, Williams JW Jr, Mäkelä M. Antibiotics for acute maxillary sinusitis. Cochrane Database Syst Rev 2008;CD000243. [PMID: 18425861]

Allergic Rhinitis

- ■ Essentials of Diagnosis
  - • Seasonal or perennial occurrence of clear nasal discharge, sneezing, itching of eyes and nose
  - • Pale, boggy mucous membranes with conjunctival injection
  - • Environmental allergen exposure; presence of allergen-specific IgE

- ■ Differential Diagnosis
  - • Upper respiratory viral infections
  - • Chronic sinusitis
  - • Vasomotor or nonallergic rhinitis

- ■ Treatment
  - • Oral or nasal antihistamines; oral decongestants
  - • Intranasal corticosteroids
  - • Nasal saline irrigation
  - • Adjunctive measures: Antileukotriene medications, intranasal anticholinergic agents, cromolyn sodium
  - • Avoiding or reducing exposure to allergens
  - • For cases refractory to medications, referral to allergist for consideration of immunotherapy may be appropriate

- ■ Pearl

A Wright's—not Gram's—flambé of secretions is the best way to demonstrate eosinophils: stain the smear, ignite it, decolorize it, and the cells stand out at low power.

Reference

Marple BF, Stankiewicz JA, Baroody FM, et al; American Academy of Otolaryngic Allergy Working Group on Chronic Rhinosinusitis. Diagnosis and management of chronic rhinosinusitis in adults. Postgrad Med 2009;121:121. [PMID: 19940423]

Benign Paroxysmal Positional Vertigo

- **Essentials of Diagnosis**
  - Acute onset of vertigo with or without nausea, lasting for seconds to a minute
  - Provoked by changes in head positioning rather than by maintenance of a particular posture, often provoked by rolling over in bed
  - Rotatory nystagmus with positive Dix-Hallpike test (delayed onset of symptoms by movement of head with habituation and fatigue of symptoms)
  - Caused by dislocated otoconia (from labyrinth of the inner ear) that cause abnormal stimulation

- **Differential Diagnosis**
  - Endolymphatic hydrops
  - Vestibular neuronitis
  - Posterior fossa tumor
  - Vertebrobasilar insufficiency
  - Migraines

- **Treatment**
  - Possible spontaneous recovery in weeks to months
  - Medical treatment with anti-vertigo medications may be helpful in the acute setting for a severe exacerbation of BPPV
  - Otolaryngologic referral for persistent symptoms or other neurologic abnormalities
  - Epley maneuver to reposition otoconia highly successful
  - Surgery to occlude posterior semicircular canal or singular nerve sectioning considered for refractory cases

- **Pearl**

Learn this well—it's the most common cause of an otherwise potentially serious symptom in primary care settings.

Reference

Halker RB, Barrs DM, Wellik KE, Wingerchuk DM, Demaerschalk BM. Establishing a diagnosis of benign paroxysmal positional vertigo through the dix-hallpike and side-lying maneuvers: a critically appraised topic. Neurologist 2008;14:201. [PMID: 18469678]

Chronic Serous Otitis Media

- **Essentials of Diagnosis**
  - Due to obstruction of the eustachian tube, resulting in transudation of fluid
  - More common in children, but can occur in adults after an upper respiratory tract infection, scuba diving, air travel, or eustachian tube obstruction by tumor
  - Painless hearing loss with feeling of fullness or voice reverberation in affected ear
  - Dull, immobile tympanic membrane with loss of landmarks and bubbles seen behind tympanic membrane; intact light reflex
  - Fifteen- to 20-decibel conductive hearing loss by audiometry; patient lateralizes to affected ear on Weber tuning fork examination

- **Differential Diagnosis**
  - Acute otitis media
  - Nasopharyngeal tumor (as causative agent)

- **Treatment**
  - Oral decongestants, antihistamines, oral or intranasal steroids, and antibiotics
  - Tympanotomy tubes for refractory cases with audiology and otolaryngology referral

- **Pearl**

Unilateral otitis media, especially in a patient of Asian ethnicity, may well be caused by nasopharyngeal carcinoma; mirror examination of the nasopharynx is essential for complete evaluation of unilateral serous otitis media in adults.

Reference

Pelikan Z. The role of nasal allergy in chronic secretory otitis media. Ann Allergy Asthma Immunol 2007;99:401. [PMID: 18051208]

21

Endolymphatic Hydrops (Ménière's Syndrome)

- ■ Essentials of Diagnosis
  - • Etiology is unknown
  - • Distention of the endolymphatic compartment of the inner ear is a pathologic finding
  - • Classic syndrome: Episodic vertigo and nausea (lasting minutes to hours), aural pressure, tinnitus, and fluctuating hearing loss
  - • Sensorineural hearing loss by audiometry worse in the low frequencies

- ■ Differential Diagnosis
  - • Benign paroxysmal positional vertigo
  - • Posterior fossa tumor
  - • Vestibular neuronitis
  - • Vertebrobasilar insufficiency
  - • Migraine
  - • Psychiatric disorder
  - • Multiple sclerosis
  - • Syphilis

- ■ Treatment
  - • Low-salt diet and diuretics
  - • Antihistamines, diazepam, and antiemetics for severe symptomatic relief
  - • Intratympanic corticosteroid injections
  - • Intratympanic aminoglycoside injection for ablation of unilateral vestibular function
  - • Surgical treatment in refractory cases: Decompression of endolymphatic sac, vestibular nerve section, or labyrinthectomy if profound hearing loss present

- ■ Pearl

One of the few unilateral diseases of paired organs.

Reference

Süslü N, Yilmaz T, Gürsel B. Utility of immunologic parameters in the evaluation of Meniere's disease. Acta Otolaryngol 2009;129:1160. [PMID: 19863304]

Epiglottitis

■ Essentials of Diagnosis

- More common in children but increasingly recognized in adults
- Sudden onset of stridor, odynophagia, dysphagia, and drooling
- Muffled voice, toxic-appearing and febrile patient; patients may present in a "sniffing" position
- Unlike in children, indirect laryngoscopy is generally safe to perform in adults
- Should be suspected when odynophagia is out of proportion to oropharyngeal findings
- *Haemophilus influenzae* type B was historically the most common organism, but incidence of epiglottitis has dropped dramatically due to vaccination

■ Differential Diagnosis

- Viral croup
- Foreign body in larynx
- Retropharyngeal abscess
- Lemierre's syndrome (septic thrombophlebitis of internal jugular vein)

■ Treatment

- Humidified oxygen with no manipulation of oropharynx or epiglottis
- Airway observation in a monitored setting, intubation with tracheotomy stand-by
- Children usually need intubation; adults need close airway observation
- Parenteral antibiotics active against *Haemophilus influenzae* and Streptococcus pneumoniae, plus a short course of systemic corticosteroids

■ Pearl

The patient with hoarseness, drooling, and a severe sore throat, whose physical exam is unimpressive, has epiglottitis until proven otherwise.

Reference

Mathoera RB, Wever PC, van Dorsten FR, Balter SG, de Jager CP. Epiglottitis in the adult patient. Neth J Med 2008;66:373. [PMID: 18931398]

21

Epistaxis

- **Essentials of Diagnosis**
    - Bleeding is most commonly from the anterior septum (Kiesselbach's plexus)
    - Precipitating factors: Nasal trauma, mucosal dryness, hypertension, anticoagulation, inhaled drug use, and hereditary hemorrhagic telangiectasia

- **Differential Diagnosis**
    - In recurrent and/or persistent cases, consider endoscopic examination to evaluate for nasal masses or mucosal disease that may result in repeated bleeding episodes

- **Treatment**
    - Treat underlying causes (ie, control blood pressure if hypertensive)
    - Direct pressure to nares continuously for 15 minutes
    - Topical nasal decongestant spray (phenylephrine, oxymetazoline, Neo-Synephrine)
    - If visible, bleeding site can be cauterized with silver nitrate
    - If bleeding continues despite pressure, nasal packing should be placed (gauze ribbon, compressed sponge, epistaxis balloon catheter)
    - Posterior epistaxis balloons generally have separate anterior and posterior balloons
    - Endovascular embolization and surgical cauterization and/or vessel ligation are considerations for refractory persistent bleeding

- **Pearl**

Patients with posterior nasal packs should be admitted for monitoring; reflex bradydysrhythmia can develop because of stimulation of the deep posterior oropharynx by the packing.

Reference

Schlosser RJ. Clinical practice. Epistaxis. N Engl J Med 2009;360:784. [PMID: 19228621]

Viral Rhinitis

- **Essentials of Diagnosis**
  - Headache, nasal congestion, clear rhinorrhea, sneezing, scratchy throat, and malaise
  - Due to a variety of viruses, including rhinovirus and adenovirus
  - Examination of the nares reveals erythematous mucosa and clear discharge

- **Differential Diagnosis**
  - Acute sinusitis
  - Allergic rhinitis
  - Bacterial pharyngitis

- **Treatment**
  - Supportive treatment only: Anti-inflammatories, antihistamines, decongestants
  - Phenylephrine nasal sprays (should not be used for more than 5 days), saline nasal spray
  - Secondary bacterial infection suggested by a change of rhinorrhea from clear to yellow or green; cultures are useful to guide antimicrobial therapy

- **Pearl**

To date, no cure has been discovered for the common cold; physicians should not anticipate one and resist the temptation to give antibiotics— though this remains difficult in insistent patients.

Reference

Simasek M, Blandino DA. Treatment of the common cold. Am Fam Physician 2007;75:515. [PMID: 17323712]

21

22

Poisoning

Acetaminophen (Tylenol; Many Others)

- **Essentials of Diagnosis**
  - Most widely used antipyretic/analgesic makes it the most common cause of acute hepatic failure in the United States
  - First 24 hours: May be asymptomatic or have generalized malaise
  - 24–48 hours: Increased transaminases, right upper quadrant pain, vomiting
  - 72–96 hours: Enzymes peak, hepatic failure, encephalopathy, renal failure possible
  - 4 days–3 weeks: Resolution of symptoms (if they survive)
  - Toxic dose: 150 mg/kg (children) or 7.5 g (adults)
  - Peak levels occur 30–60 minutes after ingestion
  - Measure serum acetaminophen level 4 hours postingestion
  - Plot on nomogram and treat if level above lower limit (> 150 μg/mL); if lab units in milligrams per deciliter, multiply by 10
  - Detectable serum acetaminophen level or elevated transaminases require treatment if presentation after 24 hours
  - Patients may not realize that combination analgesics (eg, Percocet, Vicodin, Darvocet) contain acetaminophen

- **Differential Diagnosis**
  - Viral hepatitis, pancreatitis, peptic ulcer disease

- **Treatment**
  - Activated charcoal with N-acetylcysteine (NAC; see below)
  - Gastric lavage if less than 1 hour since ingestion or large ingestion
  - NAC: repeat dose of NAC if vomited within 1 hour of administration
  - If given within 8 hours of ingestion, NAC nearly 100% protective
  - Intravenous NAC may be given when oral route not possible

- **Pearl**

In childhood overdose, it is usually the second-born who suffers it; the taller sibling may reach the medicine chest and feed the unknowing younger one.

Reference

Waring WS, et al. Lower incidence of anaphylactoid reactions to N-acetylcysteine in patients with high acetaminophen concentrations after overdose. Clin Toxicol (Phila) 2008;46:496. [PMID: 18584360]

Amphetamines, Ecstasy, Cocaine

■ Essentials of Diagnosis

- Sympathomimetic clinical scenario: Anxiety, tremulousness, agitation, tachycardia, hypertension, diaphoresis, dilated pupils, muscular hyperactivity, hyperthermia
- Psychosis and seizures can occur, 2–6 hours postingestion if severe
- Metabolic acidosis may occur
- With cocaine in particular, hemorrhagic stroke and myocardial infarction
- Ecstasy (MDMA) associated with serotonin syndrome (see antidepressants), hyponatremia, and malignant hyperthermia
- Obtain rectal temperature
- Studies include glucose, chemistry panel, renal panel, urinalysis, ECG, cardiac monitoring, prothrombin time (PT) /partial thromboplastin time (PTT)

■ Differential Diagnosis

- Anticholinergic poisoning
- Functional psychosis
- Heat stroke
- Other stimulant overdose (eg, ephedrine, phenylpropanolamine)

■ Treatment

- Activated charcoal for oral ingestions if airway is protected or secure; may not be effective because most are rapidly absorbed
- Gastric lavage if less than 1 hour since ingestion
- For agitation or psychosis: Sedation with benzodiazepines may need large doses; titrate rapidly in first 30 minutes; neuroleptics lower seizure threshold and may worsen the clinical outcome
- For hyperthermia: Remove clothing, cool mist spray, cooling blanket, benzodiazepines for muscle rigidity
- For hypertension: Benzodiazepines; if refractory, start nitroprusside infusion; avoid beta-blockers, as they may worsen hypertension due to unopposed alpha stimulation
- For chest pain: Benzodiazepines, aspirin, nitroglycerin; give morphine if not responsive

■ Pearl

These remain common clinical problems, and amphetamine abuse in particular should be considered in a hyperadrenergic patient.

Reference

Dutra L, Stathopoulou G, Basden SL, Leyro TM, Powers MB, Otto MW. A meta-analytic review of psychosocial interventions for substance use disorders. Am J Psychiatry 2008;165:179. [PMID: 18198270]

22

Anticholinergics
(Atropine, Scopolamine, Antihistamines)

■ Essentials of Diagnosis

- Contained in antihistamines, antipsychotics, antispasmodics, belladonna alkaloids, cyclic antidepressants, mushrooms, and some plants
- Anticholinergic toxidrome: "Hot as Hades" (hyperthermia), "blind as a bat" (mydriasis), "dry as a bone" (dry mucous membranes, thirst), "red as a beet" (flushed, dry skin), and "mad as a hatter" (agitation)
- Also can see myoclonus, decreased gut motility, distended bladder, seizures
- Prolonged QT interval and torsade de pointes with nonsedating antihistamines
- Useful studies include electrolyte panel, creatinine, calcium, glucose, urinalysis, creatinine kinase, and ECG

■ Differential Diagnosis

- Sympathomimetic overdose
- LSD or other hallucinogen ingestion
- Delirium tremens, acute psychosis
- Hyperthyroidism
- Jimsonweed or other ingestion of an anticholinergic-containing plant

■ Treatment

- Single-dose activated charcoal (repeated doses may cause abdominal distention)
- Consider gastric lavage if less than 1 hour since ingestion
- In those with hyperthermia, benzodiazepines, cooling fan, ice water bath, intravenous hydration
- Despite being the reversal agent, the use of physostigmine is controversial and limited to severe symptomatology (tachycardia with hypotension, repeat seizures, severe agitation or seizures) as it can cause asystole; it is contraindicated if conduction abnormalities are seen on ECG or tricyclic coingestion is suspected

■ Pearl

To distinguish anticholinergic toxicity from sympathomimetic toxicity, check for skin moisture (eg, sweating in the axilla); anticholinergic toxicity yields a hot but dry axilla.

Reference

Lin TJ, Nelson LS, Tsai JL, Hung DZ, Hu SC, Chan HM, Deng JF. Common toxidromes of plant poisonings in Taiwan. Clin Toxicol (Phila) 2009;47:161. [PMID: 18788001]

Antidepressants: Atypical Agents (Serotonin Syndrome)

- ## Essentials of Diagnosis
  - Trazodone, bupropion, venlafaxine, and the SSRIs (fluoxetine, sertraline, paroxetine, fluvoxamine, escitalopram, citalopram); well-tolerated in pure overdoses, high toxic:therapeutic ratios
  - Nausea, vomiting, dizziness, blurred vision, sinus tachycardia; citalopram may cause ECG changes
  - Serotonin syndrome (by overdose or interaction with other medications): Mental status changes, agitation, autonomic instability, myoclonus, hyperreflexia, diaphoresis, tremor, diarrhea, incoordination, fever
  - Useful studies include ECG, chemistry panel, urinalysis

- ## Differential Diagnosis
  - Alcohol withdrawal
  - Heatstroke
  - Hypoglycemia, hyperthyroidism
  - Neuroleptic malignant syndrome

- ## Treatment
  - Activated charcoal
  - Gastric lavage if less than 1 hour since large ingestion or if a mixed drug ingestion
  - In those with hyperthermia, aggressive cooling, intravenous fluids, and benzodiazepines useful
  - Cardiac monitoring and ECG based on specific agent (eg, citalopram)
  - Benzodiazepines initially; bupropion, venlafaxine, and SSRIs associated with seizures
  - Serotonin syndrome typically self-limited within 24–36 hours; stop all offending agents
  - Cyproheptadine (an antiserotonergic agent) in serotonin syndrome has unproven benefit; consider only after cooling and sedation initiated

- ## Pearl

Remember that rave participants increase the risk by taking an SSRI ("preloading") followed by ecstasy.

Reference

Nelson LS, Erdman AR, Booze LL, et al. Selective serotonin reuptake inhibitor poisoning: an evidence-based consensus guideline for out-of-hospital management. Clin Toxicol (Phila) 2007;45:315. [PMID: 17486478]

Antidepressants: Tricyclics

- ■ Essentials of Diagnosis
  - Hypotension, tachydysrhythmia, and seizures are the most life-threatening presentation and develop within 2 hours of ingestion; other symptoms due to anticholinergic effects
  - Peripheral antimuscarinic: Dry mouth, dry skin, muscle twitching, decreased bowel activity, dilated pupils
  - Central antimuscarinic: Agitation, delirium, confusion, hallucinations, slurred speech, ataxia, sedation, coma
  - Cardiac: QRS-interval widening, large R-wave in aVR, terminal right axis deviation, prolonged QTc interval, sinus tachycardia
  - Generalized seizures from $GABA_A$-receptor antagonism
  - Toxicity can occur at therapeutic doses in combination with other drugs (antihistamines, antipsychotics)
  - Useful studies include ECG and telemetric monitoring, chemistry panel, renal panel, glucose, urinalysis, qualitative tricyclic determination, complete blood count

- ■ Differential Diagnosis
  - Other drug ingestions: Carbamazepine, antihistamines, class Ia and Ic antiarrhythmics, propranolol, lithium, cocaine
  - Hyperkalemia
  - Hypocalcemia

- ■ Treatment
  - Activated charcoal
  - Gastric lavage if less than 1 hour since ingestion
  - Alkalinize serum with sodium bicarbonate for QRS > 100 milliseconds, refractory hypotension, or ventricular dysrhythmia (to reach goal serum pH 7.50–7.55)
  - Seizures usually respond to benzodiazepines; phenytoin not recommended for refractory seizures due to possible prodysrhythmic effects
  - Hypotension must be rapidly corrected with intravenous fluids and vasopressors if necessary (eg, norepinephrine)

- ■ Pearl

TCAs are responsible for a high percentage of overdose-related deaths; development of newer and perhaps safer antidepressants holds hope for ameliorating this.

Reference

Pierog JE, Kane KE, Kane BG, Donovan JW, Helmick T. Tricyclic antidepressant toxicity treated with massive sodium bicarbonate. Am J Emerg Med 2009;27:1168.e3. [PMID: 19931778]

Arsenic

- **Essentials of Diagnosis**
  - Symptoms appear within 1 hour after ingestion but may last as long as 12 hours
  - Symptoms depend on amount, time, and form ingested
  - A garlic smell may be noticed on breath or from body fluids
  - Acute ingestion: Nausea, vomiting, abdominal pain, diarrhea, dysrhythmias, hypotension, seizures
  - Acute hemolytic anemia may develop, leading to hemoglobinuria
  - Chronic ingestion: Headache, encephalopathy, dermatitis, neuropathy, peripheral edema, leukopenia
  - Useful studies include abdominal x-ray (may demonstrate metallic ingestion), spot urine for arsenic, complete blood count (basophilic stippling of red cells), renal panel, liver panel, urinalysis, 24-hour urine, ECG

- **Differential Diagnosis**
  - Gastroenteritis
  - Septic shock
  - Other heavy metal toxicities, including thallium, iron, lead, and mercury
  - Other peripheral neuropathies, including Guillain-Barré syndrome
  - Addison's disease

- **Treatment**
  - Intravenous fluids and vasopressors, if necessary, for hypotension
  - Dysrhythmias: Lidocaine or defibrillation for ventricular tachycardia; intravenous magnesium or isoproterenol, overdrive pacing for torsade de pointes
  - Benzodiazepines for seizures
  - Chelation therapy should begin as soon as acute arsenic toxicity is suspected
  - If radiopaque material visible on abdominal films, bowel decontamination recommended (gastric lavage followed by activated charcoal followed by whole-bowel irrigation until abdominal films are clear)

- **Pearl**

Although the point has been made repeatedly on stage and screen, it is still wise to suspect this poisoning in a widowed woman with psychiatric problems, especially if it has happened more than once.

Reference

Rahman MM, Ng JC, Naidu R. Chronic exposure of arsenic via drinking water and its adverse health impacts on humans. Environ Geochem Health 2009;31(suppl 1):189. [PMID: 19190988]

Benzodiazepines

- **Essentials of Diagnosis**
  - Primarily CNS effects, including drowsiness, slurred speech, confusion, ataxia, respiratory depression, hypotension, coma
  - Isolated benzodiazepine ingestion rarely results in death; mixed ingestions (alcohol, narcotics, other sedatives) increase morbidity and mortality

- **Differential Diagnosis**
  - Other sedative-hypnotic agents (eg, chloral hydrate, barbiturates)
  - Toxic alcohols
  - Opioid ingestion
  - Metabolic encephalopathy
  - Encephalitis, meningitis, other medical diseases of the CNS

- **Treatment**
  - Patients who are unresponsive or confused should receive dextrose, thiamine, and naloxone
  - Respiratory depression should be monitored closely; intubate if necessary
  - Activated charcoal
  - Flumazenil, the reversal agent, has an extremely limited role in patients with acute overdose due to the possibility of severe side effects (eg, seizures)

- **Pearl**

Obtain the toxicology screen before giving benzodiazepines for any suspected withdrawal syndrome.

Reference

Charlson F, Degenhardt L, McLaren J, Hall W, Lynskey M. A systematic review of research examining benzodiazepine-related mortality. Pharmacoepidemiol Drug Saf 2009;18:93. [PMID: 19125401]

Beta-Blockers

- **Essentials of Diagnosis**
  - Hypotension, bradycardia, atrioventricular block, cardiogenic shock, torsade de pointes (due to sotalol)
  - Altered mental status, psychosis, seizures, and coma, most often in the setting of hypotension and hypoglycemia, but may also occur with propranolol and other lipophilic agents
  - Onset of symptoms typically within 2 hours of overdose
  - Useful studies include ECG (bradycardia, prolonged PR interval, AV block, widened QRS interval), serum digoxin level, chemistry panel

- **Differential Diagnosis**
  - Calcium antagonist and digitalis overdose
  - Cardiogenic shock
  - Tricyclic antidepressant toxicity
  - Cholinergic toxicity

- **Treatment**
  - If endotracheal intubation or gastric lavage required, pretreat with atropine to limit vagal stimulation
  - Gastric lavage is recommended for large overdoses, provided the patient presents within 1 hour of ingestion (even if asymptomatic)
  - Multidose activated charcoal for sustained-release preparations
  - Supportive therapy for bradycardia and hypotension, including crystalloid infusion and atropine
  - Administration of glucagon can be diagnostic and therapeutic
  - If the above fails, then epinephrine, isoproterenol, or dobutamine infusion, aortic balloon pump
  - High-dose insulin with glucose therapy effective in refractory cases of beta-blocker overdose

- **Pearl**

Beta-blocker toxicity commonly has mental status changes, whereas calcium channel blocker toxicity doesn't.

Reference

Kerns W 2nd. Management of beta-adrenergic blocker and calcium channel antagonist toxicity. Emerg Med Clin North Am 2007;25:309; abstract viii. [PMID: 17482022]

Calcium Antagonists (Calcium Channel Blockers)

- ■ Essentials of Diagnosis
  - Bradycardia, hypotension, atrioventricular block, hyperglycemia
  - Cardiogenic shock or cardiac arrest leading to pulmonary edema
  - Decreased cerebral perfusion leads to confusion or agitation, dizziness, lethargy, seizures
  - Useful studies include ECG, serum digoxin level, chemistry panel, and ionized calcium

- ■ Differential Diagnosis
  - Beta-blocker or digitalis toxicity
  - Tricyclic antidepressant toxicity
  - Acute myocardial infarction with cardiogenic shock
  - Hypotensive, bradycardic shock typically distinct from hyperdynamic shock of hypovolemia or sepsis

- ■ Treatment
  - Gastric lavage often used
  - Activated charcoal if airway is protected and/or secure
  - Whole-bowel irrigation for sustained-release preparations
  - Supportive therapy for coma, hypotension, and seizures
  - To combat cardiotoxic effects: Fluid boluses and atropine
  - Calcium chloride is the reversal agent if refractory
  - Glucagon bolus: 2–5 mg over 60 seconds, repeat up to total of 10 mg; then begin intravenous infusion
  - High-dose insulin with glucose therapy may be effective when above measures have failed

- ■ Pearl

Verapamil is the most potent negative inotrope among calcium blockers; severe cardiac failure may ensue with overdose.

Reference

Arroyo AM, Kao LW. Calcium channel blocker toxicity. Pediatr Emerg Care 2009;25:532. [PMID: 19687715]

Carbon Monoxide

- ■ Essentials of Diagnosis
  - • May result from exposure to any incomplete combustion of any carbonaceous fossil fuel (eg, automobile exhaust, smoke inhalation, improperly vented gas heater)
  - • Causes tissue hypoxia and thus affects the organs with highest oxygen demand (heart, brain)
  - • Symptoms nonspecific and flulike: Fatigue, headache, dizziness, abdominal pain, nausea, confusion
  - • With more severe intoxication, lethargy, syncope, seizures, coma
  - • Secondary injury from ischemia: Myocardial infarction, rhabdomyolysis, noncardiogenic pulmonary edema, retinal hemorrhages, neurologic deficits
  - • Survivors of severe poisoning may have permanent neurologic deficits
  - • Useful studies include carboxyhemoglobin level (can be venous), ECG, chemistry panel, renal panel, arterial blood gas; pulse oximetry can be falsely normal

- ■ Differential Diagnosis
  - • Cyanide poisoning; depressant drug ingestion
  - • Acute coronary syndrome; meningitis; encephalitis

- ■ Treatment
  - • Remove from exposure
  - • Maintain airway and assist ventilation; intubation may be necessary
  - • 100% oxygen by nonrebreathing facemask decreases carboxyhemoglobin half-life to 80 minutes from 4–6 hours
  - • Hyperbaric oxygen (decreases carboxyhemoglobin half-life to 20 minutes) considered in patients with syncope, coma, seizures, Glasgow Coma Scale score < 15, myocardial ischemia, ventricular dysrhythmias, neurologic deficits or persistent headache, ataxia after 2–4 hours of oxygen treatment, or pregnant women

- ■ Pearl

Think of carbon monoxide poisoning if several family members present with nonspecific symptoms during the winter months; indoor combustion of firewood may be responsible.

Reference

Wolf SJ, et al. Critical issues in the management of adult patients presenting to the emergency department with acute carbon monoxide poisoning. Ann Emerg Med 2008;51:138. [PMID: 18206551]

Cardiac Glycosides (Digitalis)

- ■ Essentials of Diagnosis
  - Accidental ingestion, common in children
  - May be due to plant ingestions: Oleander, foxglove, lily of the valley, red squill, dogbane
  - Age, coexisting disease, electrolyte disturbance (hypokalemia, hypomagnesemia, hypercalcemia), hypoxemia, and other cardiac medications (including diuretics) increase potential for digitalis toxicity
  - Acute overdose: Nausea, vomiting, severe hyperkalemia, visual disturbances, syncope, confusion, delirium, bradycardia, supraventricular or ventricular dysrhythmias, atrioventricular block
  - Chronic toxicity: Nausea, vomiting, ventricular arrhythmias
  - Elevated serum digoxin level in acute overdose; level may be normal with chronic toxicity
  - Useful studies include: ECG, serum digoxin level, chemistry panel, magnesium, calcium, renal panel

- ■ Differential Diagnosis
  - Beta-blocker or calcium channel blocker toxicity
  - Tricyclic antidepressant ingestion
  - Clonidine overdose
  - Organophosphate insecticide poisoning

- ■ Treatment
  - Activated charcoal; multiple doses may be required due to enterohepatic circulation of digoxin
  - Gastric lavage if less than 1 hour since ingestion
  - Maintain adequate airway and assist ventilation as necessary
  - Correct hypomagnesemia, hypoxia, hypoglycemia, hyperkalemia or hypokalemia; calcium is contraindicated, as it may generate ventricular arrhythmias
  - Lidocaine, phenytoin, magnesium for ventricular arrhythmias
  - Atropine, pacemaker for bradycardia or atrioventricular block
  - Digoxin-specific antibody indicated if: Severe ventricular dysrhythmias, bradycardia unresponsive to atropine, digoxin level > 15 ng/mL, ingestion of > 10 mg in previously healthy adult, and serum potassium > 5 mEq/L

- ■ Pearl

Think of this immediately with exceptionally high levels of potassium without very obvious other explanation.

Reference

Vivo RP, Krim SR, Perez J, Inklab M, Tenner T Jr, Hodgson J. Digoxin: current use and approach to toxicity. Am J Med Sci 2008;336:423. [PMID: 19011400]

Cyanide

- ■ Essentials of Diagnosis
  - • Laboratory or industrial exposure (plastics, solvents, glues, fabrics), smoke inhalation in fires
  - • Byproduct of the breakdown of nitroprusside, ingestion of cyanogenic glycosides in some plant products (apricot pits, bitter almonds)
  - • Absorbed rapidly by inhalation, through skin, or gastrointestinally
  - • Symptoms shortly after inhalation or ingestion; some compounds (acetonitrile, a cosmetic nail remover) metabolize to hydrogen cyanide, and symptoms may be delayed
  - • Dose-dependent toxicity; headache, dyspnea, anxiety, nausea, confusion, bradycardia, hypotension, shock, seizures, death
  - • Disrupts the ability of tissues to use oxygen; picture mimics hypoxia, including profound lactic acidosis
  - • High oxygen saturation of venous blood; retinal vessels bright red
  - • Odor of bitter almonds on patient's breath or vomitus only sensed by 40% of population
  - • Useful studies include: Chemistry panel, renal panel, serum glucose, arterial blood gas, serum lactate level

- ■ Differential Diagnosis
  - • Carbon monoxide or hydrogen sulfide poisoning
  - • Methemoglobinemia; acute coronary syndrome
  - • Other sources of acidosis in suspected ingestion: Methanol, ethylene glycol, salicylates, iron, metformin

- ■ Treatment
  - • Remove patient from the source of exposure, decontaminate skin, 100% oxygen by face mask, intravenous fluid, cardiac monitoring
  - • For ingestion, activated charcoal
  - • Inhaled amyl nitrite or intravenous sodium nitrite plus sodium thiosulfate antidote; nitrites may exacerbate hypotension or cause massive methemoglobinemia
  - • In case of fire exposure, consider thiosulfate alone, as methemoglobinemia and carbon monoxide may cause reduced oxygen-carrying capacity

- ■ Pearl

In a patient brought in from a theater fire with lactic acidosis, this is the diagnosis.

Reference

Kerns W 2nd, Beuhler M, Tomaszewski C. Hydroxocobalamin versus thiosulfate for cyanide poisoning. Ann Emerg Med 2008;51:338. [PMID: 18282534]

22

Ethanol (Alcohol)

- ■ Essentials of Diagnosis
  - • Slurred speech, nystagmus, decreased motor coordination, respiratory depression
  - • With the development of tolerance, blood alcohol levels correlate poorly with degree of intoxication
  - • Most common cause of an osmolar gap (significant acidosis, however, should not be assumed due to ethanol alone)

- ■ Differential Diagnosis
  - • Other alcohol ingestion (methanol, isopropanol)
  - • Benzodiazepine ingestion

- ■ Treatment
  - • Supportive care including intubation for airway protection if indicated
  - • Gastric lavage indicated only for massive ingestion within 30 minutes
  - • Bedside glucose check or empiric dextrose, thiamine, folate
  - • Examination to evaluate for injuries or illness; check for hypothermia
  - • Serial observation until clinically sober; consider other causes if further deterioration in mental status
  - • Assessment and referral to treatment programs are appropriate when the patient is sober; referral to primary health care and services for housing, food, and jobs may also be appropriate

- ■ Pearl

Chronic ethanol use may cause acetaminophen toxicity at low levels; p450 induction converts it to the toxic metabolite.

Reference

McKeon A, Frye MA, Delanty N. The alcohol withdrawal syndrome. J Neurol Neurosurg Psychiatry 2008;79:854. [PMID: 17986499]

Gamma-Hydroxybutyrate

- **■ Essentials of Diagnosis**
  - An endogenous metabolite of GABA that is easily made at home, GHB is used recreationally and in involuntary intoxication (eg, date rape); it has no clinical use in the United States
  - Has been used as an anesthetic, in the treatment of alcohol withdrawal, and as an adjunctive agent for body builders
  - An odorless, colorless, nearly tasteless liquid, powder, or capsule
  - Dose-related response; euphoria, nystagmus, clonic jerking, mild hypothermia, bradycardia, nausea, vomiting, respiratory depression, coma, and seizures may occur
  - Clinical clues include abrupt onset of uncharacteristic aggressive behavior with rapidly following drowsiness and marked agitation on stimulation despite prolonged apnea and hypoxia
  - May be detectable in urine by mass spectrometry for up to 12 hours; may generate U waves on ECG

- **■ Differential Diagnosis**
  - Ethanol or other alcohol intoxication
  - Opioid ingestion
  - Other sedative-hypnotic ingestion (benzodiazepines, chloral hydrate, methaqualone)

- **■ Treatment**
  - Consider gastric lavage and activated charcoal; may be of limited value in small ingestions and due to rapid absorption
  - Supportive care including intubation if needed for airway stabilization or respiratory assistance
  - Check for mixed ingestion of alcohol or other agents
  - Consider arterial blood gas and head CT in comatose patient with unreliable history
  - Patient counseling and evidence collection in the setting of rape or assault; drug testing is also appropriate in this setting

- **■ Pearl**

Imaginative street names for this dangerous drug include "liquid ecstasy" and "Georgia home boy."

Reference

Carter LP, Pardi D, Gorsline J, Griffiths RR. Illicit gamma-hydroxybutyrate (GHB) and pharmaceutical sodium oxybate (Xyrem): differences in characteristics and misuse. Drug Alcohol Depend 2009;104:1. [PMID: 19493637]

Iron

- ■ Essentials of Diagnosis
  - • Five clinical stages of acute iron toxicity occur: (1) local GI toxicity (within 6 hours), (2) latent (6–24 hours after ingestion), (3) systemic toxicity (12–48 hours after ingestion), (4) hepatic failure (2–3 days), (5) gastric outlet obstruction (2–8 weeks)
  - • Initially, GI irritation results in vomiting, diarrhea, abdominal pain, mucosal ulceration, and bleeding (hematemesis, melena)
  - • Systemic effects begin with disruption of cellular metabolism resulting in acidosis, lethargy, hyperventilation, seizures, coma, coagulopathy, and hypovolemic shock
  - • Elevated serum iron levels correlate somewhat with toxicity, but falsely low levels may occur due to variable absorption rates and the presence of deferoxamine
  - • Radiopaque tablets may be visible on plain abdominal radiographs; negative radiographs do not exclude iron ingestion (common children's chewables are not radiopaque)
  - • In addition to serum iron levels, useful studies include blood count, abdominal x-ray, chemistry and renal panel, PT/PTT, serum glucose, blood gas, and type and screen

- ■ Differential Diagnosis
  - • Arsenic, copper salt, mercurial salt poisoning
  - • Salicylate, theophylline, or acetaminophen overdose
  - • Infectious gastroenteritis, appendicitis, sepsis

- ■ Treatment
  - • Consider GI lavage early after ingestion or if pill fragments still in stomach on abdominal x-ray
  - • Whole-bowel irrigation; endoscopic or surgical removal may be appropriate for large iron loads
  - • Aggressive intravenous fluid and pressor support; correct coagulopathy with vitamin K and fresh-frozen plasma
  - • Chelation therapy with deferoxamine for anyone with toxic appearance and/or a very high serum iron level

- ■ Pearl

The potential for a toxic reaction is based on ingestion of elemental iron; moderate toxicity at a dose of 20–60 mg/kg, severe toxicity above 60 mg/kg.

Reference

Atiq M, Dang S, Olden KW, Aduli F. Early endoscopic gastric lavage for acute iron overdose. Acta Gastroenterol Belg 2008;71:345. [PMID: 19198585]

Isoniazid (INH)

- **Essentials of Diagnosis**
  - Symptoms usually begin within 2 hours of ingestion with vomiting and photophobia
  - Common triad: Profound metabolic acidosis, persistent coma, refractory seizures
  - Hyperglycemia commonly occurs and may mimic DKA
  - Chronic therapeutic use results in peripheral neuritis, tinnitus, hepatitis, memory impairment, and hypersensitivity reactions
  - Hepatic failure the most dangerous adverse reaction to chronic use
  - Substantial genetic variability in the rate at which people metabolize INH; about half of US population are slow metabolizers

- **Differential Diagnosis**
  - Salicylate, cyanide, carbon monoxide, or anticholinergic overdose
  - In the patient with seizures, acidosis, and coma, consider sepsis, meningitis, encephalitis, diabetic ketoacidosis, head trauma
  - Hepatitis due to other cause

- **Treatment**
  - Gastric lavage and activated charcoal for large ingestion within 2 hours
  - Pyridoxine (vitamin B_6) is the reversal agent: 1 g for each gram of INH ingested; 5 g slow intravenous empiric dose will stop seizures and thus correct acidosis
  - Benzodiazepines as adjunct in seizure control, but will not work if used as sole agent
  - Supportive therapy for coma, hypotension

- **Pearl**

Ten to twenty percent of patients using INH for treatment of tuberculosis will have elevated serum aminotransferases and do not require discontinuation of the drug; 1% overall will have clinical hepatitis, especially middle-aged patients, and must stop it.

Reference

Morrow LE, Wear RE, Schuller D, Malesker M. Acute isoniazid toxicity and the need for adequate pyridoxine supplies. Pharmacotherapy 2006;26:1529. [PMID: 16999664]

22

Lead

- **Essentials of Diagnosis**
  - Results from chronic exposure; sources include solder, batteries, paint (in homes built before 1970)
  - Symptoms and signs include colicky abdominal pain, gum lead line, constipation, headache, irritability, neuropathy, learning disorders in children, episodes of gout (saturnine gout)
  - Ataxia, confusion, obtundation, seizures
  - Useful studies include complete blood count, chemistry panel, renal panel, lead level, abdominal x-ray, long bone radiographs (looking for lead lines)
  - Blood lead > 10 μg/dL toxic, > 70 mg/dL severe

- **Differential Diagnosis**
  - Other heavy metal toxicity (arsenic, mercury)
  - Tricyclic antidepressant, anticholinergic, ethylene glycol, or carbon monoxide exposure
  - Other sources of encephalopathy: Alcohol withdrawal, sedative-hypnotic medications, meningitis, encephalitis, hypoglycemia
  - Medical causes of acute abdomen (eg, porphyria, sickle cell crisis)
  - For chronic toxicity: Depression, iron deficiency anemia, learning disability
  - Idiopathic gout

- **Treatment**
  - Airway protection and ventilatory assistance as indicated; supportive therapy for coma and seizures
  - Lavage for acute ingestion; whole-bowel irrigation, endoscopy, or surgical removal if a large lead-containing object is visible on abdominal radiograph
  - Chelation therapy based on clinical presentation and blood lead levels
  - Investigate the source and test other workers or family members who might have been exposed

- **Pearl**

The prevalence of automated blood smear analysis may make the diagnosis of lead intoxication difficult: virtually all cases have extensive basophilic stippling in red cells.

Reference

Sanders T, Liu Y, Buchner V, Tchounwou PB. Neurotoxic effects and biomarkers of lead exposure: a review. Rev Environ Health 2009;24:15. [PMID: 19476290]

Lithium

- **Essentials of Diagnosis**
    - Acute ingestion (high serum, low tissue burden): Dystonia, ataxia, tremor, hyperreflexia, nausea, vomiting, abdominal cramping
    - Chronic ingestion (high tissue [ie, neurologic] burden): Confusion, which may progress to seizures and/or coma if unrecognized and patient continues lithium ingestion
    - Ventricular dysrhythmia, sinus arrest, asystole, sinus bradycardia, nephrogenic diabetes insipidus
    - Elevated serum lithium levels (> 1.5 mEq/L); acute ingestions lead to higher serum levels than chronic overdose
    - U waves, flattened or inverted T waves, ST depression may be seen on ECG
    - Multiple medications increase the risk of lithium toxicity (angiotensin-converting enzyme inhibitors, loop diuretics, NSAIDs, phenothiazines), as do renal failure, volume depletion, gastroenteritis, and decreased sodium intake
    - Useful studies: Chemistry panel (a decreased anion gap may be seen), renal panel, urinalysis, ECG

- **Differential Diagnosis**
    - Neurologic disease (cerebrovascular accident, postictal state, meningitis, parkinsonism, tardive dyskinesia)
    - Other psychotropic drug intoxication; neuroleptic malignant syndrome

- **Treatment**
    - Airway protection, ventilatory and hemodynamic support as indicated
    - Gastric lavage if within first hour of ingestion
    - Activated charcoal not useful for lithium overdose, but may be useful for other ingested medications; whole-bowel irrigation for sustained-release preparations
    - Sodium polystyrene sulfonate (Kayexalate) may be useful to bind lithium (monitor potassium if used)
    - Aggressive normal saline hydration with close management of volume and electrolytes to enhance lithium excretion
    - Indications for hemodialysis in acute ingestions: Decreased level of consciousness, seizures, renal failure with inability to excrete lithium, or lithium level > 4 mEq/L; chronic ingestions: symptomatic patient with lithium level > 2.5 mEq/L

- **Pearl**

Lithium is metabolized in the kidney identically to sodium: in volume-depleted states both sodium and lithium are retained—toxicity may thus occur without overdose.

Reference

Grandjean EM, Aubry JM. Lithium: updated human knowledge using an evidence-based approach. CNS Drugs 2009;23:397. [PMID: 19453201]

22

Methanol, Ethylene Glycol, and Isopropanol

- ■ Essentials of Diagnosis
  - • Morbidity and mortality from metabolites of methanol and ethylene glycol; before breakdown, they all depress the central nervous system
  - • Methanol: Windshield washer fluid, carburetor fluid, glass cleaners, lacquers, adhesives, inks; formic acid (metabolite) causes visual loss and metabolic acidosis
  - • Ethylene glycol: Antifreeze, deicing solutions, solvents; oxalic acid (metabolite) causes renal failure
  - • Isopropanol: Rubbing alcohol, nail polish removers
  - • Anion gap, renal dysfunction, osmolal gap, abnormal ECG may be seen
  - • Urine fluoresces under Wood's lamp with ethylene glycol

- ■ Differential Diagnosis
  - • Ethanol ingestion
  - • Other causes of an anion gap acidosis
  - • Hypoglycemia

- ■ Treatment
  - • Gastric lavage only if patient presented within 30 minutes; activated charcoal will not bind alcohols
  - • Maintain adequate airway and assist ventilation
  - • Supportive therapy for coma and seizures
  - • Fomepizole (Antizol) in any symptomatic adult or child, and in an asymptomatic adult with methanol or ethylene glycol levels > 20 mg/dL; ethanol an alternative, blocks formation of metabolites
  - • Methanol: 50 mg of leucovorin (folinic acid)
  - • Ethylene glycol: Thiamine and pyridoxine
  - • Hemodialysis for metabolic acidosis, renal, visual symptoms (methanol); deterioration despite intensive supportive care, electrolyte imbalances unresponsive to conventional therapy, levels > 25 mg/dL for ethylene glycol and isopropanol
  - • Isopropanol: Supportive

- ■ Pearl

Ethylene glycol is colorless; antifreeze is dyed greenish brown to discourage ingestion.

Reference

Kraut JA, Kurtz I. Toxic alcohol ingestions: clinical features, diagnosis, and management. Clin J Am Soc Nephrol 2008;3:208. [PMID: 18045860]

Methemoglobinemia

■ Essentials of Diagnosis

- Cyanosis unresponsive to oxygen is hallmark of methemoglobinemia
- Seen in infants, especially after diarrheal illness
- Drugs that can oxidize normal ferrous (Fe^{2+}) hemoglobin to abnormal ferric (Fe^{3+}) hemoglobin (methemoglobin) include local anesthetics (lidocaine, benzocaine), aniline dyes, nitrates and nitrites, nitrogen oxides, chloroquine, trimethoprim, dapsone, and phenazopyridine
- Methemoglobin cannot bind oxygen and decreases delivery of oxygen bound to normal heme (shifting the oxyhemoglobin dissociation curve to the left)
- Dizziness, nausea, headache, dyspnea, anxiety, tachycardia, and weakness at low levels, to myocardial ischemia, arrhythmias, decreased mentation, seizures, coma
- Saturation fixed at 85% even in severe hypoxemia
- Definitive diagnosis is by co-oximetry (may be from a venous sample); routine blood gas analysis may be falsely normal
- Blood may appear chocolate brown

■ Differential Diagnosis

- Hypoxemia
- Sulfhemoglobinemia
- Carbon monoxide or hydrogen sulfide poisoning

■ Treatment

- Activated charcoal for recent ingestion
- Discontinue offending agent; high-flow oxygen
- Intravenous methylene blue for symptomatic patients with high methemoglobin levels or methemoglobin levels > 30%; contraindicated in patients with G6PD deficiency
- If methylene blue therapy fails or is contraindicated, then exchange transfusion or hyperbaric oxygen

■ Pearl

An in vitro phenomenon unrelated to cardiopulmonary disease; oxygen saturation is fixed at 85%.

Reference

do Nascimento TS, Pereira RO, de Mello HL, Costa J. Methemoglobinemia: from diagnosis to treatment. Rev Bras Anestesiol 2008;58:657. [PMID: 19082413]

Opioids

- **Essentials of Diagnosis**
  - Respiratory depression, miosis, altered mental status
  - Signs of intravenous drug abuse (needle marks, a tourniquet)
  - Some (propoxyphene, tramadol, dextromethorphan, meperidine) may cause seizures
  - Noncardiogenic pulmonary edema
  - Meperidine or dextromethorphan plus a monoamine oxidase inhibitor may produce serotonin syndrome

- **Differential Diagnosis**
  - Alcohol or sedative-hypnotic overdose
  - Clonidine overdose
  - Phenothiazine overdose
  - Organophosphate or carbamate insecticide exposure
  - Gamma-hydroxybutyrate overdose
  - Congestive heart failure
  - Infectious or metabolic encephalopathy
  - Hypoglycemia, hypoxia, postictal state

- **Treatment**
  - Naloxone for suspected overdose (0.4 mg IV for mildly sedated patients suspected of opioid overdose; 2 mg IV for severely sedated or comatose patient, repeat dose up to 10 mg IV)
  - Naloxone will last for approximately 45 minutes if administered intravenously, which is much shorter than the half-life of many opioid preparations; consider subcutaneous or intramuscular depot injection when patient is stable
  - Gastric lavage for very large ingestions presenting within 1 hour
  - Activated charcoal for oral ingestion if airway is protected or secure
  - Maintain adequate airway and assist ventilation, including intubation
  - Supportive therapy for coma, hypothermia, and hypotension
  - Benzodiazepines for seizures
  - Acetaminophen level
  - Update tetanus for IV drug users

- **Pearl**

Fixed doses of acetaminophen and codeine may result in altered mental status in hospitalized patients with intercurrent illness causing renal insufficiency and reduced opioid clearance.

Reference

Aquina CT, Marques-Baptista A, Bridgeman P, Merlin MA. OxyContin abuse and overdose. Postgrad Med 2009;121:163. [PMID: 19332974]

Organophosphates and Carbamates

■ Essentials of Diagnosis

- Insecticides (eg, Orthene, malathion, parathion) and agents of chemical warfare (sarin) inhibit red blood cell acetylcholinesterase (AchE) and plasma cholinesterase and may be inhaled, ingested, or absorbed through the skin
- Organophosphates permanently inactivate AchE; carbamates will dissociate from AchE within 24 hours
- Clinical manifestations secondary to cholinergic stimulation ("SLUDGE"): Salivation, lacrimation, urination, defecation, gastrointestinal distress, emesis
- Miosis, bradycardia, bronchospasm, bronchorrhea may also be observed

■ Differential Diagnosis

- Curare or neuromuscular blocker poisoning
- Hypothyroidism
- Pulmonary edema
- Asthma or chronic obstructive pulmonary disease (COPD) exacerbation

■ Treatment

- Decontaminate skin if exposed and avoid secondary exposure to health providers
- Nasogastric tube suction if within 1 hour, charcoal if possible; however, administration may be difficult if patient is persistently vomiting
- 100% oxygen; maintain adequate airway and assist ventilation as necessary, avoid succinylcholine if intubation required (use a nondepolarizing agent)
- Atropine (2–4 mg IV doses in adults, 0.05 mg/kg doses in children) doubling dose every 5–10 minutes until secretions stop; may require *very* large repeated doses or infusion
- Pralidoxime 1–2 g over 30 minutes, may repeat in 1 hour and every 4–8 hours

■ Pearl

Carbamates are reversible inhibitors of cholinesterases; cholinergic crises are shorter than with organophosphates, and atropine is the antidote of choice.

Reference

Leibson T, Lifshitz M. Organophosphate and carbamate poisoning: review of the current literature and summary of clinical and laboratory experience in southern Israel. Isr Med Assoc J 2008;10:767. [PMID: 19070283]

22

Salicylates

- **Essentials of Diagnosis**
  - Many over-the-counter products other than aspirin contain salicylates, including Pepto-Bismol, various liniments
  - Mild acute ingestion: Hyperpnea, lethargy, tinnitus
  - Moderate intoxication: Severe hyperpnea, neurologic disturbances, severe lethargy
  - Severe intoxication: Fever, agitation, confusion, severe hyperpnea, seizures
  - Chronic pediatric ingestion: Hyperventilation, volume depletion, acidosis, hypokalemia, metabolic acidosis, respiratory alkalosis; in adults: hyperventilation, confusion, tremor, paranoia, memory deficits

- **Differential Diagnosis**
  - Any cause of anion gap metabolic acidosis
  - Sepsis; carbon monoxide poisoning

- **Treatment**
  - Elevated serum salicylate level; treatment should always consider both serum level and clinical condition
  - Gastrointestinal lavage or whole-bowel irrigation for early, large, or sustained-release ingestions; activated charcoal
  - Maintain adequate airway and assist ventilation, remembering that these patients require extremely high minute ventilation to combat metabolic acidosis
  - Supportive therapy for coma, hyperthermia, hypotension, and seizures; correct hypoglycemia and hypokalemia
  - Intravenous fluid resuscitation with normal saline to maintain urine output at 2–3 mL/kg per hour; urinary alkalinization with sodium bicarbonate to enhance salicylate excretion (urine pH 7.5–8)
  - Indications for hemodialysis: (1) serum salicylate levels > 100 mg/dL in acute ingestions (60 mg/dL in chronic ingestions), coma, seizures, renal or hepatic failure, and pulmonary edema; (2) severe acid–base imbalance; (3) rising serum salicylate levels; or (4) failure to respond to conservative treatment

- **Pearl**

Another of the "triple ripples" in medicine: gap acidosis, contraction alkalosis, and respiratory alkalosis.

Reference

Pearlman BL, Gambhir R. Salicylate intoxication: a clinical review. Postgrad Med 2009;121:162. [PMID: 19641282]

Theophylline

■ Essentials of Diagnosis

- Mild: Nausea, vomiting, tachycardia, tremor
- Severe: Any tachyarrhythmia, hypokalemia, hyperglycemia, metabolic acidosis, hallucinations, hypotension, seizures
- Chronic: Vomiting, tachycardia, and seizures (may be the first and only sign of chronic toxicity), but no hypokalemia or hyperglycemia
- Wide pulse pressure early
- Theophylline level is essential to care

■ Differential Diagnosis

- Salicylate overdose
- Caffeine overdose
- Iron toxicity
- Sympathomimetic poisoning
- Anticholinergic toxicity
- Thyroid storm
- Alcohol or other drug withdrawal

■ Treatment

- Gastric lavage if presentation within 1 hour
- Activated charcoal mainstay of therapy
- Whole-bowel irrigation if no charcoal response, or if sustained release preparation is taken
- Oxygen; maintain adequate airway and assist ventilation
- Monitor for arrhythmias; correct hypokalemia
- Treat seizures with benzodiazepines
- Hypotension and tachycardia may respond to beta-blockade
- Indications for hemodialysis or hemoperfusion: Acute theophylline level > 90 mg/L or rapidly approaching it; level of > 40 mg/L chronically in a patient with a poor response to oral activated charcoal and any patient with ongoing seizures, ventricular dysrhythmias, poorly responsive hypotension

■ Pearl

Less commonly used than it once was in COPD; if inappropriate sinus tachycardia occurs in patients receiving this drug, beware of toxic levels: once seizures occur, the prognosis is far worse.

Reference

Charytan D, Jansen K. Severe metabolic complications from theophylline intoxication. Nephrology (Carlton) 2003;8:239. [PMID: 15012710]

22

Index